W0043536

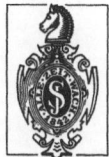

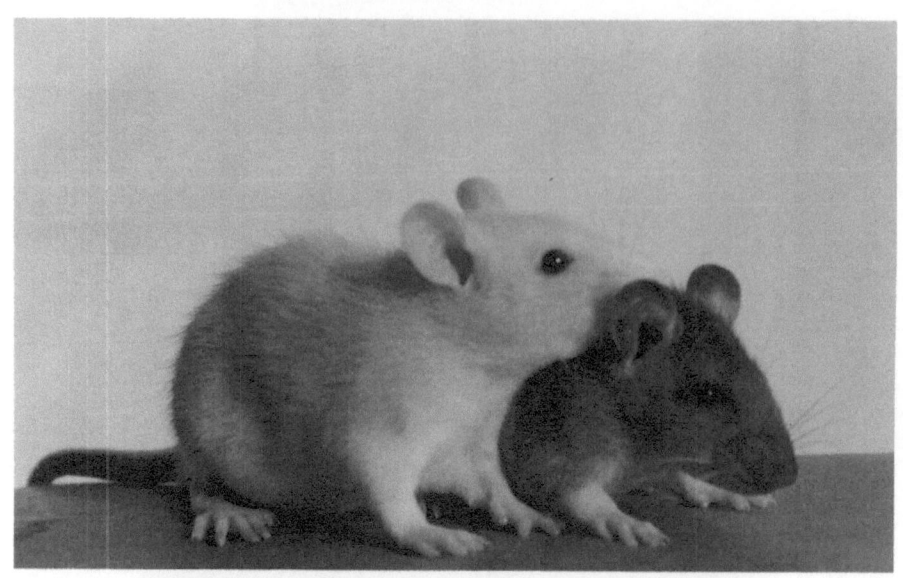

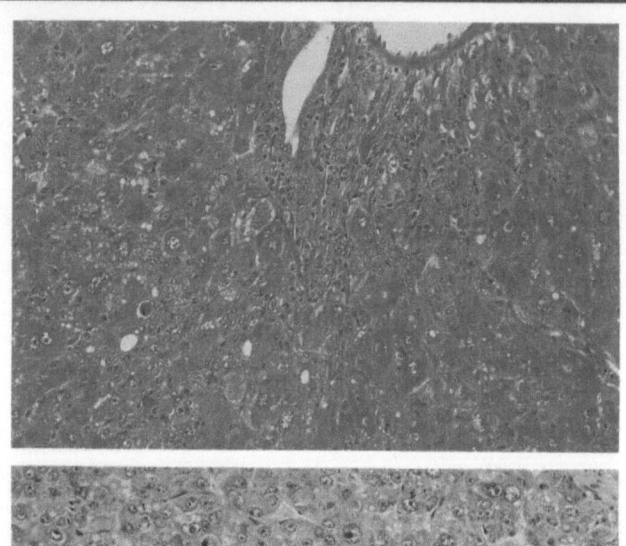

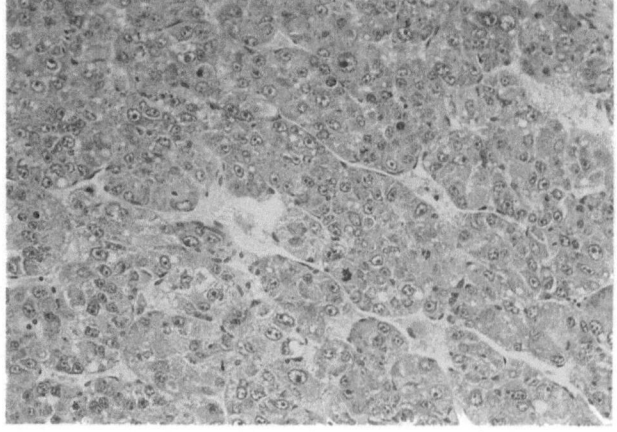

M. Mori · M.C. Yoshida
N. Takeichi · N. Taniguchi (Eds.)

The LEC Rat

A New Model for Hepatitis and
Liver Cancer

With 158 Illustrations, 2 in Color

Springer-Verlag
Tokyo Berlin Heidelberg
New York London Paris
Hong Kong Barcelona

Michio Mori, M.D., Ph.D.
Department of Pathology, Sapporo Medical College, Minami 1, Nishi 17, Chuo-ku, Sapporo, 060 Japan

Michihiro C. Yoshida, D.Si., Ph.D.
Chromosome Research Unit, Faculty of Science, Hokkaido University, Kita 10, Nishi 8, Kita-ku Sapporo, 060 Japan

Noritoshi Takeichi, M.D., Ph.D.
Laboratory of Pathology, Cancer Institute, Hokkaido University School of Medicine, Kita 15, Nishi 7, Kita-ku, Sapporo, 060 Japan

Naoyuki Taniguchi, M.D., Ph.D.
Department of Biochemistry, Osaka University Medical School, 2-2 Yamadaoka, Suita, Osaka, 565 Japan

ISBN-13: 978-4-431-68155-7   e-ISBN-13: 978-4-431-68153-3
DOI: 10.1007/ 978-4-431-68153-3

© Springer-Verlag Tokyo 1991
Softcover reprint of the hardcover 1st edition 1991

Typesetting: Best-set Typesetter Ltd., Hong Kong

Foreword

The LEC strain of rats, which spontaneously develop acute hepatitis associated with jaundice, chronic hepatitis, and ultimately hepatocellular carcinomas, was established by scientists in Sapporo, Japan. Careful observation and breeding led to the initial discovery of this characteristic, inherited liver disease in rats. Subsequent collaboration between scientists in Sapporo and other centers has revealed an autosomal recessive nature of inheritance, along with a variety of histopathological and biochemical findings.

The causative mechanism(s) underlying this abnormality remained a mystery for some time, providing a challenge for many scientists who were attracted to the quest for clues to this enigma. In particular, the mechanism of spontaneous development of hepatocellular carcinomas in rats overcoming the acute phase of hepatitis and surviving with chronic hepatitis proved extremely interesting, because the involvement of a causative virus had been excluded in the early stages of investigation.

Professor Michio Mori of Sapporo Medical College played a key role in the study of LEC rats, especially in the elucidation of the pathogenesis of hepatitis and hepatocellular carcinoma. He is one of the editors of this monograph which is composed of original contributions by the many scientists who have carried out their own studies on LEC rats.

Of the various histopathological and biochemical alterations which have been reported, some are clearly secondary or tertiary events sequential to the primary change caused by gene mutation.

Exciting information has recently emerged from Prof. Kobayashi's laboratory at Hokkaido University School of Medicine. Marked accumulation of copper in the liver and significant deprivation of ceruloplasmin in the serum were demonstrated, with hepatitis being provoked when certain levels of copper are reached in the liver. It is suspected that deficiency of serum ceruloplasmin followed by accumulation of copper in hepatocytes triggers the death of hepatocytes, thereby inducing regenerative proliferation of hepatic cells. In a much earlier phase of the studies, it was noted that infiltration of inflammatory cells was not prevalent in LEC rat hepatitis, in accordance with this newly elucidated mechanism. The pathogenesis of LEC rat liver disorders probably mimics that in Wilson's disease in humans which is known to be caused by an abnormality of copper metabolism.

It is becoming increasingly well documented that human cancers are produced by accumulations of genetic alterations, including those involving oncogenes and anti-oncogenes. Such changes at the gene level are the result of DNA damage produced by xenobiotics as well as by endogenous autobiotics. DNA damage caused by active oxygen is an unavoidable outcome of oxidative metabolism, mutations similar to those caused by nitrosamine and nitric oxide with involvement of nitric oxide synthetase occurring continuously in the human body. Any factors which evoke cell-proliferation should yield more opportunities for fixation of modified DNA bases as mutations. From the above descriptions, hepatocellular carcinomas of LEC rats, which are produced without viral infection and without any obvious excess burden of environmental mutagens, should provide a good model for human hepatocarcinogenesis. After hepatitis virus infection, especially in the case of hepatitis C in which genetic integration has not been confirmed, hepatomas occur frequently. The striking similarities to the course of events in LEC rats cannot be stressed too often. Aspects other than simple proliferation which deserve consideration include the fact that accumulation of copper may produce active oxygen species. It is also reported that LEC rats are particularly susceptible to hepatocarcinogens. Various factors are presumably acting in a mutually complementary manner in elevating the development of so-called spontaneous hepatocellular carcinomas. Molecular analysis of mutated oncogenes and altered anti-oncogenes in LEC rats in comparison with those in human hepatomas should shed further light on the carcinogenic mechanism(s), hopefully leading us to new approaches to the prevention or arrest of the neoplastic process.

This monograph reflects the present state of the art regarding our understanding of LEC rats and the pathophysiology of events occurring during their life span. The documented information relevant to hepatic neoplasia should be invaluable for scientists from different research disciplines, including pathology, oncology, and molecular biology and for physicians and surgeons working in the clinical field as well.

Takashi Sugimura
President
National Cancer Center
Japan

Preface

Hepatitis affects more than 200 million people worldwide, and liver cancer is one of the most common fatal malignancies, with 250,000–500,000 new cases reported each year. Although it is well known that liver cancer often develops in association with chronic liver diseases, the etiologic roles of chronic hepatitis in liver carcinogenesis remain undetermined.

The LEC rat is a new mutant strain recently established at the Center for Experimental Plants and Animals of Hokkaido University, Sapporo, Japan. The LEC rat suffers from hereditary hepatitis and subsequent liver cancer at a high frequency, and it is a most suitable and unique animal model for the study of hepatitis and liver cancer.

This monograph describes the characteristic features of LEC rats from the standpoints of biochemistry, immunology, genetics, veterinary science, oncology, and pathology. We hope that the book will provide an understanding of how the LEC rat can be used in studies of liver carcinogenesis, prevention and treatment of hepatitis, and many other fields of medicine, biology, immunology, and pharmacology.

Difficulties in breeding and maintaining this animal strain mean that approximately 40% of animals die of fulminant hepatitis around 4 months after birth. Distribution of LEC rats has therefore been limited to researchers in Japan. However, worldwide distribution of LEC rats will begin through the Charles-River Japan Inc., by the time this book is published.

The editors are indebted to the contributors for submitting their extremely informative manuscripts on time. We are grateful to Dr. Takashi Sugimura, the president of the National Cancer Center, Tokyo, for his encouragement of the LEC rat studies and for writing the foreword to this book. The book was supported in part by a Grant-in-Aid for Publication of Scientific Research Result from the Ministry of Education, Science, and Culture of Japan. We also extend our appreciation to the publishers, Springer-Verlag Tokyo.

We are grateful to Emeritus Prof. Masamichi Sasaki, who was director of the Experimental Animal Laboratory of Hokkaido University in which the

LEC rat strain was established. We sincerely thank Mrs. Kazuko Kagami, Mr. Ryuji Nagao, and Mr. Eiji Kamimura for their careful and skillful handling of the rats. Without their devotion, the LEC rat could not have been established. Financial support from Otsuka Pharmaceutical Co. Ltd. assisted in maintaining the rats. We also thank Prof. Mitsuhiko Hisada, of the Center for Experimental Plants and Animals of Hokkaido University, for his work as chairman of the LEC rat maintenance committee.

Michio Mori
Michihiro C. Yoshida
Noritoshi Takeichi
Naoyuki Taniguchi

Contents

Part 1 Establishment and Natural History

Part 2   Hepatitis

List of Contributors

Glossary

LEC: An inbred mutant strain of rat with hereditary hepatitis isolated from randomly bred Long-Evans rats originating from Kobe University. Inbreeding was started in 1976 at Hokkaido University. The LEC rat has a cinnamon-like colored coat and is maintained at the Center for Experimental Plants and Animals, Hokkaido University, Sapporo Japan.

LEA: An inbred strain of rat with an agouti-like coat that was isolated simultaneously from the randomly bred Long-Evans rats from which the LEC rat was established. This strain is often used as a control for the LEC rat and is also maintained at the Center for Experimental Plants and Animals, Hokkaido University, Sapporo Japan.

PART I Establishment and Natural History

1 — Origin of the LEC Strain with a New Mutation Causing Hereditary Hepatitis

MICHIHIRO C. YOSHIDA[1], MOTOMICHI SASAKI[2], and RYUICHI MASUDA[1]

Over the last 10 years, a large number of animal models for human diseases has been discovered in laboratory mice and rats. Such model animals have become an indispensable tool in many fields of biological and medical research. During the isolating of substrains with different coat colors from non-inbred Long-Evans rats, we established a new mutant LEC strain causing hereditary hepatitis [1,2]. The clinical signs of hepatitis in LEC rats are similar to human liver disease. Furthermore, liver cancer appears in long-surviving rats after recovery from jaundice. Therefore, LEC rats provide a pertinent model useful for basic and clinical studies of hepatitis and liver cancer, including its experimental therapy, because the treatment and prevention of hepatitis and subsequent liver cancer are current problems of humans. In this introductory chapter, we review the history of the LEC strain.

Establishment of the LEC Strain

Spontaneous hepatitis associated with severe jaundice was first found in 1983 in an LEC inbred strain maintained at the Center for Experimental Plants and Animals, Hokkaido University (Hokkaido, Japan). The establishment of this LEC strain dates back to October, 1975 when we obtained several non-inbred Long-Evans rats from a closed colony maintained by Professor Taketoshi Sugiyama, formerly of Kobe University (Kobe, Japan), who is devoted to the cytogenetic study of leukemia using the Long-Evans strain. At that time, each rat had a different coat color of hooded brown (or cinnamon-like), black-brown, or agouti with a white or cream belly, so we adopted a sibmating system to achieve segregation of each coat color. We

[1] Chromosome Research Unit, Faculty of Science, Hokkaido University, Sapporo, 060 Japan
[2] Sasaki Cancer Institute, Chiyoda-ku, Tokyo, 101 Japan

maintained these rats at the Experimental Animal Laboratory, the predecessor of the Center, in which over 30 inbred strains of rats and mice were kept. This Experimental Animal Laboratory was founded by Prof. Sajiro Makino in 1957 as a breeding and resource center of inbred strains of rats and mice. From this Laboratory, the Center developed in 1981 as an integral facility center to breed and culture wide varieties of biological materials, including the inbred rodent strains. Before moving to the Center, inbreeding of the Long-Evans rats had been started by the breeder, Mrs. Kazuko Kagami, under the direction of one of the authors (M.S.) who was the Director of the Laboratory. Although female infertility occurred at around the 10th–12th generations of inbreeding, due to progressive genic homozygosity, several strains with different coat colors were developed over 20 generations by full-sibmatings as of 1982. However, because of limited facilities only two strains, LEA and LEC, were maintained. The LEA had a hooded agoutic coat color, and the LEC coat color was hooded brown or diluted agouti, both with a white or cream belly.

Discovery of Hepatitis and Natural History

During the routine inbreeding of LEC rats, severe jaundice appeared in an adult male LEC rat, 149 days after birth, among six siblings of a litter in the 24th generation (early February, 1984). Even though LEC rats had a brown coat color, the discovery of jaundice came from its strongly yellowish skin, ears, tail, and genital region. The jaundiced rat died within 1 week after the onset of jaundice. No other littermates developed jaundice. This first affected rat had already sired a litter of F_{25} before the onset of jaundice. This litter and further offsprings were sibmated by our usual breeding program without any particular selection for jaundice. After the first finding of the jaundice, LEC rats between the F_{25} and F_{31} generations were examined daily from birth to ascertain any development of jaundice.

Actually, jaundice was found in every generation, and the frequency of appearance of jaundiced rats increased in successive generations (Table 1). Jaundice appeared in the offspring of both jaundiced and nonjaundiced parents. Detailed analysis of affected rats revealed that they were characterized by several symptoms of hepatitis, such as severe jaundice, subcutaneous bleeding, oliguria, bilirubinuria, and loss of body weight. These symptoms did not appear in young rats (before they were approximately 3–4 months of age), but they did appear suddenly and unpredictably in adult rats between 88 and 149 days of age (average: 4 months). Most jaundiced rats had a very poor prognosis and showed a prompt decrease in body weight as well as in intake of food and water. Death usually occurred within 1 week in severely affected rats, most probably as a result of rapid progression of the hepatitis. At autopsy, jaundiced rats showed golden yellow subcutaneous tissues, atrophic liver, slightly enlarged spleen, and yellowish kidneys.

Table 1. Frequency of jaundiced LEC rats in eight successive generations[a].

Generation	No. of litters	No. of offspring Total	No. of offspring Jaundice	Jaundice Male	Jaundice Female	Frequency of jaundiced rats (%)	Onset of jaundice (days after birth)
F_{24}[b]	1	6	1	1	0	16.7	149
F_{25}	1	8	4	1	3	50.0	89
F_{26}	1	6	6	3	3	100.0	139
F_{27}	3	21	14	4	10	66.7	88
F_{28}	3	20	19	10	9	95.0	129
F_{29}	5	35	31	12	19	88.6	110
F_{30}	8	57	50	24	26	87.7	111
F_{31}	4	33	25	12	13	75.8	103

[a] Jaundiced rats were diagnosed by the following clinical signs of jaundice: anemia, oliguria, subcutaneous bleeding and loss of body weight (From [2] with permission)
[b] The first jaundiced rat appeared in the F_{24} generation

Litter size in each generation did not show any significant change, and individuals in each litter had no reduced growth rate before the onset of hepatitis. There was no apparent sex difference in the incidence of hepatitis. Since hepatitis always appeared in adult rats after their having produced at least one litter, the progeny could be easily maintained by routine sibmating before the onset of hepatitis.

Since all jaundiced rats from the F_{24} to F_{28} generations were sacrificed for histopathological analysis, an exact rate for recovery and survival could not be obtained. Therefore, survival of all individuals from the F_{30} generation was checked without sacrificing them after the onset of hepatitis. Of a total of 57 rats obtained from eight litters, jaundice was observed in 50 rats (Table 1), of which 16 (32%) died and 34 recovered and survived for more than 1 year with an increase in their weight. The remaining seven asymptomatic (not jaundiced) rats also survived for more than 1 year. However, it is not clear why such a difference in the appearance of jaundice existed in the same litter.

Although mutants causing jaundice have been reported in laboratory rats [3,4] and mice [5,6], these animals did not show hepatitis. Therefore, LEC rats are a quite unique strain in which hepatitis associated with severe jaundice is present, with a possibility that genetic factor(s) may be related to the occurrence of the disease.

Inheritance

Under the hypothesis that the LEC strain itself is mutant for hepatitis and that the mutation is caused by a single autosomal recessive gene, it followed that all rats must be carriers. This was verified by mating LEC rats to rats of LEA, LEJ, and WKAH strains maintained at Hokkaido University,

Table 2. Mode of inheritance of the hepatitis. (From [2, 7] with permission).

| Cross (female: male) | Tested (n) | Hepatitis rats[a] | | P^c |
		Observed (n)	Expected[b] (n)	
LEC × LEC	32	32	32	NS
(LEC × LEA) F$_1$	32	0	0	NS
(LEA × LEC) F$_1$	13	0	0	NS
(LEC × LEJ) F$_1$	9	0	0	NS
(LEJ × LEC) F$_1$	6	0	0	NS
(LEC × LEA) F$_2$	45	14	11.3	NS
(LEA × LEC) F$_2$	38	13	9.5	NS
(LEC × LEJ) F$_2$	21	4	5.3	NS
(LEJ × LEC) F$_2$	21	3	5.3	NS
(WKAH × LEC) F$_2$	12	3	3.0	NS
(LEC × LEA) F$_1$ × LEC	30	12	15.0	NS
(LEA × LEC) F$_1$ × LEC	40	17	20.0	NS
(LEC × LEJ) F$_1$ × LEC	21	10	10.5	NS
(LEJ × LEC) F$_1$ × LEC	13	5	6.5	NS

[a] Hepatitis was diagnosed by histological examinations
[b] Calculated number of hepatitis rats supposing that the inheritance mode of hepatitis is autosomal recessive
[c] NS, not significant in X^2-test ($P > 0.1$)

and crossing the F$_1$s to produce F$_2$s and backcross hybrids [2,7]. The presence of hepatitis was diagnosed by histological examinations. None of the F$_1$ hybrids developed hepatitis within 8 months after birth, while approximately 25% of F$_2$ rats and 50% of backcrossed rats developed the disease while the remaining rats were normal. These proportions were not significantly different from the expected numbers ($P > 0.1$) (Table 2). No evidence was obtained for the sex ratio deviating from 1:1 in mutant or normal rats. Therefore, the new mutation causing hepatitis in LEC rats fits the inheritance pattern of a single autosomal recessive gene, and so the gene symbol, *hts*, for the mutation was proposed [7]. From these genetic analyses, it was concluded that only rats with the genotype *hts/hts* among F$_2$ and backcrossed rats could develop hepatitis, whereas heterozygotes (*hts/+*) of F$_1$, F$_2$, and backcrossed rats could have normal livers.

From the present crossing tests, it was possible to determine the linkage of hepatitis with coat color. The coat color of LEC rats hooded diluted-agouti (*AAhhpp*) and that of LEJ rats was hooded black (*aahhPP*). In LEC × LEJ and LEJ × LEC, all F$_1$ rats were hooded agouti. Although the segregation of the coat color phenotypes of hooded diluted-agouti, agouti, and black occurred in F$_2$ rats, these phenotypes were not related with the appearance of hepatitis, indicating that hepatitis is not linked to the *a* or *p* coat color loci.

Since hepatitis was not found in rats within 3 months of age, the *hts* gene may not be operative in young rats. How hepatitis occurs suddenly in adult rats raises an interesting question. At present, the function of the mutant *hts* gene has not been clarified. However, it may have a pleiotropic effect on the cause of hepatitis and subsequent hepatic lesions. As described below, increased levels of serum glutamic oxaloacetic transaminase (GOT), glutamic pyruvic transaminase (GPT), and bilirubin as characteristics of hepatitis were observed in parallel with histological changes of the liver [1]. In F_2 and backcrossed rats, similar features of hepatitis were seen to those seen in LEC rats. Histological characters were an enlargement of hepatocytes with huge nuclei, the appearance of some Councilman bodies in sinusoids, and a decrease of hepatic lobules as a result of the collapse of hepatocytes. Moreover, preneoplastic foci which were seen in the long-surviving LEC rats were also found in the affected hybrid rats which were surviving at 8 months.

General Features of Physiological Characters

Some physiological traits were compared in LEC and LEA rats [1,2], and their details will be reviewed in the following chapter. In brief, the urine of all of the jaundiced rats was strongly positive for bilirubin. The affected rats showed an approximately 40-fold increase of total serum bilirubin levels compared with those of the LEC rats before the onset of hepatitis and of the age-matched LEA rats. An increase in each level of GOT and GPT also was observed, whereas those of GOT and GPT in LEC rats before the onset of hepatitis as well as in LEA rats were always low. Other enzymes of serum levels of alkaline phosphatase and urea nitrogen increased markedly, while levels of choline esterase, acid phosphatase, and albumin decreased in proportion to the stage and severity of the hepatitis [1]. These physiological characteristics were also strikingly similar to those seen in fulminant hepatitis in humans.

Daily observations and monitoring of LEC rats indicated that the onset of hepatitis was sudden and occurred in affected siblings in each litter within a few days. Daily measurements of body weight and food and water intake gave no clear warning of impending hepatitis, even during the preceding week, when compared with the age- and sex-matched LEA rats. The only possible indicator of susceptibility was the bilirubinuria that was sometimes noticed several days before the appearance of jaundice. Marked hyperbilirubinemia occurred within a few days of the onset of the disease, and was associated with oliguria and dehydration.

General Histological Features

Histological observations of the liver of LEC rats have been presented by Yoshida et al. [2]. A detailed description of the histology of the liver of LEC rats will be reviewed in the following chapter. A brief report by Yoshida et al. [2] mentioned that no histological abnormality was found in the liver of young LEC rats during the first 3 months after birth during which time jaundice usually did not appear. After 3 months, the initial change in the liver was an enlargement of most hepatocytes with huge nuclei which sometimes contained several nucleoli as well as nuclear pseudo-inclusions. Degeneration with a pyknotic nucleus in scanty cytoplasm was found in some hepatocytes, and the appearance of Councilman bodies was also noted. Further progression of the liver lesion was found in jaundiced rats. A marked increase in Councilman bodies and bile pigments in activated Kupffer's cells was observed. The area of hepatic lobules in the jaundiced rats, as a result of the collapse of hepatocytes, was smaller than that of normal rats. Inflammatory cell infiltration by lymphocytes or neutrophils occurred slightly. Mononuclear phagocytes containing erythrocytes were often found in the sinusoids. Regeneration of hepatocytes and proliferation of collagen fibers were never observed. Histological sections of the autopsied livers showed similar features to those found in sacrificed rats which had focal coagulative necrosis of the hepatocytes, in addition to a large number of Councilman bodies. Regeneration of hepatocytes was never observed in autopsied livers.

The liver of asymptomatic or recovered rats at 6–8 months of age showed a chronic (mild) hepatitis responsible for regeneration in the periportal areas of the hepatic lobules with small hepatocytes and small cells with an oval nucleus and scan cytoplasm, similar to cholangiolar cells, the so-called oval cells. These areas contained some cell types intermediate between small hepatocytes and cholangiolar cells. Some of the intermediate cells reacted positively with immunohistochemical staining for alpha-fetoprotein, indicating a transient appearance of a regeneration of hepatocytes from the cholangiolar cells, similar to those found in the early stages of azo-dye hepatocarcinogenesis [8].

These rats, which survived for more than 8 months, had hyperplastic foci composed of small hepatocytes with vacuolar or basophilic cytoplasm and small round nuclei. Mitotic figures were sometimes detected in the foci. The size of these foci increased with age, becoming larger than the hepatic lobules. These large whitish lesions appeared to be histologically identical with the hyperplastic nodules that were found in rat liver with hepatocarcinogenesis.

In rats that had survived for more than 1 year, large liver tumors with whitish and/or reddish colors, associated with necrosis, were often observed. Histological characteristics of the tumor cells represented well-differentiated hepatocelluar carcinomas with typical trabecular structures [2]. Thus, these results revealed that LEC rats have a remarkably high susceptibility to the spontaneous development of liver neoplasia.

Conclusions

The LEC rat is quite a unique mutant strain causing hepatitis and subsequent hepatic lesions including liver cancer. The characteristics of the mutation in the LEC strain clearly distinguish it from previously described mutations causing jaundice in rats [3,4] and mice [5,6]. Therefore, the animal model of hepatitis represented by the LEC rat has proved its value in various fields of medical research. This model had been of great benefit to the understanding and elucidation of hepatitis as well as of hepato-carcinogenesis.

Although the LEC strain is an autosomal recessive mutant, the mutant *hts* gene has not yet been determined. The appearance of hepatitis in adult rats suggests that the expression of the liver lesion is subject to developmental modification. Certain biochemical defects are known in the Gunn rat which is deficient in glucuronyl transfer [3], and in the mutant Wistar rat that has impaired hepatic anion transport to bile [4]. Obviously, biochemical pathways need to be studied in the LEC rat, and an approach to resolve the mechanism(s) for the cause of the hepatitis is necessary. Sugiyama et al. [9] examined several drug-metabolizing enzymes in the liver of LEC rats, and demonstrated no enzyme deficiency, although they did find low content of cytochrome P-450 in young LEC rats before the development of hepatitis. It is assumed that the decrease in the content of P-450 may lead to the inhibition of excretion of bile acids and certain endogeneous steroids from hepatocytes, and that accumulation of their metabolites in the liver may account for the cause of hepatitis. Very recently, heritable low levels of plasma ceruloplasmin and hepatic copper accumulation were found in LEC rats. These impaired copper metabolisms may be etiologically associated with hepatic lesions in LEC rats. Therefore, as described in the following chapters, the potential of the LEC strain for various fields of investigation is considerable.

Acknowledgments. We wish to thank Mrs. Kazuko Kagami and Mr. Eikichi Kamimura of the Center for Experimental Plants and Animals of Hokkaido University for their assistance. We also acknowledge Dr. Noritoshi Takeichi and Prof. Hiroshi Kobayashi, Hokkaido University School of Medicine, and Dr. Kimimaro Dempo and Prof. Michio Mori, Sapporo Medical College for their early studies of LEC rats. This work was partly supported by Grants-in-Aid for Scientific Research from the Ministry of Education, Science and Culture, and of Health and Welfare of Japan.

References

1. Sasaki M, Yoshida MC, Kagami K, Takeichi N, Kobayashi H, Dempo K, Mori M (1985) Spontaneous hepatitis in an inbred strain of Long-Evans rats. Rat News Lett. 14:4–6
2. Yoshida MC, Masuda R, Sasaki M, Takeichi N, Kobayashi H, Dempo K, Mori M (1987) New mutation causing hereditary hepatitis in the laboratory rat. J Hered 78:361–365

3. Gunn CH (1938) Hereditary acholuric jaundice in new mutant strain of rats. J Hered 29:137–139
4. Jansen PL, Peter WH, Lamers WH (1985) Hereditary chronic conjugated hyperbilirubinemia in mutant rats caused by defective hepatic anion transport. Hepatology 5:573–579
5. Russell ES, Bernstein SE (1968) Blood and blood formation. In: Biology of the laboratory mouse. Green ER (ed) Dover, New York, pp 351–372
6. Saxton AM, Eisen EJ, Johnson BH, Burkhart JG (1985) New mutation causing jaundice in mice. J Hered 76:441–446
7. Masuda R, Yoshida MC, Sasaki M, Dempo K, Mori M (1988) Hereditary hepatitis of LEC rats is controlled by a single autosomal recessive gene. Lab Anim 22:166–169
8. Dempo K, Chisaka N, Yoshida Y, Kaneko A, Onoe T (1975) Immunofluorescent studies on alpha-fetoprotein-producing cells in the early stage of 3'-methyl-4-dimethylaminoazobenzene carcinogenesis. Cancer Res 35:1282–1287
9. Sugiyama T, Takeichi N, Kobayashi H, Yoshida MC, Sasaki M, Taniguchi N (1988) Metabolic predisposition of a novel mutant (LEC rats) to hereditary hepatitis and hepatoma: Alterations of the drug metabolizing enzymes. Carcinogenesis 9:1569–1572

2 — Reproductive Performance and Effects of Pregnancy on the Acute Phase of Hepatitis in LEC Rats

NORIYUKI KASAI[1], EIKICHI KAMIMURA[2], ICHIRO MIYOSHI[1], and MICHIHIRO C. YOSHIDA[3]

Introduction

LEC rats have been established as a mutant strain that suffers from fulminant hepatitis and severe jaundice at about 4 months of age [1,2]. The clinical symptoms of hepatitis include severe jaundice, a bleeding tendency, oliguria, loss of body weight, and elevation of the serum levels of bilirubin and hepatic enzymes, such as glutamic oxaloacetic transaminase (GOT) and glutamic pyruvic transaminase (GPT). About one-half-of the animals die within 1 week after the onset of jaundice and, in survivors, hepatocellular carcinoma spontaneously appears after 1 or 1.5 years of age [3]. Recently we described clinico-pathological studies of LEC rats in the acute phase of hepatitis, and made it clear that this phase started 3–4 weeks before the onset of fulminant hepatitis [4]. On the other hand, the sexual maturity of the LEC rat is usually achieved by around the age at which the hepatitis occurs. Therefore, the breeding of LEC rats seems to be highly influenced by a decrease of breeding rate due to the hepatitis.

In this paper, we describe the reproductive performance of LEC rats from data obtained during their maintenance and breeding, and the relation of breeding to the clinico-pathological characteristics of hepatitis in the LEC rat.

Reproductive Efficiency

Reproductive performance of the first two matings of LEC rats and two normal control inbred strains, LEA and WKAH, is shown in Table 1. The LEA is one of two inbred strains, LEA and LEC, which were established

---

[1] The Institute for Animal Experimentation, School of Medicine,
[2] The Center for Experimental Plants and Animals, and
[3] Chromosome Research Unit, Faculty of Science, Hokkaido University, Sapporo, 060 Japan

Table 1. The reproductive efficiency of LEC rats compared with those of inbred strains LEA and WKAH[a].

Strains	LEC	LEA	WKAH
Observed females (n)	73	23	24
1st Pregnancy			
Pregnant females (n)	67 (91.8%)*	23 (100%)*	24 (100%)*
Neonates (n)	483	221	167
Litter size	7.2	9.6	7.0
Nursing dams (n)	52 (77.6%)**	21 (91.3%)**	21 (87.5%)**
Weanlings (n)	397	205	165
Weaning rate	82.2%	92.8%	98.8%
Reproductive rate***	5.4	8.9	6.9
Females dead by 2nd pregnancy (n)	26 (35.6%)	0	0
2nd Pregnancy			
Pregnant females (n)	33 (45.2%)*	23 (100%)*	24 (100%)*
Neonates (n)	284	296	218
Litter size	8.6	12.9	9.1
Nursing dams (n)	24 (72.3%)*	22 (95.7%)*	23 (95.8%)**
Weanlings (n)	200	252	200
Weaning rate	70.4%	85.1%	91.7%
Reproductive rate***	2.7	11.0	8.3
Females dead after 2nd pregnancy (n)	11	0	0
Total no. of weanlings	597	457	365
Final reproductive rate***	8.2	19.9	22.1
Total no. of females dead due to fulminant hepatitis	34 (46.6%)	0	0

[a] Data were summarized from the nucleus colonies of F_{47-49} for LEC, F_{42-48} for LEA, and $F_{243-250}$ for WKAH
* Percentage was calculated as the number of pregnant females divided by the number of observed females × 100
** Percentage was calculated as the number of nursing dams divided by the number of pregnant females × 100
*** Reproductive rate was calculated as the number of weanlings divided by the number of observed females

from a closed colony of randomly bred Long-Evans rats. The WKAH is an inbred strain maintained over 240 generations in our laboratory, and had originally come from a closed colony of Wistar-King A rats. The rats were maintained under conventional conditions, and fed a regular diet and water ad libitum in an air-conditioned animal room at 22° ± 3°C with a relative humidity of 55% ± 5%. The cages, made of poly-carbonate with the dimensions of 310 mm × 360 mm × 175 mm, were bedded with wooden chips. The rats were bred by sibmating and one female was paired with one male at 8–9 weeks of age.

One-hundred percent of observed females of both control strains became pregnant from the two matings. In LEC rats, even though over 90% of the females became pregnant from the first mating, the pregnancy rate dropped drastically to 45% of the original group at the second pregnancy, because 26 rats or 35.5% of the original group died, and 14 rats or 19.2% became infertile due to fulminant hepatitis by the time of the second mating. In addition, the ratio of dams that nursed neonates after parturition to pregnant females was also lower than that of control strains, and it was decreased from 78% at the first pregnancy to 73% at the second pregnancy, although this ratio slightly increased at the second pregnancy in normal inbred strains. Therefore, the weaning rate of LEC rats was poorer than that of control strains. However, average litter sizes in both pregnancies of LEC females, 7.2 and 8.6, were not very small when compared with normal controls. In addition, primiparous females generally have smaller litters, and the number of the young in the litters increases later with repeated conception [5]. In LEC rats as well, the second litter was larger than the first. Therefore, hepatitis did not seem to influence the litter size of LEC females. Thus, the reproductive rate, the ratio of the number of weanlings to the number of observed females, drastically dropped from 5.4 for the first parturition to 2.7 for the second parturition. We terminated the mating after the first delivery to obtain economical reproductive efficiency. Therefore, we could expect only 5.4 pups per female in LEC rats in a commercial reproductive plant. In the normal control strains, however, expected reproductive capacity is six or mroe litters during the life of the rat with a 100% pregnancy rate in females. Therefore, we could expect 60 or more pups per dam in a reproductive colony. The economic reproductive efficiency of LEC rats is only one-sixth or one-eighth that of normal rats.

Clinico-pathology of the Hepatitis and Sexual Maturity of LEC Rats

The glutamic pyruvic transaminase (GPT) and glutamic oxaloacetic transaminase (GOT) activities in the sera of 24 LEC rats (12 females and 12 males) were measured once a week starting from 10 to 30 weeks of age. Six of the female rats and five of the male rats died at around 18 weeks of age because of fulminant hepatitis with severe jaundice. Figure 1 shows the time course of individual GPT activities of the surviving rats and the process of general sexual maturity of the rat. The process of maturation of LEC rats was believed to be the same as that of other inbred strains since the first pregnancy occurred at around 11 weeks of age (Table 2). Therefore, we let the rats mate at 8–9 weeks of age. Normal LEC female rats became pregnant at 10–13 weeks of age with the pregnancy lasting until 13–16 weeks of age. However, the GPT activities of female LEC rats were elevated from 15 weeks of age until 19 or 20 weeks of age.

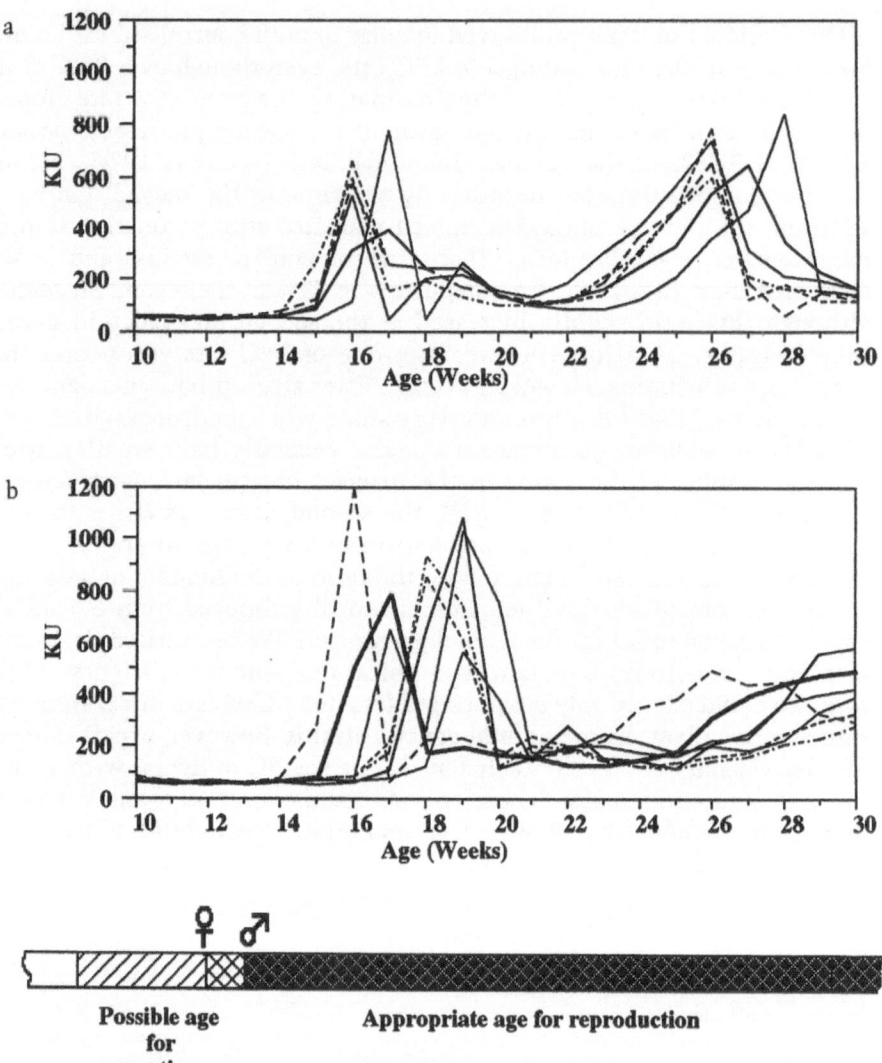

Fig. 1. The time course of GPT activities in sera of LEC rats and sexual maturity. **a** The GTP of six female rats and **b** seven male rats were measured from 10 to 30 weeks of age and plotted individually. The *bar* shows the general time course of sexual maturity in rat

Figure 2 shows the changes of the quantitative microscopical features of liver with serum GPT activities of female rats according to age. The rats were sacrificed under ether and/or sodium pentobarbital anesthesia, after which the livers were excised and paraffin sections were prepared as described previously [4]. For quantitative analyses of histology, the numbers of enlarged hepatic nuclei, Councilman bodies (eosinophilic degeneration

Table 2. The age at onset of fulminant hepatitis in virgin and multiparous females of LEC rats[a].

	Virgin rats		Multiparous rats
Number of observed females	12		17
Age at first pregnancy (weeks)			11.5 ± 1.6***
Number of females suffering from jaundice (percent)	12 (100%)	N.S.*	13 (76.5%)
Age of females at onset of jaundice (weeks)	16.5 ± 1.0***	$P < 0.01$**	22.2 ± 3.7***
Number of females dead due to fulminant hepatitis (death rate)	6 (50.0%)	N.S.*	11 (64.7%)

[a] All the observed rats were from the F_{43} generation
Statistical analyses were performed by the *chi-square test or **Student's t-test for comparison between virgin and multiparous rats. *** mean ±SD; N.S., not significant

of hepatocytes) in the sinusoid, microgranulomas in the sinusoid, and hepatocytes in mitosis were counted in all areas of each liver section as indexes (detailed in [4]). The number of large nuclei in the liver began to increase in females at 14 weeks of age despite the fact that elevation of serum GPT activities was first observed at 17 weeks of age, indicating that the hepatitis started histologically 3 or 4 weeks prior to the fulminant hepatitis. However, since sexual maturity was achieved just before the onset of hepatitis, the LEC females were able to become pregnant normally. Once the rats became pregnant, the hepatitis seemed to be delayed as described below.

In contrast, the sexual maturity of male rats was 1 week later than that of female rats, and the fulminant hepatitis occurred 1 or 2 weeks later in males (Fig. 1). The death rate of male rats due to fulminant hepatitis, 25%, was lower than that of female rats (Table 3). In addition, fertility (the reproductive ability) of male rats was not lost after surviving from fulminant hepatitis. Therefore, the influence of hepatitis on male reproductive performance was much less than that in females.

Pregnancy Delayed the Occurrence of Fulminant Hepatitis

Table 2 shows the ages at the onset of jaundice of virgin and multiparous LEC rats. All of the rats used in this observation were from the litters of F_{43}. Jaundice occurred just after the peak of the first elevation of serum GPT activities in LEC rats [4]. Therefore, jaundice was one of the symptoms of fulminant hepatitis in LEC rats. One-hundred percent of the virgin females suffered from jaundice at around 16.5 weeks of age and one-half of them died after jaundice appeared. In contrast, the multiparous females were first pregnant at about 11.5 weeks of age, and the incidence of

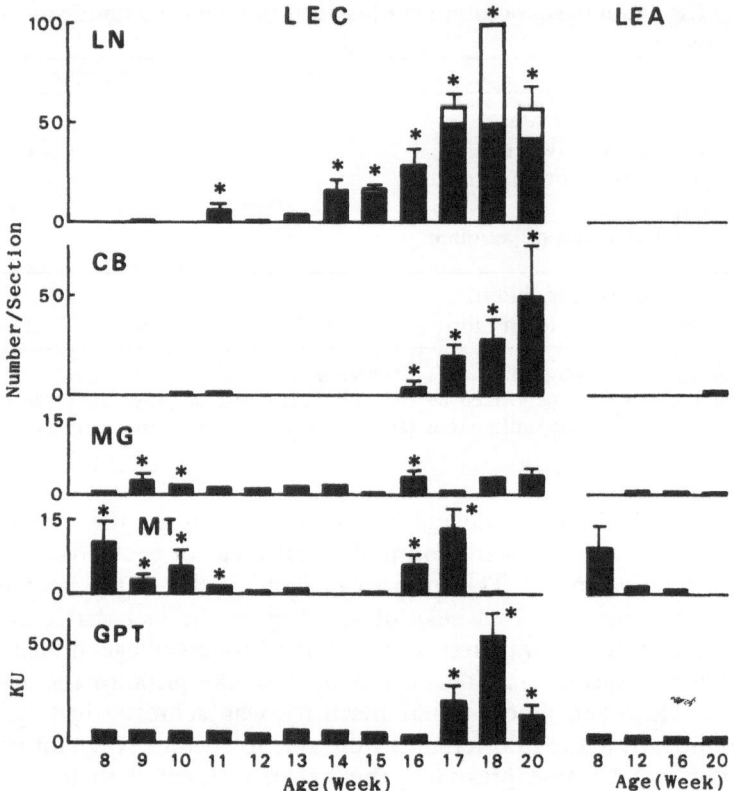

Fig. 2. The scores for histological changes of LEC rat livers with their ages in the acute phase of hepatitis. Five females were examined weekly. As controls, five female LEA rats were examined at age 8, 12, 16, and 20 weeks. *LN* large nuclei, *CB* Councilman bodies, *MG* microgranulomas, *MT* hepatocytes in mitosis, *GPT* serum GPT activities. The *open bars* in large nuclei (*LN*) show the numbers of nuclei with diameters larger than 20 μm and the *closed bars* show the numbers of nuclei with diameters between 15 and 20 μm. Values shown in the figures are for mean ± SE. Statistical analyses were performed by Wilcoxon rank-sum test (*, $P < 0.05$). (See [4])

jaundice and the death rate were not significantly different from those of virgin rats. However, the age at which jaundice began was delayed from 16.5 to 22.2 weeks, an average of 5.7 weeks, in multiparous rats. This indicates that LEC females became pregnant just before the progression to fulminant hepatitis, as mentioned in the previous section, and, once pregnant, the progression of hepatitis in LEC females was delayed for about 6 weeks. This period of time is consistent with the period of pregnancy and ensuing lactation. This phenomenon was, of course, nonexistent in LEC males, and suggests that female sex hormones secreted during pregnancy and lactation somehow suppress the progression of hepatitis.

Table 3. Average maximum GPT activities, the ages at which GPT activities reached maximum, and the survival rates of groups receiving different treatments.

Animals	Number tested	Age at peak (weeks)	Death rate (%)
		Female	
Untreated	18	16.3 ± 0.5[a]	50.0
Ovariectomized	8	18.8 ± 0.7*	87.5
Ova + Testosterone[b]	10	17.8 ± 0.4*	0.0*
Ova + Estradiol[c]	9	20.3 ± 1.3*	66.7
		Male	
Untreated	16	18.0 ± 1.1	25.0
Orchidectomized	7	18.6 ± 0.5	85.7*
Orc + Testosterone[d]	9	19.5 ± 0.5	11.1
Orc + Estradiol[e]	12	24.3 ± 2.3*	100.0*

[a] Average values are means ± SD
[b] Rats were ovariectomized and administrated testosterone.
[c] Rats were ovariectomized and administrated estradiol.
[d] Rats were orchidectomized and administrated testosterone.
[e] Rats were orchidectomized and administrated estradiol.
Statistical analyses were performed by Student's t-test for average values of age and by chi-square test for the survival rate by comparing data of each group with those of untreated rats in each sex (*, $P < 0.05$)

Effects of Sex Hormones on Fulminant Hepatitis of the Rats

We examined the effects of sex hormones on fulminant hepatitis by administering exogenous sex hormones to ovariectomized or orchidectomized LEC rats. The animals underwent these surgical procedures at 4 or 5 weeks of age. Testosterone propionate or β-estradiol 3-benzoate, was dissolved in sesame oil at 3 mg/ml and 0.3 mg/ml, respectively, and 0.1 ml aliquots of each were administered subcutaneously twice a week from 12 weeks to 25 weeks of age. Table 3 shows the age at which serum GPT activity reached maximum levels and the death rate from the first attack of fulminant hepatitis. A 4-week delay was shown in ovariectomized and estradiol-administered females, whereas other treatments caused delays of only 1.5–2.5 weeks. In addition, administration of the same dose of estradiol to orchidectomized male rats also delayed the first serum GPT elevation for 6 weeks. However, the death rate was slightly but not significantly higher for the delivering dams or the rats given estradiol than for virgin females or untreated females. This demonstrates that estradiol did not cure the hepatitis but suppressed the deterioration and delayed the occurrence of fulminant hepatitis. Adult female rat-liver cytosol was found to have a substantial number of estrogen receptors [6–8]. Therefore, it is thought that estrogen directly affects the liver.

Testosterone, however, seemed not to affect the onset of hepatitis but enabled the rats to survive the disease. During pregnancy, high levels of estrogen and testosterone are continuously secreted from the corpus luteum and/or placenta of non-pregnant females [9]. Therefore, estrogen and testosterone work well against the hepatitis of LEC rats. Progesterone is also thought to be one of the hormones which delays the occurrence of hepatitis, because it is also continuously elevated during pregnancy and lactation in the rat [9]. Thus, more detailed research into the effects of these hormones on LEC-rats hepatitis is warranted.

Conclusions

We described the reproductive performance and the effects of pregnancy on hepatitis using the monitored laboratory data of LEC rats, and elucidated the role of sex hormones in delaying the progression of hepatitis.

Over 90% of the females became pregnant at the first mating but this figure dropped to 45% of the original group at the second pregnancy because of the death and infertility of 55% of the dams due to fulminant hepatitis after the first pregnancy. With a low weaning rate, the reproductive rate, i.e., the ratio of the number of weanlings to the number of their dams, was 5.4 for the first parturition and 2.7 for the second parturition.

According to the mating data and microscopical observations, sexual maturity was shown to be achieved just before the onset of hepatitis. Therefore, female LEC rats were able to become pregnant normally.

Once the females became pregnant, the progression of hepatitis was delayed for 6 weeks. This included the periods of pregnancy and lactation. This fact suggests that female sex hormones secreted during pregnancy and lactation somehow suppress the progression of hepatitis.

We examined the effects of sex hormones on fulminant hepatitis by the administration of exogenous sex hormones to ovariectomized and orchidectomized LEC rats. The hepatitis was delayed 4 and 6 weeks for ovariectomized females and orchidectomized males, respectively, when compared with untreated LEC rats. This phenomenon may explain the delay of the onset of hepatitis in pregnant females and contribute to the continuation of the first pregnancy and lactation. The mechanism of the effect of sex hormones on hepatitis remains to be resolved, and its elucidation may help disclose the mechanism of the disease as well as indicate possible medical treatments. The role of pregnancy is to maintain the species, and so powerful is this process that even fulminant hepatitis is suppressed by it in the LEC rat.

References

1. Sasaki M, Yoshida MC, Kagami K, Takeichi H, Kobayashi K, Dempo K, Mori M, (1989) Spontaneous hepatitis in an inbred strain of Long-Evans rats. Rat News Lett 14:4–6

2. Yoshida MC, Masuda R, Sasaki M, Takeichi N, Kobayashi H, Dempo K, Mori M, (1988) New mutation causing hereditary hepatitis in the laboratory rat. J Hered 78:361–365
3. Masuda R, Yoshida MC, Sasaki M, Dempo K, Mori M, (1988) High susceptibility to hepatocellular carcinoma development in LEC rats with hepatitis. Jpn J Cancer Res 79:828–835
4. Kasai N, Osanai T, Miyoshi I, Kamimura E, Yoshida MC, Dempo K, (1990) Clinico-pathological studies of LEC rats with hereditary hepatitis and hepatoma in the acute phase of hepatitis. Lab Anim Sci 40:502–505
5. Weihe WH (1987) The laboratory rat. In: Poole B (ed) The UFAW handbook on the care and management of laboratory animals. London Scientific and Technical, London, pp 309–330
6. Eisenfeld AJ, Aten RF, Weinberger M, Haselbacher G, Halpern K (1976) Estrogen receptor in the mammalian liver. Science 191:862–865
7. Eisenfeld AJ, Aten RF (1987) Estrogen receptors and androgen receptors in the mammalian liver. J Steroid Biochem 27:1109–1118
8. Dickson RB, Aten RF, Eisenfeld AJ (1978) An unusual sex steroid binding protein in mature male rat liver cytosol. Endocrinology 103:1636–1646
9. Taya K, Komura H, Watanabe G, Sasamoto S (1989) Peripheral blood levels of immunoreactive inhibin during pseudopregnancy, pregnancy and lactation in the rat. J Endocrinol 121:545–552

3 — Differences in the Course of Hereditary Hepatitis Between Males and Females, and Between Virgins and Parous Female LEC Rats

Kazuto Yamazaki, Masaaki Nakayama, Koji Tomobe, Hiroshi Ohyama, Yumi Sawada, Tsuneo Wakabayashi[1], and Noritoshi Takeichi[2]

Introduction

A strain of Long-Evans rats (LEC), a new autosomal recessive mutant with hepatitis and severe jaundice [1–3], was established at the Cancer Institute, Hokkaido University School of Medicine, Sapporo, Japan. The mutant shows a sudden development of jaundice with a high rate of lethality around 4 months of age. The onset of jaundice is characterized by hyperbilirubinemia, elevation of serum glutamic oxaloacetic transaminase (GOT) and glutamic pyruvic transaminase (GPT) activities, with massive necrosis of hepatocytes. These clinical signs are almost identical with those of human fulminant hepatitis. It is also reported that survivors spontaneously develop liver cancer with time [4–6].

We had the opportunity of breeding LEC rats at our laboratories after their discovery at Hokkaido University. In this paper, we report differences in the course of hepatitis between sexes, and between virgin and parous females.

Materials and Methods

Animals

Three male and three female LEC rats (aged 7–9 weeks) were originally introduced by the Hokkaido Laboratory group. We maintained the animals under conventional conditions at the Eisai Tsukuba Research Laboratories, Ibaraki, Japan. The rats were fed a commercial diet (CE-2, Nihon CLEA Inc., Tokyo) and sterilized water ad libitum under a temperature-, hu-

[1] Laboratory Animal Research Center, Tsukuba Research Laboratories, Eisai Co., Ltd., Tsukuba, 300–26 Japan
[2] Laboratory of Pathology, Cancer Institute, Hokkaido University School of Medicine, Sapporo, 060 Japan

midity-, and light-controlled regime (22 ± 1°C, 55 ± 5%, and 12-h light/ dark cycle with lights on at 07:00). The animals were housed in Econ cages (Nihon CLEA Inc.) bedded with wood shavings (White Flake, Charles River Japan Inc., Kanagawa, Japan). Matings were set up at 10 weeks of age. The progeny were weaned at the age of 4 weeks. The rats between the F_1 and F_3 generations were used to obtain data on natural history and life span (males, $n = 40$; virgin females, $n = 41$; parous females, $n = 23$). We biochemically and pathologically examined the rats between the F_2 and F_5 generations.

Biochemical Examinations

Sixteen males and 20 virgin females were examined at ages 4, 8, 12, 14, 16–35, 40, 44, 48, and 52 weeks. Blood was drawn from the caudal vein, collected through heparinized tubes, and centrifugated at 3,000 rpm to obtain plasma samples. Activities of plasma glutamic oxaloacetic transaminase (GOT) and plasma glutamic pyruvic transaminase (GPT) were measured by a commercial kit (Transaminase C-test Wako, Wako Pure Pharmaceutical, Osaka, Japan).

Blood coagulation time was measured by Hepaplastintest (Eisai Co., Ltd., Tokyo). Blood samples were from whole blood drawn from the caudal vein.

Pathological Examinations

The rats we used were those with a clinically normal appearance at 6 and 12 weeks of age, with fulminant hepatitis at 18 weeks of age, and asymptomatic or recovered rats at 1–1.5 years of age. The liver, spleen, and thymus were fixed in 10% neutralized buffered formalin solution (pH 7.4) and embedded in paraffin. Sections of 4 μm thickness were made and observed by light microscopy after staining with hematoxylin and eosin, and periodic acid-Schiff.

Results

Reproduction Records

LEC female rats were able to reproduce before the onset of jaundice, and gave birth to first–third litters. The fourth parturition was observed in one case, and this litter was not weaned. A few females recovered from jaundice during pregnancy and were delivered of litters. The litter sizes of the F_1–F_3 generations at first–third parturitions are indicated in Table 1. No significant differences were noted between the parturitions. From Feburary 24, 1988 to November 27, 1990, the generation of LEC rats reached F_8. Table 2 shows mean litter sizes of each generation.

Table 1. Litter sizes of LEC rats of F_1–F_3 generations at first–third parturitions.

	Mean ± SEM	n
First	9.1 ± 0.5	17
Second	8.6 ± 0.6	10
Third	10.1 ± 0.9	9

Table 2. Litter sizes of LEC female rats at F_1–F_8 generations.

Generation	Mean ± SEM	n
F_1	8.8 ± 1.0	8
F_2	9.0 ± 0.6	13
F_3	9.6 ± 0.6	15
F_4	7.8 ± 0.6	17
F_5	8.2 ± 0.7	11
F_6	7.9 ± 0.7	13
F_7	6.6 ± 0.7	10
F_8	9.0 ± 0.0	2

Clinical Signs and Macroscopic Findings at Autopsies

Male LEC rats began to show jaundice in their ears, tails, and genitalia, and bilirubinuria, anemia, and loss of body weight at around 5 months of age. Thirty-five of the 40 males (87.5%) developed jaundice at 5–7 months of age. Seven of the 36 jaundiced males recovered, and 29 rats died with coma within a week after onset of the jaundice. In the course of the examination, 4 out of the 40 males (10.0%) were asymptomatic.

The ages at the onset of jaundice were different between virgin and parous female LEC rats. All 41 virgin females developed jaundice at 4–6 months after birth, and died within 1 week after onset of the condition. On the other hand, parous females were affected later than the virgins. Eleven of the 23 parous females (47.8%) were jaundiced at 5–7 months of age, and 4 out of 11 jaundiced females recovered. At 8–10 months after birth, 12 remaining females had jaundice, and one of them recovered. Table 3 shows the ages when jaundice was first recognized. There were significant differences between the onset ages of males, and the virgin and parous females ($P < 0.001$).

Table 4 summarizes the natural history of the LEC rat. The rates of fulminant hepatitis rats and recovered rats were examined by the Fisher's exact probability test between males, virgin females, and parous females. The following results were obtained: males vs virgin females, $P < 0.01$; males vs parous females, not significant; virgin females vs parous females, $P < 0.01$.

Table 3. Age (days) when jaundice was first observed in LEC male, and virgin and parous female rats.

Sex	n	Range	Mean ± SEM		
Male	36	140–239	173.1 ± 3.7	***	
Female					***
Virgin	41	118–182	148.6 ± 2.1	***	
Parous	23	142–301	216.9 ± 9.5		

Asterisks indicate significant differences at $p < 0.001$ by Aspin-Welch's test

Table 4. Natural history of LEC male, and virgin and parous female rats.

Sex	n	Jaundiced		Asymptomatic
		Fulminant	Recovered	
Male	40	29	7	4
		(72.5%)	(17.5%)	(10.0%)
Female				
Virgin	41	41	0	0
		(100%)		
Parous	23	18	5	0
		(78.3%)	(21.7%)	

Figure 1 shows the distribution of age at death of LEC rats, and Table 5 summarizes the life spans of the rats. The χ^2-test was conducted to derive the proportions shown in Table 5. When comparisons were made between males and virgin females, and between virgin and parous females, rats whose ages of death were 30≦ and <60 weeks, and ≧60 weeks, were pooled. The results were as follows: males vs virgin females, $\chi^2_1 = 13.0$, $P < 0.001$; males vs parous females, $\chi^2_2 = 31.4$, $P < 0.001$, and virgin females vs parous females, $\chi^2_1 = 41.3$, $P < 0.001$.

At autopsies, bilirubin deposition was observed in visceral organs of the rats which died of fulminant hepatitis. Livers retained lobule structure and their surfaces were smooth. Slight enlargement of spleens was noted. In the cases of asymptomatic or recovered rats at 1–1.5 years of age, nodular white spots 1–2 mm in diameter were scattered all over the surface of the livers.

Biochemical Examinations

Changes of plasma GOT and GPT activities are indicated in Figs. 2 and 3, respectively. Plasma activities of GOT and GPT in both sexes were almost constant from 4 to 17 weeks of age, except for the levels of GOT at 4

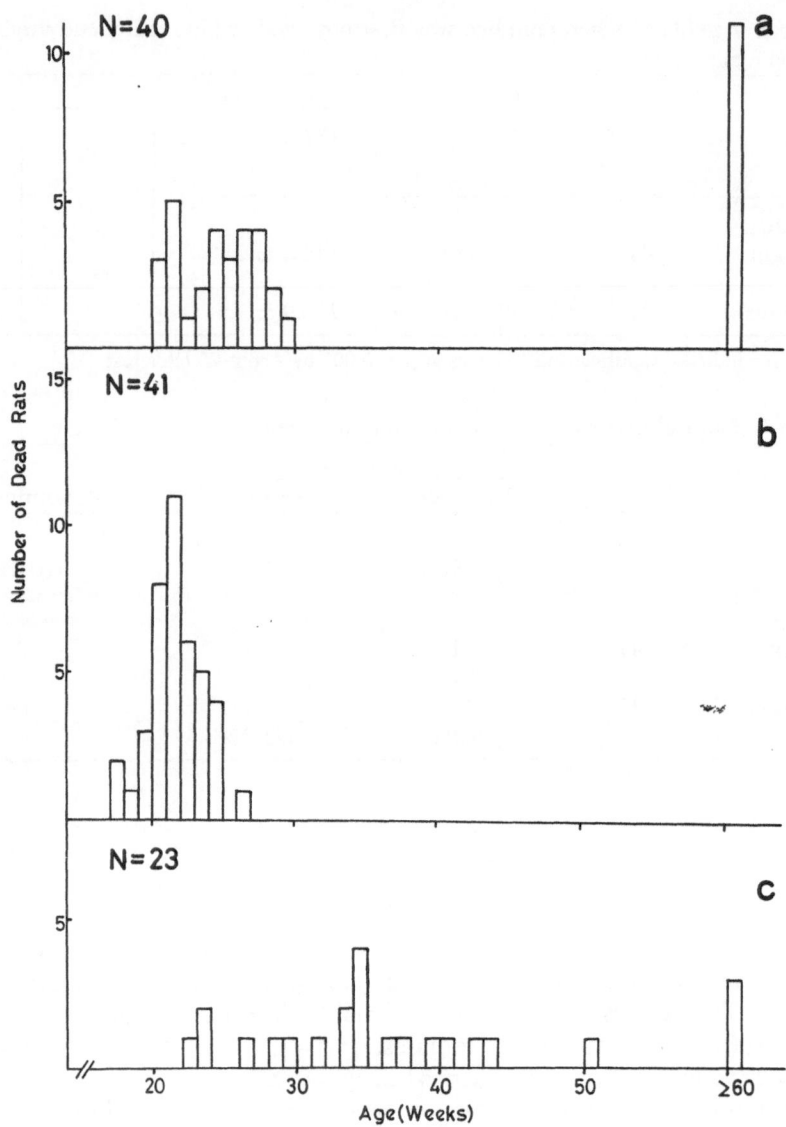

Fig. 1. Distribution of ages when the LEC rats died. **a** males, **b** virgin females, **c** parous females

weeks which were slightly higher. The activities began to elevate from about 18 weeks after birth, and reached their peaks during the presence of jaundice. Means ±SEM of plasma GOT and GPT activities during jaundice were as follows: 16 males, GOT (467 ± 65 Karmen units), GPT (208 ± 126 Karmen units) and 20 females, GOT (423 ± 39 Karmen units), GPT (165 ± 25 Karmen units).

Table 5. Summary of life spans of LEC male, and virgin and parous female rats.

Sex	n	Life span (weeks)		
		<30	30 ≦ <60	≧60
Male	40	29 (72.5%)	0	11 (27.5%)
Female				
Virgin	41	41 (100%)	0	0
Parous	23	6 (26.1%)	14 (60.9%)	3 (13.0%)

Elevation of plasma GOT and GPT activities and jaundice was observed earlier in females than in males. Death of both sexes occurred from 20 weeks of age, and all of the 20 females were dead by 24 weeks after birth. At 21 weeks of age, plasma GOT activities of 15 males and 17 females varied from 56 to 1,122 Karmen units (an average ± standard error of the mean (SEM) of 147 ± 67 Karmen units), and from 66 to 657 Karmen units (an average ± SEM of 298 ± 45 Karmen units), respectively. Plasma GPT activities of the same males and females were 22–185 Karmen units (an average ± SEM of 50 ± 10 Karmen units), and 22–313 Karmen units (an average ± SEM of 127 ± 21 Karmen units), respectively.

Recovered males chronically showed high activities of plasma GOT and GPT. At 52 weeks after birth, plasma GOT and GPT activities in 8 males varied from 13 to 191 Karmen units (an average ± SEM of 131 ± 13 Karmen units), and from 61 to 99 Karmen units (an average ± SEM of 74 ± 4 Karmen units), respectively.

Blood coagulation times in both sexes were constantly about 30 s before onset of the jaundice. During jaundice, the times were prolonged to 40–50 s. Two exceptional males showed >100 s of the time. The times in recovered males were within 30–40 s.

Pathological examinations

No pathological changes were found in livers of either males or females at 6 weeks after birth. Punctate necrosis, enlarged nuclei of hepatocytes, and activated Kupffer's cells were slightly evident at 12 weeks of age, and were prominent at 18 weeks of age. Underdevelopment of the medulla was detected in the thymus.

In the rats with fulminant hepatitis, many small vacuoles were scattered all over the liver lobules where central necrosis and enlargement of nuclei of hepatocytes and oval cells were detected without infiltration of inflammatory cells. No pathological differences were observed between the sexes. In the spleens, a severely atrophied white medulla and an extramedullary hematopoiesis were seen.

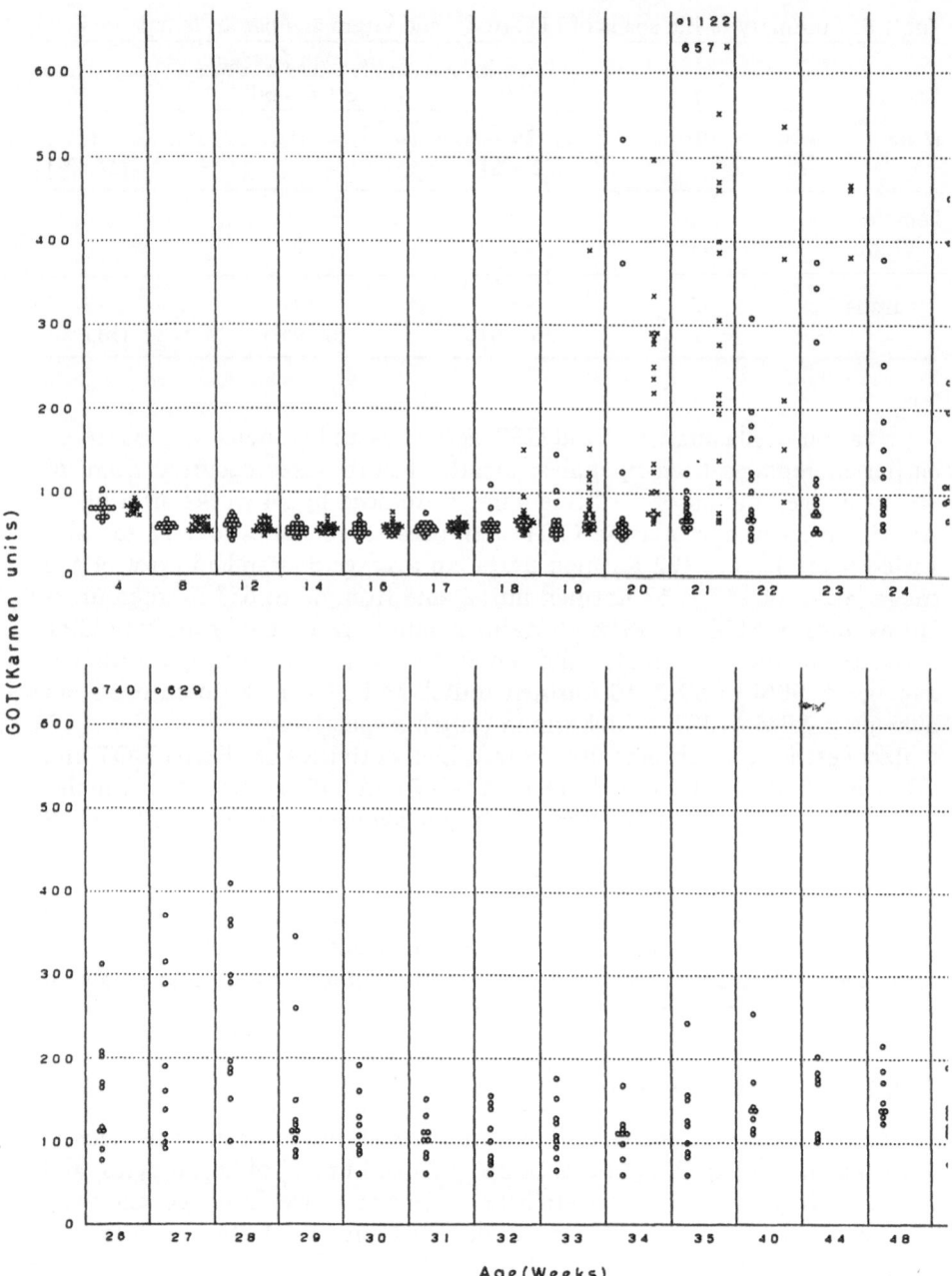

Fig. 2. Changes of activity of plasma GOT with age in LEC rats. *Circles* and *crosses* indicate individual values for males and females, respectively. *Number* next to *circles* and *crosses* are values of activity >600 Karmen units

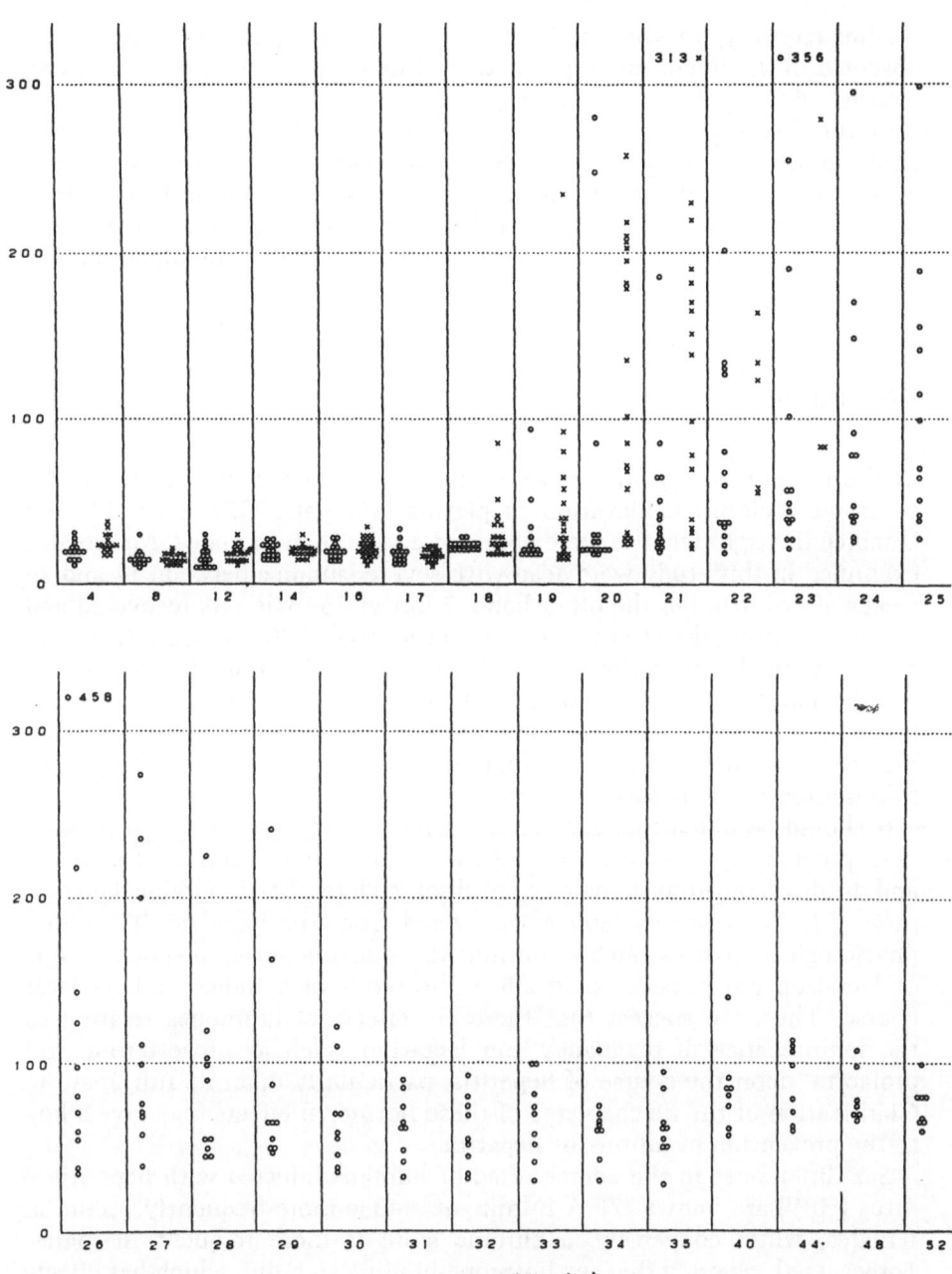

Fig. 3. Changes of activity of plasma GPT with age in LEC rats. *Circles* and *crosses* indicate individual values for males and females, respectively. *Numbers* next to *circles* and *crosses* are values of activity >300 Karmen units

After recovery, vacuoles and enlarged nuclei of hepatocytes were rarely observed in the livers, and regeneration of hepatocytes with oval cells was recognized.

In the livers of asymptomatic or recovered rats aged 52–56 weeks, cholangiofibrosis, conglomerates of macrophages, granuromatosis, heterogeneity and enlargement of nuclei of the hepatocytes, and mitotic figures were revealed, indicating hepatocirrhosis. Apparent hepatocellular carcinoma was not detected in this study. Extramedullary hematopoiesis was prominent in the thymus.

Discussion

In the present study, differences in the course of hepatitis between the sexes were clarified. Elevation of plasma GOT and GPT activities and jaundice in virgin females were observed earlier than in males. All females examined in this study were dead with severe jaundice between 17 and 26 weeks after birth. On the other hand, 7 out of 36 male rats recovered and survived >60 weeks of age, and 4 out of a total of 40 rats were clinically normal with the exception of chronic hepatitis. Accordingly, LEC virgin females had a more severe course of hepatitis than males, which suggests that virgin females were more suitable as a model of fulminant hepatitis. We speculate that it is possible that testosterone has an effect that delays fulmination of the hepatitis.

It should be noted that there were clinical differences between females with previous pregnancies and those without. The appearance of jaundice and the death of parous females were observed later than in virgins. Furthermore, 21.7% of parous females recovered from the jaundice. Therefore, physiological changes, such as hormonal, occurring during pregnancy and/ or lactation are considered to affect the onset of jaundice and its later course. Thus, we suggest that there are effects of hormones relating to the maintenance of pregnancy and lactation, such as progesterone and prolactin, upon the course of hepatitis, particularly upon its fulmination. Clarification of the mechanisms of these hormonal effects may give a key to the prevention of fulminant hepatitis.

Sex differences in the course of adult humans infected with hepatitis B virus (HBV) are known [7]. A fulminant course more frequently occurs in females, while conversely, a chronic state is more frequent in males. Forbes, et al. reported that sex hormone-binding globulin, which has effects on the balance of free sex hormones, was elevated in females with fulminant HBV infection, and suggested that the hormonal environment is important in determining the course of HBV infection [7]. We thus speculated that the course of hepatitis of LEC rats is influenced by the hormonal environment as is that of HBV infection, although hepatitis of LEC rats is not viral.

Conclusion

We investigated the course of hepatitis in the LEC rat clinically and biochemically, and revealed differences in the course between males and females, and between virgin and parous females. Plasma GOT and plasma GPT were elevated, and jaundice was recognized earlier in virgin females than in males. All of the 41 virgin females were dead (100%) with severe jandice by the age of 26 weeks, while 7 rats recovered (17.5%) and 4 rats were asymptomatic (10.0%) among the 40 males. The onset of jaundice in parous females was significantly later than in virgin females. All 23 parous females were jaundiced (100%), as were the 41 virgin females, but 5 out of the former recovered (21.7%). Therefore, we speculated what were the effects of pregnancy, and possibly of lactation as well, on the course of the hepatitis. It seems that sex hormones do effect the course of hepatitis, particularly upon its fulmination.

References

1. Sasaki M, Yoshida MC, Kagami K, Takeichi N, Kobayashi H, Dempo K, Mori M (1985) Spontaneous hepatitis in an inbred strain of Long-Evans rats. Rat News Lett: 14:4–6
2. Yoshida MC, Masuda R, Sasaki M, Takeichi N, Kobayashi H, Dempo K, Mori M (1987) New mutation causing hereditary hepatitis in the laboratory rat. J Hered 78:361–365
3. Masuda R, Yoshida MC, Sasaki M, Dempo K, Mori M (1988) Hereditary hepatitis of LEC rat strain controlled by a single autosomal recessive gene. Lab Anim 22:166–169
4. Masuda R, Yoshida MC, Sasaki M, Dempo K, Mori M (1988) High susceptibility to hepatocellular carcinoma development in LEC rats with hereditary hepatitis. Jpn J Cancer Res: 79:828–835
5. Oyamada M, Dempo K, Fujimoto Y, Takahashi H, Satoh MI, Mori M, Masuda R, Yoshida MC, Satoh K, Sato K (1988) Spontaneous occurrence of placental glutathione S-transferase-positive foci in the livers of LEC rats. Jpn J Cancer Res: 79:5–8
6. Takahashi H, Oyamada M, Fujimoto Y, Satoh MI, Hattori, A, Dempo K, Mori M, Tanaka T, Watabe H, Masuda R, Yoshida MC (1988) Elevation of serum alpha-fetoprotein and proliferation of oval cells in the livers of LEC rats. Jpn J Cancer Res: 79:821–827
7. Forbes A, Alexander GJM, Smith HM, Williams R (1988) Elevation of serum sex hormone-binding globulin in females with fulminant hepatitis B virus infection. J Med Virol: 26:93–98

4 — Pathological and Laboratory Findings of "LEC/Otk" Rats Maintained Under SPF Conditions

KAZUYA KAWANO, TSUKASA HIRASHIMA, SHIGEHITO MORI, SUMIO BANDO, KENICHI YONEMOTO, FUMIKO ABE, HIROHIKO GOTO, and TAKASHI NATORI[1]

Introduction

A mutant strain of rats, LEC, that develops spontaneous hepatic injury associated with severe jaundice was developed in 1987 [1]. In this LEC strain, isolated and established as an inbred strain by sibmating, almost 90% of the animals show hereditary hepatic injury in conventional conditions [2,3]. Genetic analysis indicated that at least one autosomal recessive gene is responsible for this disease [4]. Thus, the LEC strain is a useful model for studies on liver cell injury and liver cancer. Hepatocellular carcinomas have been found in LEC rats surviving for a long time after recovery from jaundice [2,5]. Hepatocellular carcinomas were also found in all cases in the present study, as will be reported in detail (Chap. III, p. 2).

We placed LEC rats at the F_{40} generation in specific pathogen-free (SPF) conditions, obtained the next generation by Caesarean operation, and raised them in SPF conditions. These SPF-LEC rats named (LEC/Otk) are now in the 9th generation. This paper describes the pathological, biochemical, and immunological characteristics of the SPF-LEC/Otk rats.

Materials and Methods

Animals

A total of 140 SPF-LEC/Otk rats (70 male, 70 female) were used in kinetic studies, and groups of 10 animals (5 males, 5 females) were sacrificed at 5, 10, 15, 18, 26, 40, and 60 weeks of age. The remaining rats were sacrificed for histological studies at 90 weeks of age. The LETO strain, an inbred strain of rats, derived from outbred Long-Evans/Crc rats, was used as a control strain. All rats were kept in our SPF facilities under controlled

[1] Tokushima Research Institute, Otsuka Pharmaceutical Co. Ltd., Tokushima, 771-01 Japan

temperature (23 ± 2°C), humidity (55 ± 5%), and lighting (7:00–19:00). All rats were given a laboratory diet CRF-1 (Oriental Yeast Co., Tokyo) and tap water ad libitum.

Clinical and Histopathological Examinations

The body weights of all of the animals were measured. Hematological examinations including WBC, RBC, and platelet counts, and measurements of the hemoglobin (Hb) and hematocrit (Hct) were made on the day of sacrifice using a Hematology Analyzer Ortho ELT-8/ds (Ortho Diagnostic System Co., Mass., USA). Plasma glutamic pyruvic transaminase (Monotest GPT, Behringer-Mannheim Co., Mannheim, Germany) were examined at various ages with a Bichromatic Analyzer ABBOTT VP (Japan Abbott Co., Tokyo). Serum proteins were analyzed by electrophoresis on cellulose-acetate membranes in Electra HR buffer pH 8.6–9.0 (Helena Laboratories, Texas, USA). The organs were weighed, and then fixed in 10% neutralized formalin. Paraffin sections were stained with hematoxylin and eosin (H and E) by the routine method.

Immunological Examinations

Lymphocyte subsets of peripheral, splenic, and lymph node cells were determined in rats 5, 10, and 15 weeks old, using the monoclonal antibodies OX-6, OX-33, OX-8, and fluorescein isothiocyanate (FITC)-conjugated OX-19 (Serotec, Co., Oxford, UK). For this evaluation, samples of 5×10^5 cells were incubated with 100 μl of monoclonal antibody (OX-6, OX-33, OX-8) for 60 min at 4°C, washed with 0.1%-bovine serum albumin (BSA) in phosphate-buffer saline (PBS) and incubated with phycoerythrin (PE)-conjugated rabbit anti-mouse immunoglobulin-G (IgG) for 60 min at 4°C. The cells were then washed and treated with FITC-OX-19 for 60 min at 4°C. Then, the cells were washed again, suspended in 1 ml 0.1% BSA-PBS, and analyzed in a fluorescence-activated cell sorter (FACS; Ortho Spectrum III, Ortho Diagnostic System Co., Mass., USA). The background fluorescence, taken as that of cells incubated without the first antibody, was less than 1.0%. Statistical analysis of the data was performed by Student's t-test (two-tailed).

Serum immunoglobulin subclasses were determined with "Mouse and Rat Monoclonal Typing Kits" (Serotec, Co., Oxford, UK). Quantitative analyses were made with radial immunodiffusion kits (The Binding Site Co., Birmingham, UK).

Segregation Analysis

(LEC/Otk × F₃₄₄/Ducrj) F_1 and F_2 hybrids were used to determined whether there was any genetic association between spontaneous hepatic injury and immunological disorders, such as IgG1 deficiency and T lymphopenia. The

Table 1. Onset and recovery of spontaneous hepatic injury in LEC/Otk rats (F_{40} + 2, 3).

Item	Male	Female
Symptom at onset	Jaundice	Jaundice
No. of Diseased rats*/no. of rats examined (%)	48/50 (96.0)	50/50 (100)
Age at onset (weeks)	17.3 ± 1.5**	15.9 ± 1.1
No. of Recoveries/no. of diseased rats (%)	38/48 (79.2)	36/50 (72.0)
Days for recovery after onset of diseases	6.8 ± 2.1	7.5 ± 1.7
No. of Deaths/no. of diseased rats (%)	10/48 (20.8)	14/50 (28.0)
Day of death after onset	2.2 ± 1.0	2.7 ± 1.1
No. of Recurrences/no. of remissions (%)	1/38 (2.6)	21/36 (58.3)

* All rats were jaundiced; ** Mean ±S.D.

IgG1 and lymphocyte contents of the offspring were determined at 10 weeks of age, and the animals were sacrificed at 25 weeks of age to determine their plasma GPT levels as well as for preparations of histological sections of the liver stained with H and E.

Results

Rate of Onset and Clinical Course of the Disease

Jaundice developed abruptly at 16 or 17 weeks of age in 96% of the male LEC/Otk rats and in 100% of the females (Table 1). Rats with jaundice showed weakness and exhibited a mucosal or subcutaneous hemorrhagic tendency. Some of these rats (28% of the females and 20% of the males) died of consumption within 3 days after the onset of jaundice. Rats that recovered within a week had a pale pink skin. Some of the rats that had recovered suffered from less severe jaundice again 9 weeks after the first attack (58.3% of the females, 2.6% of the males). All of the rats that had recovered from the second attack of jaundice survived without residual signs of the disease.

Laboratory Findings (Table 2)

At the time of onset of jaundice, the RBC, Hb, and Hct values decreased markedly and the platelets count increased slightly. The plasma bilirubin level increased markedly at the onset of jaundice and returned to the normal range during remission. Both the plasma alkaline phosphatase (ALP) and blood urea nitrogen (BUN) levels increased during the stage of jaundice. The BUN level later returned to the normal range, whereas the ALP level remained slightly higher than that in LETO rats. The plasma albumin level decreased markedly at the onset of jaundice and remained lower than that of control rats during remission. The α-1 globulin fraction

Table 2. Clinical features of LEC/Otk rats with hepatic injury and LETO rats.

Strain	LEC/Otk					LETO		
Animal No.	#4642	#4668	#3025	#3026	#3054	#21601	#21602	#21603
Age (weeks)	15	16	27	27	27	16	16	16
Sex	Female	Female	Male	Male	Male	Male	Male	Male
Symptoms at onset	Jaundice Bilirubinuria	Jaundice Bilirubinuria	None	None	None	None	None	None
Hepatic injury	Fulminant	Fulminant	Chronic	Chronic	Chronic	None	None	None
Hematological parameters								
WBC ($\times 10^3$/mm^3)	18.5	11.0	10.3	10.8	9.6	7.2	7.7	7.6
RBC (10^6/mm^3)	2.6	5.3	10.4	9.7	10.3	7.3	7.9	8.2
Hematocrit (%)	13.6	23.1	44.0	40.0	42.6	37.7	41.1	41.9
Platelets ($\times 10^3$/mm^3)	1569	926	1090	1024	1133	871	953	1104
*Biochemical parameters**								
P-Albumin (g/dl)	2.95	2.83	3.43	3.46	3.51	3.70	3.85	3.66
P-GOT (IU/L)	876	774	488	423	400	88	96	108
P-GPT (U/L)	262	620	425	396	388	22	23	23
P-ALP (IU/L)	375	406	567	437	434	233	229	229
P-Total bilirubin (mg/dl)	44.7	3.6	0.4	0.4	0.3	0.1	0.2	0.1
BUN (mg/dl)	56.0	18.2	18.4	15.8	18.3	16.9	19.7	17.8
Autopsy								
Body wt. (g)	110	160	218	245	259	360	350	402
Liver wt. (g)	3.93	5.00	5.70	6.45	6.57	9.77	9.09	11.10
Spleen wt. (mg)	375	318	375	393	380	647	605	734
Thymus wt. (mg)	38	53	37	86	68	379	328	410

* Assay method: P-Albumin (BCG method), P-GOT, P-GPT (UV method), P-ALP (para-nitrophenylphosphate method), P-Total bilirubin (Michaelson's method), BUN (urease indophenol method)

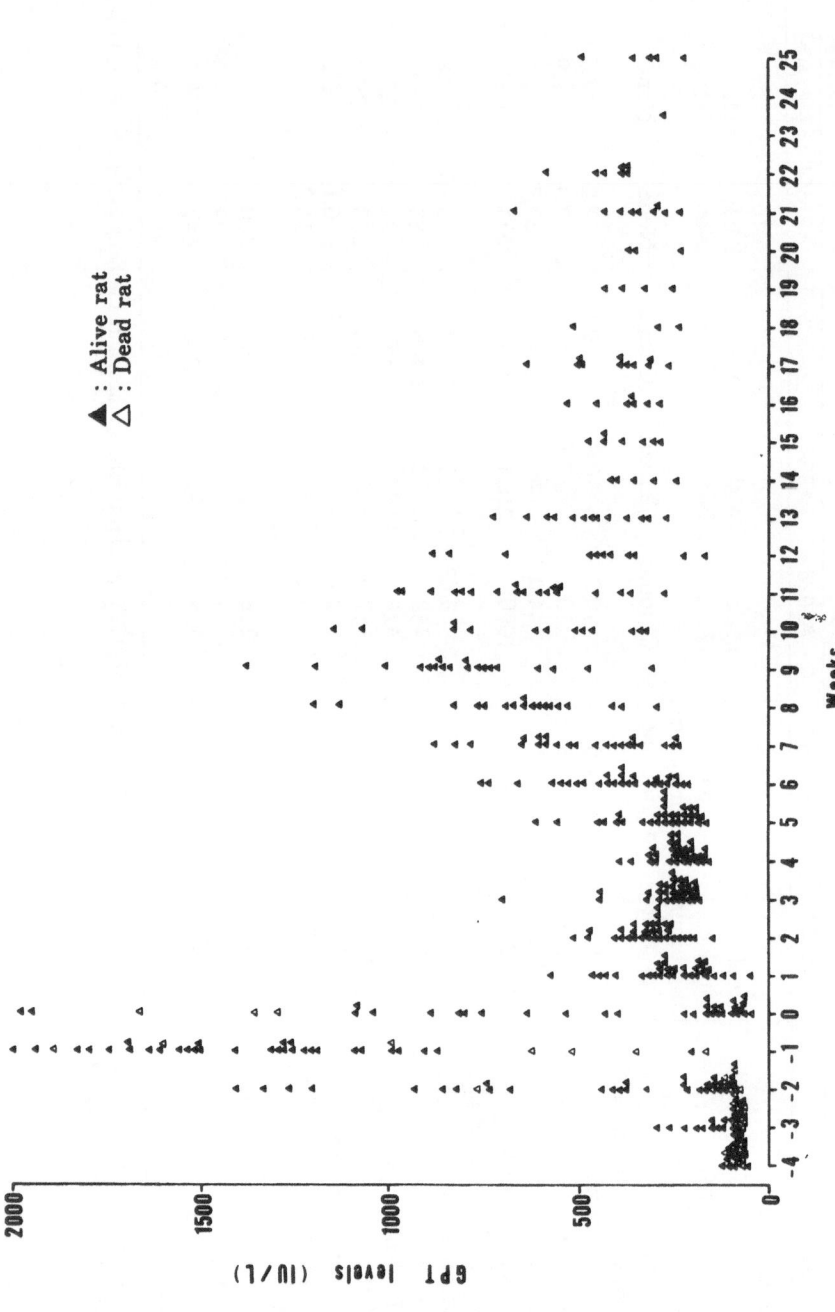

Fig. 1. Plasma GPT levels in male LEC/Otk rats before (−*n* weeks) and after (*n* weeks) the onset of jaundice (day 0). *n* = 55, ▲: rats that died with jaundice. ▲: rats that recovered from jaundice. Control rats (LETO) showed a normal range of GPT (30–60IU/L) without any increase with age

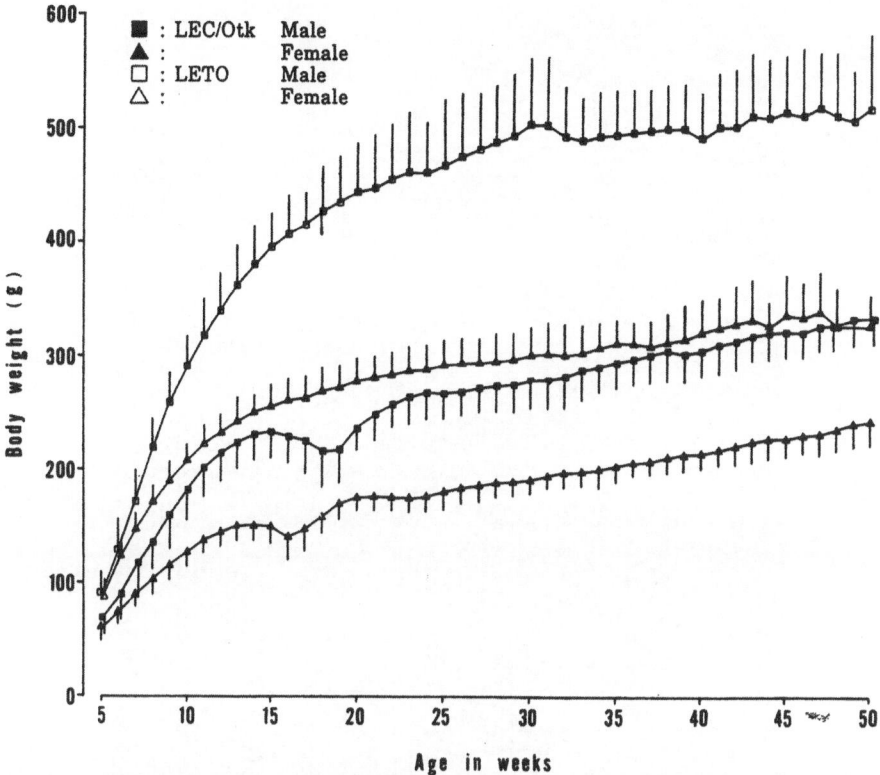

Fig. 2. Body weight changes in LEC/Otk and LETO rats. Values are means ±S.D.

of LEC rats appeared to be significantly lower than that of control animals throughout their lives.

The plasma GPT level correlated well with the clinical course of the disease. As shown in Fig. 1, P-GPT levels started to increase 1–2 weeks before the onset of jaundice, reached a peak during jaundice, and then decreased rapidly. P-GPT showed a second, lower increase correlated with jaundice. After the second increase of P-GPT, its plasma level decreased gradually. The body weight was inversely correlated with both the P-GPT level and the clinical course of the disease (Fig. 2). Animals without jaundice showed slight P-GPT elevations with slight decreases in body weight and water intake. In the control LETO rats. P-GPT levels remained within the normal range throughout life.

Histopathological Changes

The livers of 5-week-old LEC/Otk rats showed a normal architecture. Significant changes, such as uneven-sized nuclei, cells with two nuclei, fat droplets, and occasional mitoses, were observed in the livers of rats of

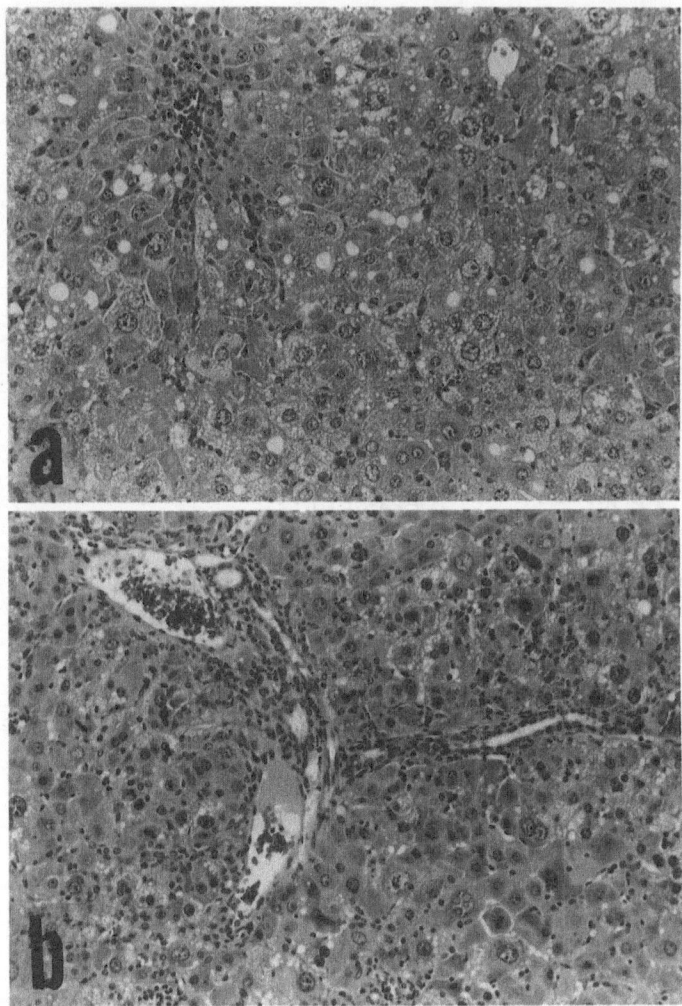

Fig. 3. a A histological section of the liver of a LEC/Otk rat with severe jaundice. Focal liver cell necrosis with minimal inflammatory reactions is present. A fine fatty accumulation is observed in the cytoplasm of liver cells, which show characteristic microvesicular fatty changes. The nuclei are extremely large, some containing pseudo-inclusion bodies, with Councilman bodies observed in sinusoidal areas, and activated Kupffer's cells (H and E, × 50). **b** Section of the liver of a LEC/Otk rat in the chronic stage. The periportal areas of hepatic lobules are occupied by small hepatocytes and cholangio-epithelial cells with oval nuclei (oval cells) with scanty cytoplasm, H and E, × 50

10–15 weeks old. No liver cell necrosis or inflammatory cell infiltration was seen. In rats of over 15 weeks of age, liver cell changes became prominent. Fine fatty droplets were observed in the cytoplasm of enlarged liver cells that showed characteristic microvesicular fatty changes. The nuclei became extremely large, sometimes containing pseudo-inclusion bodies. Councilman bodies were observed in the sinusoidal area and Kupffer's cells were activated. Multiple focal to submassive liver cell necroses were frequently observed, but inflammatory reactions were slight (Fig. 3a). After 18 weeks of age, the livers showed bi-directional changes: degenerative changes indicated by decrease in volume of hepatic lobules as the result of liver cell necrosis, and residual liver cells with huge nuclei, Councilman bodies, and other regenerative changes including small hepa-tocytes, cholangioepithelial cells with oval nuclei (oval cells) with scanty cytoplasm, and hyperplastic pseudo-bile ducts (Fig. 3b). The regenerative changes gradually became predominant throughout the liver after 26 weeks of age. Foci of small hepatocytes with basophilic cytoplasm and small round nuclei (hyperplastic foci) were seen. With age, these foci developed into hyperplastic nodules that were larger than the hepatic lobules. Fibrotic changes also slowly extended to surrounding liver tissue, and became grossly visible as whitish nodules from the size of a pinhead to a rice grain. The nodules markedly increased in size and hardness from 40 weeks of age, frequently occupying almost the entire surface of the liver. Histo-logically, they resembled cholangiofibrotic tissue, consisting of columnar or cuboidal epithelial cells forming glandular structures with fibrotic stroma. In rats that had survived for more than 1 year, soft, reddish tumors as well as hard whitish nodules developed. The reddish nodules consisted of well-developed and differentiated cells closely resembling the surround-ing liver cells with trabecular structures. No atypism was seen. The tumors were hyperplastic nodules or benign adenomas. No cirrhosis or inflam-matory change was seen.

Flow Cytometric Analysis

Subsets of peripheral blood lymphocytes (PBL) were analyzed by flore-scence-activated cell sorter (FACS) with various monoclonal antibodies, and the results are shown in Fig. 4. The proportion of T cells, especially helper T cell (OX-19$^+$/OX-8$^-$), was much lower in the PBL of LEC rats than in those of LETO rats: the proportion of T cells in LEC rats remained within 15% regardless of age, whereas that in LETO rats ranged from 50% at 10 weeks to 60% at 15 weeks. The proportions of helper T cell and suppressor/cytotoxic T cell (OX-19$^+$/OX-8$^+$) were 40% and 20%, respect-ively, in controls, but 6.0 ± 2.0 and $4.6 \pm 1.3\%$, respectively, in LEC rats. The T_H/Tc/s T cell ratio was 1.5–3.5 in LETO rats and 1.0–1.5 in LEC rats, indicating a relative reduction in helper T cells. In contrast to helper T cell and suppressor/cytotoxic T cell, a significant increase of NK cells

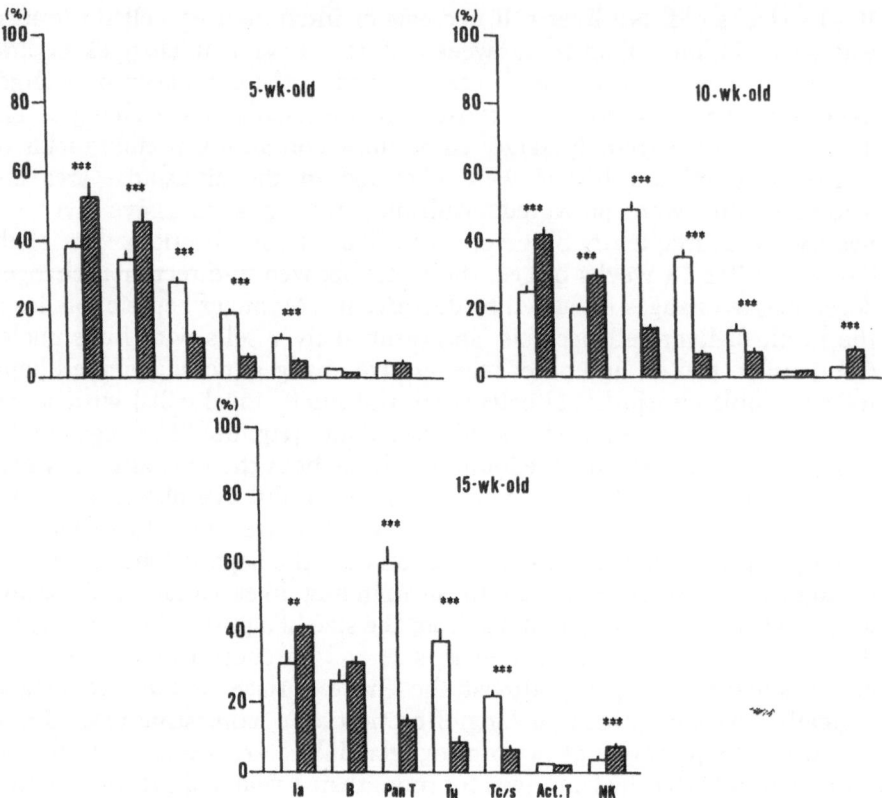

Fig. 4. Proportions of peripheral blood lymphocyte subsets in LEC/Otk and LETO rats. *Open bars;* LETO rats; *shaded bars,* LEC/Otk rats. *Columns* and *bars* show means ±S.D. (*n* = 8). Significance of difference from value for LETO rats: ***P < 0.001, **P < 0.01

(OX-19⁻/OX-8⁺) was evident in LEC rats, i.e., 8.2% at 10 weeks, and 7.5% at 15 weeks, whereas that in LETO rats was 2%–3%.

Serum Immunoglobulin Subclasses

The serum immunoglobulin levels in LEC rats of various ages were monitored by the Ouchterlony method. A significant decrease of the IgG1 subclass of immunoglobulins was observed in LEC rats, even at 5 weeks of age, and only a faint band of precipitate with anti-IgG1 antiserum was obtained with serum of 15-week old LEC rats.

Segregation Analysis

Phenotypes such as histological "hepatic injury", the serum IgG1 content, and numbers of helper T cells in the (LEC/Otk × F₃₄₄/Ducrj) F₂ hybrids were examined. No significant association was found between histological changes and immunological disorders.

Discussion

In this work, the clinical features of the LEC/Otk strain in SPF conditions, such as kinetic changes in jaundice and the P-GPT level, histopathological changes, and immunological disorders, were characterized. The characteristic features of the strain were found to be as follows: (1) jaundice developed in almost all rats with an increased P-GPT level, (2) the animals showed episodes of jaundice, high P-GPT levels, and liver cell necrosis, but only slight inflammatory cell infiltration, (3) as indicated by kinetic studies, P-GPT levels increased twice, first at 18 weeks, and then at 25 weeks of age, and (4) the animals showed immunological disorders, such as deficiency of immunoglobulins, especially IgGl, and of helper T cells.

Almost all of the rats had high levels of P-GPT, usually associated with jaundice, at 16–17 weeks of age. The rats of onset and remission of the disease were higher than those reported for conventional LEC rats (88%) [2]. Moreover, a characteristic feature of SPF-LEC rats was a second increase of P-GPT about 9 weeks after the first increase. These results indicate that SPF-LEC rats show a more concentrated form of the disease than conventional LEC rats.

Three possible explanations for the pathogenesis of spontaneous hepatic injury in LEC rats may be considered: it may be (1) due to viral agents, (2) an autoimmune type hepatic injury due to immunological disorders, or (3) a metabolic disorder that is genetically controlled by an autosomal recessive gene.

The first possibility is supported by the clinical features of the disease, such as its late onset (16–17 weeks), chronic change (70%), and final high incidences of liver malignancies closely resembling those in human B-type hepatitis. However, we could not detect any viral particles by electron microscopy (unpublished data). Moreover, tissue homogenates of affected animals did not induce the disease in weanling rats (data not shown). These results indicate that viral agents are not responsible for the pathogenesis of the disease.

A characteristic feature of LEC rats is that they are deficient in a subclass of immunoglobulin (IgGl) and a subset of helper T cells from an early age. However, these immunological disorders were not genetically associated with the onset of liver disease in LEC rats, thus, the second possibility is unlikely to apply to them.

The third possibility is supported by the following circumstantial evidence: (1) accumulation of fine fatty droplets, which is a characteristic pathological change in drug-induced liver injury (e.g., that by tetracycline) [6,7], (2) a significant decrease in cytochrome p-450, (3) increased γ-GTP activity [8], (4) high susceptibility to D-galactosamine, (5) prominent quantitative increase of liver cell DNA, which reaches a maximum of 62N, and giant nuclei [9], and (6) significantly increased deposition of copper [10].

These findings support the idea that the abnormality is a metabolic disorder that is genetically governed by an autosomal recessive gene. However, no direct information on the mechanism of liver cell necrosis in LEC rats is available at present.

Acknowledgments. Tables and figures are reprinted from the original article (Journal of Gastroenterology and hepatology, 6:53–58, 1991), by the coutesy of Blackwell Scientific Publications (Australia) PTY Ltd.

References

1. Sasaki M, Yoshida MC, Kagami K, Takeichi N, Kobayashi H, Dempo K, Mori M (1985) Spontaneous hepatitis in an inbred strain of Long-Evans rats, Rat News Lett 14:4–6
2. Yoshida MC, Masuda R, Sasaki M, Takeichi N, Kobayashi H, Dempo K, Mori M (1987) New mutation causing hereditary hepatitis in the laboratory rat. J Hered 78:361–365
3. Takeichi N, Kobayashi H, Yoshida MC, Sasaki M, Dempo K, Mori M (1988) Spontaneous hepatitis in Long-Evans rats. A potential animal model for fulminant hepatitis in man, Acta Pathol Jpn 38:1369–1375
4. Masuda R, Yoshida MC, Sasaki M, Dempo K, Mori M (1988) Hereditary hepatitis of LEC rats is controlled by a single autosomal recessive gene. Lab Anim 22:166–169
5. Dempo K, Oyamada M, Fujimoto Y, Takahashi H, Satoh M, Hattori A, Mori M (1988) Pathological changes of the liver in LEC rats with hereditary hepatitis. J Toxicol Pathol 1:53–60
6. Kunelis CT, Peters RL, Edmondson HA (1965) Fatty liver of pregnancy and its relationship to tetracycline therapy. Am J Med 38:359–377
7. Dawling HF, Lepper MA (1964) Hepatic reactions to tetracycline. JAMA 188: 307–309
8. Sugiyama T, Takeichi N, Kobayashi H, Yoshida MC, Sasaki M Taniguchi N (1988) Metabolic predisposition of a novel mutant (LEC rats) to hereditary hepatitis and hepatoma: Alterations of the drug metabolizing enzymes. Carcinogenesis 9:1569–1572
9. Fujimoto Y, Oyamada M, Hattori A, Takahashi H, Sawaki M, Dempo K, Mori M, Nagao M (1989) Accumulation of abnormally high ploidy in the liver of LEC rats developing spontaneous hepatitis. Jpn J Cancer Res 80:45–50
10. Li Y, Togashi Y, Satoh S, Emoto T, Kang J-H, Takeichi N, Kobayashi H, Kojima Y, Une Y, Uchino J (1991) Spontaneous hepatic copper accumulation in Long-Evans cinnamon rats with hereditary hepatitis. J Clin Invest 87:1858–1861

5 — Clinical and Pathological Characteristics of LEC Rats with Spontaneous Hepatitis

TSUTOMU NAMIENO[1,2], NORITOSHI TAKEICHI[2], MOTOMICHI SASAKI[3], KIMIMARO DEMPO[4], MICHIO MORI[4], JUN-ICHI UCHINO[2], and HIROSHI KOBAYASHI[1]

Introduction

Currently, there are very few available animal models for the research of human hepatitis. We have known for many years that the marmoset and the chimpanzee are sensitive to hepatitis A and B viruses, respectively. It has been reported that the woodchunk *(Marmota monax)* shows a high incidence of persistent infection with woodchuck hepatitis virus (WHV), one of the hepadna viruses, and that the incidence of hepatocellular carcinomas in WHV-positive woodchucks is extremely high [1].

However, marmosets, chimpanzees, and woodchucks are difficult to obtain, and they are not generally used in experiments due to the high cost and the difficulty of raising them in captivity. We have succeeded in isolating LEC rats which spontaneously developed acute hepatitis 4–5 months after birth, about 80% of which showed clinical and histopathological findings similar to those of human fulminant hepatitis and which died within 2 weeks from the onset of the disease. We also observed that liver cancer occurred spontaneously in long-surviving LEC rats [2,3].

In this paper we present clinical and histopathological characteristics of an inbred strain of LEC rats with spontaneous hepatitis.

Materials and Methods

Rats

Among the LEC and LEA rats isolated according to coat color from a closed colony of Long-Evans rats (provided in 1975 by Professor Taketoshi Sugiyama, Kobe University School of Medicine, Kobe, Japan) Hokkaido

---

[1] Laboratory of Pathology, Cancer Institute,
[2] First Department of Surgery, School of Medicine,
[3] Sasaki Cancer Institute, Chiyoda-ku, Tokyo, 565 Japan
[4] Department of Pathology, Sapporo Medical College, Sapporo, 060 Japan

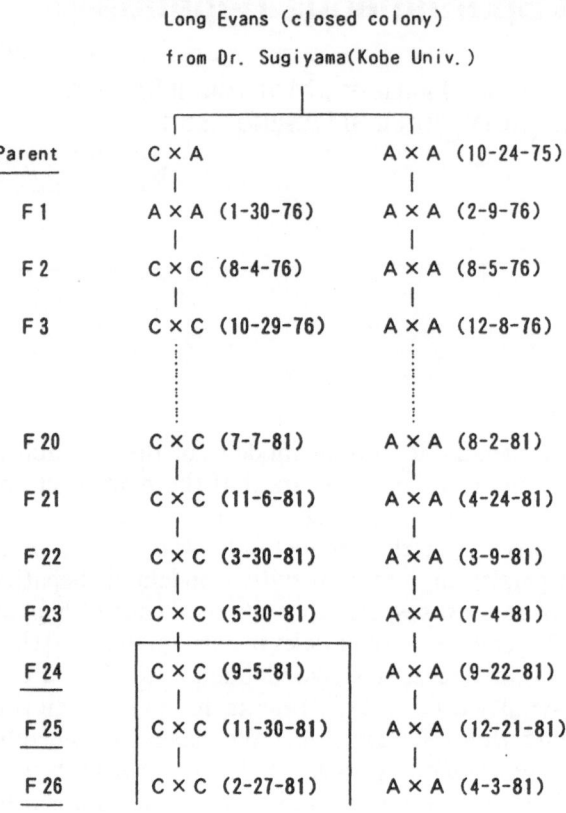

Fig. 1. Pedigree record of LEC and LEA rats. The LEC rats from the 24th generation develop hepatitis spontaneously

Parent	C × A	A × A (10-24-75)
F 1	A × A (1-30-76)	A × A (2-9-76)
F 2	C × C (8-4-76)	A × A (8-5-76)
F 3	C × C (10-29-76)	A × A (12-8-76)
F 20	C × C (7-7-81)	A × A (8-2-81)
F 21	C × C (11-6-81)	A × A (4-24-81)
F 22	C × C (3-30-81)	A × A (3-9-81)
F 23	C × C (5-30-81)	A × A (7-4-81)
F 24	C × C (9-5-81)	A × A (9-22-81)
F 25	C × C (11-30-81)	A × A (12-21-81)
F 26	C × C (2-27-81)	A × A (4-3-81)

University, only the LEC rats developed acute hepatitis spontaneously from the 24th generation onwards (Fig. 1). Accordingly, in this experiment we used mainly the 29th generation rats. Both of the strains are now in the 32nd-33rd generation.

Qualitative Chemical Urinalysis

A Multisticks III Kit (Miles-Sankyo Co., Ltd., Tokyo) was used for testing bilirubin, protein, and other substances in the urine.

Hematological Tests

The left or right jugular vein of each rat (LEC rats before developing acute hepatitis: $n = 20$, LEC rats with acute hepatitis: $n = 20$, LEA rats: $n = 16$) was punctured, and about 3 ml of peripheral blood was removed. About 1 ml of the blood was divided into containers to which EDTA-2K salt was added, which was used for hemocytometry. The serum of the remaining blood was removed and used for general biochemical tests. Hemocytometry and other tests were carried out by an automatic cell counter (Sysmex E-4000: resistance type, TOA Electronics Ltd., Tokyo).

Biochemical Tests

The serum was prepared as described above. Total bilirubin and direct/indirect bilirubin in serum were measured by the San Test Kit (Sanko Junyaku K.K., Tokyo), and the levels of glutamic oxaloacetic transaminase (SGOT) and glutamic pyruvic transaminase SGPT were measured by Gliford (GOT, GPT) reagent (Gliford Co., USA). The serum protein fractions of the LEC and LEA rats were measured by cellulose acetate membrane electrophoresis (Karl Zeiss Co., Ltd.).

Histopathological Tests

The organs removed at the post-mortem examination were fixed with 10% formalin solution and prepared in 4-μm sections, and H and E staining was carried out for examining the sections under a light microscope.

Statistical Analysis

The results were expressed as mean values ± standard deviation, and Student's t-test and the χ^2-test were carried out.

Only the LEC rats spontaneously developed hepatitis and the LEA rats showed no abnormalities at all in the clinical, histopathological, or biochemical tests. Therefore, we carried out our study using the LEA rats as a control group.

Results

Clinical Course

Among the LEC and LEA rats from the 24th to 31st generations of sibmating, only the LEC rats developed acute hepatitis spontaneously. Up to the present, spontaneous development of acute hepatitis has been observed in 150 (67 males and 83 females) of 186 LEC rats (about 80%) from 26 mother rats. The hepatitis was accompanied by jaundice with other clinical signs (Table 1).

The most evident characteristic of the pathological change is the sudden appearance of vital jaundice at around 4 months (about 115 days) after birth. Jaundice is distinctly observed in the ear lobes and the distal ends of the extremities. Other symptoms were loss of body weight, anemia, oliguria, subcutaneous hemorrhage, and sluggish movements. About 80% (121/150) of the LEC rats with spontaneous acute jaundice showed con-

Table 1. Freqency of incidence of jaundice (acute hepatitis) seen in a total of eight generations of LEC rats.

Generation	No. of litter	No. of offspring		Jaundice		Frequency of jaundiced rats (%)	Onset of jaundice (days after birth)
		Total	Jaundice	Male	Female		
F$_{24}$	1	6	1	1	0	16.7	149
F$_{25}$	1	8	4	1	3	50.0	89
F$_{26}$	1	6	6	3	3	100.0	139
F$_{27}$	3	21	14	4	10	66.7	88
F$_{28}$	3	20	19	10	9	95.0	129
F$_{29}$	5	35	31	12	19	88.6	110
F$_{30}$	8	57	50	24	26	87.7	111
F$_{31}$	4	33	25	12	13	75.8	103

Jaundiced rats were diagnosed by the following clinical signs of jaundice: anemia, oliguria, subcutaneous hemorrhage, and body weight loss. The diagnosis of acute hepatitis was confirmed pathologically.

current serious symptoms, and within 2 weeks after the onset of hepatitis, they showed clinical symptoms and histopathological findings similar to those of human fulminant hepatitis, and subsequently died. These animals presented marked subcutaneous deposits of bilirubin, nasal hemorrhage, and spots of subcutaneous hemorrhage. Commonly observed findings by laparotomy included bilirubin deposition under the peritoneum adjacent to the abdominal wall, intraperitoneal hemorrhage, reddish-brown atrophy of the liver, mild swelling of the spleen, and yellowing of the kidneys.

About 20% of the rats (29/150) showed remission of acute hepatitis, but about one-half of the 20% suffered recurrences in the course of remission and died. The incidences of hepatitis decreased slightly in later gener-

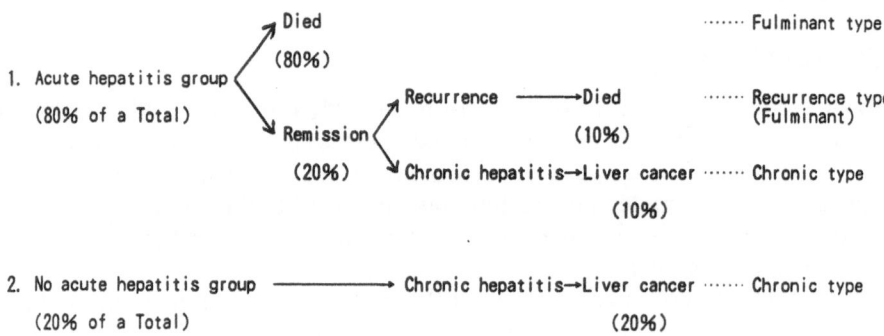

Fig. 2. Clinical course of LEC rats with spontaneous development of hepatitis (24th-31st generation). Acute hepatitis group were clinically diagnosed by systemic jaundice and definined pathologically. The incidence rate of acute hepatitis was approximately 80% of total LEC rats

ations, and by improvement of the physical conditions, 30% of the rats (52/186) survived for longer periods (Fig. 2).

Qualitative Chemical Urinalysis

Before developing hepatitis, the LEC rats ($n = 186$) showed no abnormalities compared to the LEA rats ($n = 250$). However, all of the LEC rats which developed hepatitis ($n = 150$) showed strongly positive urine bilirubin in qualitative tests, with mildly positive urinary protein and virtually normal urobilinogen levels. Therefore, based on the findings of chemical urinalysis, it appears unlikely that the jaundice is a post-hepatic lesion. No abnormalities were observed in the urinary findings of LEA rats of the same age.

Hematological Tests

Red blood counts (RBCs) in the peripheral blood were not significantly different between the LEA and the LEC rats prior to the development of acute hepatitis. However, RBCs were markedly low in the LEC rats with acute hepatitis, which showed a significant decrease ($P < 0.001$) in comparison with those of the LEA and the LEC rats prior to the development of acute hepatitis.

Furthermore, although hemoglobin (Hb) and hematocrit (Hct) levels were not significantly different between the LEA and the LEC rats prior to the development of acute hepatitis, these levels were significantly reduced ($P < 0.001$) in the LEC rats with acute hepatitis. These findings match the symptoms of anemia observed by gross examination of the palpebral conjunctiva. White blood counts (WBCs) in the peripheral blood were not significantly different between the LEA and the LEC rats prior to the development of acute hepatitis. However, WBCs rapidly increased in the LEC rats with acute hepatitis, and showed a significant difference ($P < 0.001$) compared to the LEA and the LEC rats prior to the development of acute hepatitis. Platelet counts (PLT) in the peripheral blood were not significantly different between the LEA and the LEC rats prior to the development of acute hepatitis. PLT, however, were low in the LEC rats with acute hepatitis, with a significant difference ($P < 0.001$) compared to the LEA and the LEC rats prior to the development of acute hepatitis (Table 2).

Biochemical Tests

1. Blood Bilirubin Level

Total blood bilirubin (T.Bil) showed no significant difference between the LEC ($n = 30$) and the LEA ($n = 30$) rats prior to the incidence of hepatitis, and remained within the normal range. On the other hand, T.Bil of the

Table 2. Comparison of hematological data in LEC and LEA rats.

Items	LEC Prehepatitis (n = 20)	LEC Hepatitis (n = 21)	LEA (n = 16)
WBC (/µl)	4500 ± 1600*	8200 ± 2010	4800 ± 1200
RBC (× 10^4/µl)	768 ± 65	296 ± 57	812 ± 102
Plt (× 10^4/µl)	68.6 ± 18.5	41.6 ± 21.3	71.5 ± 15.4
Hb (g/dl)	14.5 ± 5.2	6.1 ± 3.6	15.7 ± 6.3

*Mean ± standard deviation
There were no significant differences in any data from prehepatitis LEC and LEA rats. However, significant differences ($P<0.001$) were observed in the data in the above table from hepatitis LEC rats compared to those from prehepatitis LEC and LEA rats

LEC rats with acute hepatitis was markedly elevated to 36.8 ± 14.5 mg/dl ($n = 20$), with a direct bilirubin level of 19.4 ± 5.5 mg/dl and an indirect level of 17.1 ± 7.5 mg/dl: i.e., there was no significant difference between the direct and the indirect bilirubin levels. T.Bil of the LEA rats of the same age was within the normal range (Fig. 3).

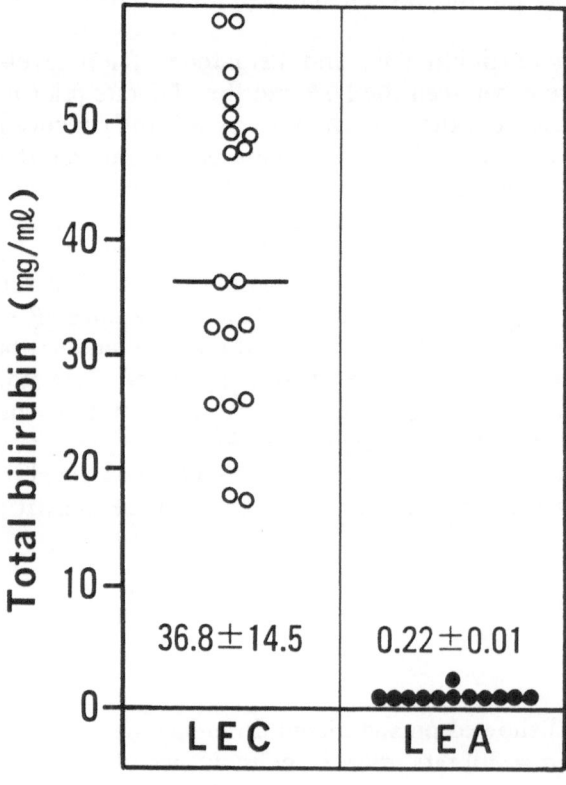

Fig. 3. Total blood bilirubin values in LEC rats with acute hepatitis and age-matched LEA rats

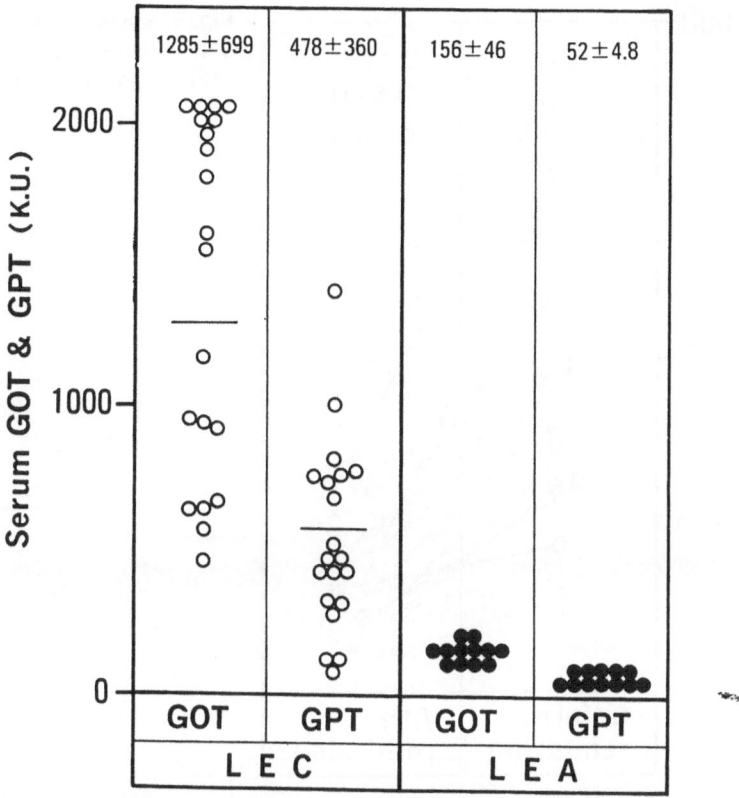

Fig. 4. SGOT and SGPT values in LEC rats with acute hepatitis and age-matched LEA rats

2. SGOT and SGPT

Both SGOT and SGPT were within the normal range prior to the incidence of hepatitis, with no significant difference between the LEA and the LEC rats. However, in the LEC rats with acute hepatitis, SGOT rose suddenly to levels of 2,000 units or more in some LEC rats. At the same time, SGPT rose significantly as well (Fig. 4).

By examining each individual case with predominance of SGOT and SGPT levels, we found that the earlier the stage of hepatitis when blood samples were taken, the higher the value of SGOT. Moreover, both SGOT and SGPT levels dropped in the LEC rats which showed remission of acute hepatitis (Fig. 5).

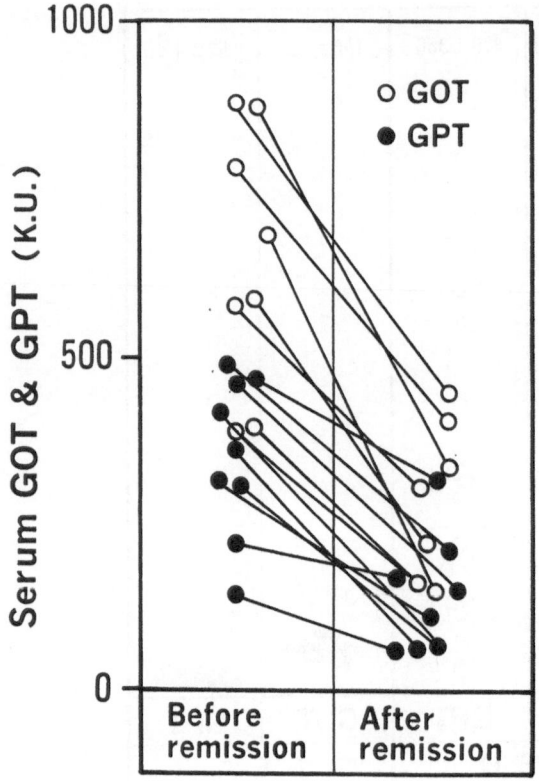

Fig. 5. Changes in SGOT and SGPT values after onset of acute hepatitis in LEC rats

3. Serum Albumin

Serum total protein and albumin showed a low level in the LEC rats compared to the LEA rats. This phenomenon is thought to be attributed to reduced protein synthesis in the liver (Fig. 6).

4. Cellulose Acetate Membrane Electrophoresis

In our investigation of cellulose acetate membrane electrophoresis using 6- and 12-week-old rats, we found that γ-globulin fractions were non-measurable in the majority of LEC rats, and that γ-globulin fractions were also at too low a level to measure.

In contrast, the γ-globulin fractions in 6- to 12-week-old LEA rats all showed definite increases (Fig. 7). The main component of γ-globulin fractions is immunoglobulin G (IgG); thus, we consider that the increase indicates that autoproduction of IgG following consumption of IgG originating from the mother is weak in the LEC rats, while it is smoothly produced in the LEA rats.

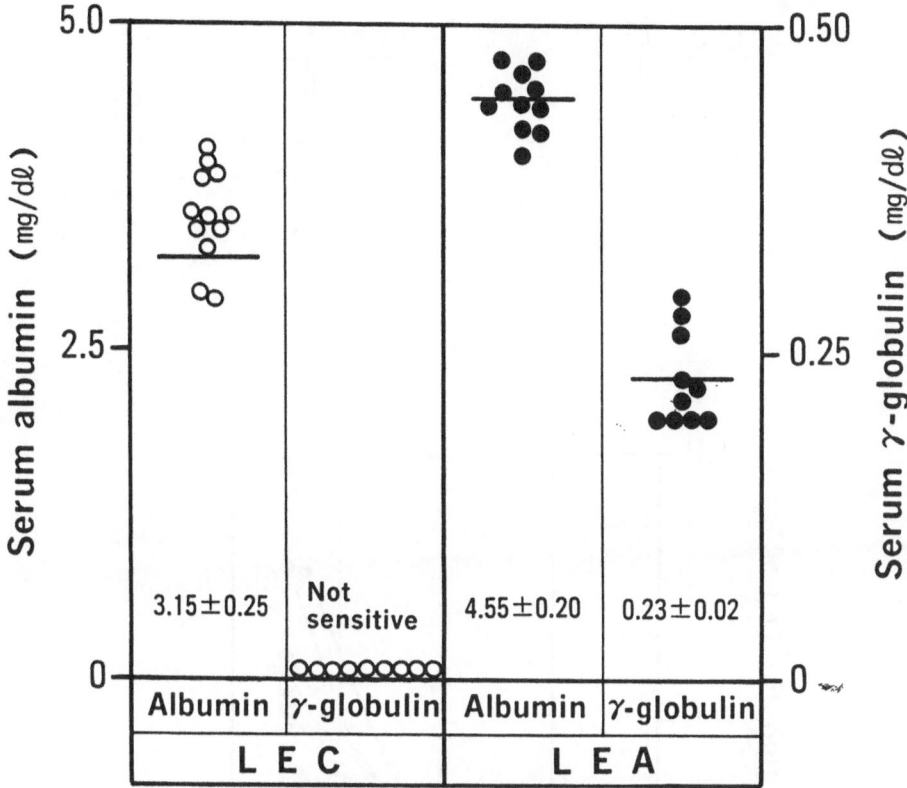

Fig. 6. Serum albumin and γ-globulin values in LEC and LEA rats

Histopathological Tests (Fig. 8)

1. Liver Tissue Findings in LEC Rats Prior to the Incidence of Acute Hepatitis

The liver tissue findings in 1-month-old LEC rats (*n* = 15) prior to the incidence of acute hepatitis were considered to be normal. Hepatocytes formed hepatic cords, arranged in a radial pattern centering around the central veins of the liver, and they made up the typical hepatic lobule. The hepatic lobule presented in a polygon form, and showed findings similar to those for human liver tissue, with Glisson's capsule observed on its edge. However, in the liver tissue of LEC rats (*n* = 20) 2–3 months after birth, the nuclear division image of liver cells was rarely seen, and inequalities in size were observed, although it was not possible to discern liver cell necrosis and inflammatory cell infiltration.

2. Liver Tissue Findings in LEC Rats with Acute Hepatitis

Numerous scattered spotty necrotic sites were observed throughout the liver tissue of all of the LEC rats, and scattered hepatocytes with giant

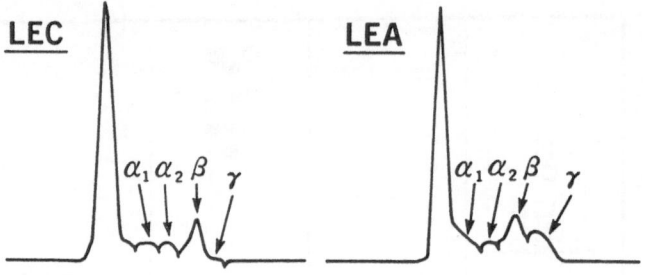

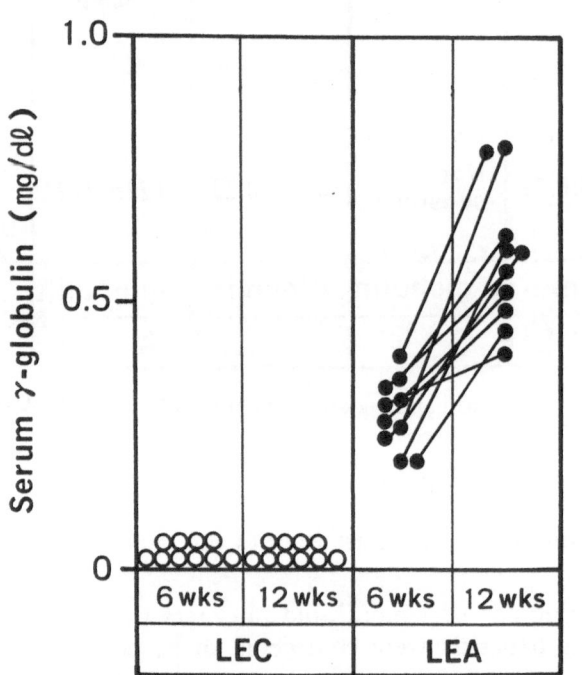

Fig. 7. Changes in serum γ-globulin values in 6- and 12-week old LEC and LEA rats. The upper figures show cellulose acetate membrane electrophoresis images of both 12-old week LEC and LEA rats, and the below figure shows changes in serum γ-globulin values in both strains

atypical nuclei were also seen. Numerous Kupffer's cells which contained englobed red blood cells and bile pigment were also observed. However, infiltration by lymphocytes and inflammatory cells was slight (Fig. 9a).

In the LEC rats which had passed the turning point from acute to fulminant hepatitis ($n = 121$), the liver tissue showed extensive necrosis

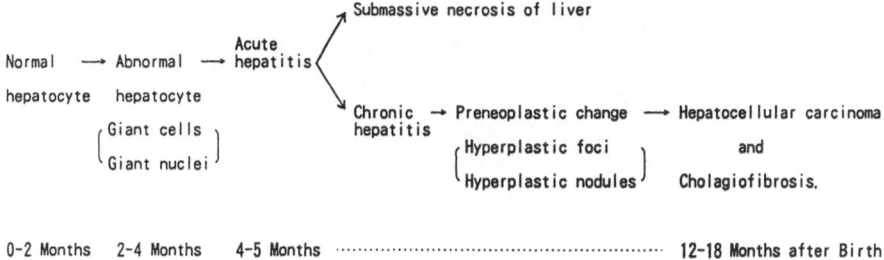

Fig. 8. Histopathological changes of the liver tissue in the LEC rats with spontaneous development of hepatitis

followed by collapse of the liver. Submassive coagulation necrosis in the hepatocytes of the interlobular region (about 90%: 108/121) was observed, and there were other cases (about 10%: 13/121) of central necrosis spreading out from the central veins of the liver, with inflammatory cell infiltration also being observed (Fig. 9b).

3. Other Findings

In the spleens (n = 56) of virtually all of the LEC rats, the red splenic pulp was enlarged, with clear hyperplasia of histiocytes which contained englobed red blood cells and hemosiderin. In the kidneys (n = 56), all of the LEC rats showed bilirubin deposition and necrosis in the renal tubules, and this is thought to be symptommatic of jaundice.

Discussion

Our findings on LEC rats constitute the first report of experimental animals showing spontaneous, high-rate, and late-developing acute and fulminant hepatitis. Moreover, LEC rats which survived for long periods (about 30% of the total) presented the clinical and histopathological picture of chronic hepatitis, and those observed for a course of 1.5 years or more after birth spontaneously developed liver cancer, whether they had a previous history of acute hepatitis or not. However, we did not observe concurrent cirrhosis of the liver in gross and histological examinations conducted during the course of this observation. Concerning jaundice in the experimental animals, the rats with hereditary jaundice (Gunn rats) reported by Gunn [4] in 1934 are well known. The Gunn rats developed nuclear icterus immediately after birth and died, and it was made clear that this was caused by a lack of an autosomal recessive inherited enzyme (UDP-glucuronyl transferase). In 1978, Summers et al. [1] reported on the incidence of hepatitis and liver cancer (hepatoma) in woodchucks which was caused by a virus similar to the human hepatitis B virus. This is the woodchuck hepatitis

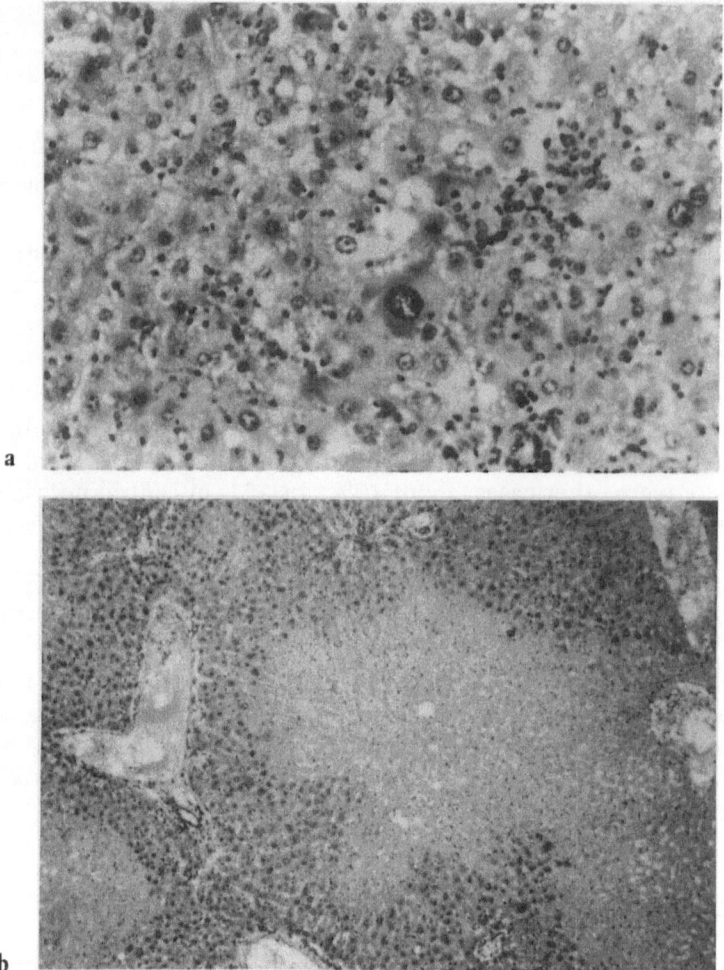

Fig. 9. a Liver tissue of LEC rat (four-months old) with acute hepatitis. Scattered spotty necrosis sites and hepatocytes with giant atypical nuclei are observed, as well as numerous Kupffer's cells (H and E, × 250). **b** Liver tissue of the LEC rat in transitional phase of fulminant hepatitis. Central necrosis is observed (H and E, × 100)

virus (WHV), one of the hepadna viruses, which has a high rate of persistent infection in woodchucks.

The mechanism of onset of acute and fulminant hepatitis in the LEC rats is assumed to be due to factors such as the influence of hepatitis viruses, hereditary elements, and abnormalities in the immune system. The LEC rats which showed remission from acute hepatitis and those which never have hepatitis accounted for about 30% of the total. There will be a need for further studies on the transition to chronic hepatitis, cirrhosis of the liver, and liver cancer in these rats when they survive over long periods of time.

Fortunately, the LEA rats, which never develop hepatitis, are simultaneously isolated and raised from the same closed colony as the LEC rats. It is likely that the causes of hepatitis in the LEC rats will be made clear by pathological, genetic, and biochemical comparative studies of these two strains of rats.

Acknowledgment. This work was supported in part by grants from the Ministry of Education, Science, and Culture of Japan.

References

1. Summers J, Smolec JM, Smyder R (1978) A virus similar to human hepatitis B virus associated with hepatitis and hepatoma in woodchucks. Proc Natl Acad Sci USA 75:4533–4537
2. Sasaki M, Yoshida MC, Kagami K, Takeichi N, Kobayashi H, Dempo K, Mori M (1985) Spontaneous hepatitis in an inbred strain of Long-Evans rats. Rat News Lett 14:4–6
3. Yoshida MC, Masuda R, Sasaki M, Takeichi N, Kobayashi H, Dempo K, Mori M (1987) New mutation causing hereditary hepatitis in the laboratory rat. J Hered 78:361–365
4. Gunn CK (1938) Hereditary acholuric jaundice in a new mutant strain of rats. J Hered 29:137–141

6 — High Susceptibility to Spontaneous Development of Hepatocellular Carcinoma in LEC Rats

Ryuichi Masuda, Michihiro C. Yoshida[1], Motomichi Sasaki[2], Kimimaro Dempo, and Michio Mori[3]

Introduction

Spontaneous hepatitis was first found in the LEC strain rat, which had been maintained conventionally at the Center for Experimental Plants and Animals, Hokkaido University [1]. The hepatitis appears suddenly in LEC rats at about 4 months after birth, and leads to a high mortality [2]. Characteristics of the disease are similar to those of fulminant hepatitis in humans, showing bilirubinuria, hyperbilirubinemia (frequently severe jaundice), subcutaneous bleeding, loss of body weight, increased levels of serum glutamic oxaloacetic transaminase, glutamic pyruvic transaminase and alkaline phosphatase, and single-cell necrosis or spotty necrosis of liver tissues with faint inflammatory cell response. Genetic analysis by crossing tests indicated that the disease has an autosomal recessive mode of inheritance, being ruled by a single gene designated *hts* (symbol for hepatitis) [3]. Many rats died of submassive necrosis in liver tissues within 1 week after the onset of hepatitis. The remaining animals survived with chronic hepatitis more than 1 year and developed preneoplastic and neoplastic lesions of the liver [2]. Electron microscopic analysis failed to reveal any viral particles in the affected liver, and intraperitoneal injections of liver homogenates of jaundiced rats did not induce hepatitis in neonatal rats of another strain [2], although viral hepatitis has been reported to be associated with hepatocarcinogenesis in humans [4,5], woodchucks [6], ground squirrels [7] and ducks [8]. Although the cause of hepatitis in LEC rats is different from that of viral hepatitis in the other cases, regenerative stimuli caused by hepatitis may promote development of liver tumors in all cases. In this report, the natural history of spontaneous hepatic lesions in LEC rats are described with regard to the anatomical and histopathological

[1] Chromosome Research Unit, Faculty of Science, Hokkaido University, Sapporo, 060 Japan
[2] Sasaki Cancer Institute, Chiyoda-ku, Tokyo, 101 Japan
[3] Department of Pathology, Sapporo Medical College, Sapporo, 060 Japan

aspects. Furthermore, establishment and characterization of a hepatocellular carcinoma (hepatoma) cell line obtained from an LEC rat are reported.

Long-term Survey of LEC Rats

LEC rats were kept for a long time after recovery from fulminat hepatitis [9]. They were housed in groups of one to three rats per cage and reared in an air-conditioned animal room at $22 \pm 2°C$ with a relative humidity of 55 $\pm$ 5%. They were fed a laboratory diet (CMF, Oriental Yeast Co., Tokyo) and water ad libitum. The diet contained water (7.0%), crude proteins (27.7%), crude fats (8.8%), ash (6.6%), crude fiber (3.5%), nonnitrogenous substances (46.4%), and vitamins.

Of 56 (28 females : 28 males) LEC rats consisting of eight litters in the F_{30} generation, 16 (8:8) rats (29%) died of fulminant hepatitis and the

Table 1. Appearance of hepatitis and subsequent hepatic lesions in LEC rats of F_{30}.

Litters	Litter size no. (♀:♂)	Dead rats by hepatitis no. (♀:♂)	Survived rats with subsequent hepatic lesions no. (♀:♂)
1	8 (4:4)	1 (1:0)	7 (3:4)
2	7 (4:3)	3 (1:2)	4 (3:1)
3	7 (4:3)	2 (1:1)	5 (3:2)
4	6 (3:3)	3 (2:1)	3 (1:2)
5	7 (3:4)	0 (0:0)	7 (3:4)
6	8 (3:5)	0 (0:0)	8 (3:5)
7	7 (3:4)	3 (1:2)	4 (2:2)
8	6 (4:2)	4 (2:2)	2 (2:0)
Total	56 (28:28)	16 (8:8)	40 (20:20)

The lethality by hepatitis is 29% (16/56)

Table 2. Appearance of hepatitis and subsequent hepatic lesions in LEC rats of F_{31}.

Litters	Litter size no. (♀:♂)	Dead rats by hepatitis no. (♀:♂)	Survived rats with subsequent hepatic lesions no. (♀:♂)
1	4 (3:1)	0 (0:0)	4 (3:1)
2	9 (7:2)	4 (4:0)	5 (3:2)
3	10 (5:5)	3 (3:0)	7 (2:5)
4	9 (4:5)	5 (1:4)	4 (3:1)
Total	32 (19:13)	12 (8:4)	20 (11:9)

The lethality by hepatitis is 38% (12/32)

Table 3. Incidence of putatively preneoplastic and neoplastic lesions and other lesions in long-survived LEC rats from F_{29} and F_{30}. [From [9]].

Generation	Survived (months*)	Survived rats no. (♀:♂)	Preneoplastic and neoplastic lesions			Cholangiofibrosis no. (♀:♂)
			Foci no. (♀:♂)	Foci and nodules no. (♀:♂)	Foci, nodules, and carcinomas no. (♀:♂)	
F_{29}	12–14	2 (2:0)			2 (2:0)	2 (2:0)
	14–16	2 (2:0)			1 (1:0)	2 (2:0)
	16–18	5 (2:3)	1 (1:0)		4 (1[a]:3)	3 (1:2)
	18–20	5 (1:4)			5 (1:4)	3 (1:2)
	24–26	2 (2:0)			2 (2[a]:0)	2 (2:0)
	26–28	4 (2:2)			4 (2:2[a])	4 (2:2)
F_{30}	12–14	8 (7:1)	1 (1:0)	2 (2:0)	2 (1:1)	8 (7:1)
	14–16	4 (2:2[b])			3 (2:1)	3 (2:1)
	16–18	23 (11:12)		5 (5:0)	18 (6:12[a,b])	21 (11:10)
	18–20	2 (0:2)			2 (0:2[b])	2 (0:2)
	22–24	3 (0:3)			3 (0:3)	2 (0:2)
Total		60 (31:29)	2 (2:0)	7 (7:0)	46 (18:28)	52 (30:22)
				92%, 55/60		87%, 52/60

* These months do not indicate actual survival age, because the rats were sacrificed when they showed palpable enlargement of livers or severe sickness

[a] One had metastasis of hepatoma in the lung or kidney

[b] One had leukemia

remaining 40 (20:20) (71%) recovered from severe conditions of the disease (Table 1). In F_{31}, 38% [12 (8:4)/32 (19:13)] died of the disease (Table 2), although F_{31} rats were not used for the long-term study. Thus, affected rats died with a mortality rate of about 30%, but the remaining animals recovered from the acute hepatitis and survived more than 12 months. Enlargement of the liver was observed in these surviving rats with the first detection made in a female at the age of 10 months, while in older rats the enlarged liver was prominently palpable. Histological examination showed that the long-surviving rats had putatively preneoplastic and neoplastic lesions in the liver. Among the 60 surviving rats in F_{29} and F_{30}, 55 rats developed hyperplastic foci, nodules, and hepatomas in a very high incidence (92%; 55/60) [9] (Table 3). Of the 55 rats, 46 (84%) had hepatomas, two had hyperplastic foci, and seven had hyperplastic foci and nodules. There was a higher incidence of hepatomas in males (97%; 28/29) than in females (58%; 18/31). Cholangiofibrosis was observed at a high incidence (87%; 52/60). Thus, most rats developed either preneoplastic or neoplastic lesions including overt hepatomas together with cholangiofibrosis in the liver; seven rats had only preneoplastic and neoplastic lesions and four females only more severe cholangiofibrosis. Chronic hepatitis occurred in nontumorous parts of each liver, showing many enlarged hepatocytes with huge nuclei.

Anatomical and Histological Examinations of Spontaneous Hepatomas

Upon gross examination, hepatomas showing multiple tumors had a smooth surface with a whitish and/or reddish color, while cholangiofibrosis showed a rough surface with a white color [9] (Fig. 1). Extensive necrosis was often observed in relatively large hepatomas. Among the 46 rats with hepatomas, four showed metastasis in the lung or kidney, and two developed leukemia with enlarged lymph nodes of the mesentery (Table 3). A 14-month-old male rat had only leukemia with no sign of putatively preneoplastic lesions, cholangiofibrosis, or other neoplasms. Occasionally, hepatomas were larger in males than in females even though the animals were from the same litter. On the other hand, cholangiofibrosis, covering most parts of the abdomen in some severe cases, was more extensive in females than in males.

Histologically, the initial change in the liver of 3-month-old LEC rats was an enlargement of hepatocytes [9]. A faint inflammatory response was seen in the portal triads and sinusoids. Following that, single cell necrosis or spotty necrosis occurred everywhere in hepatic lobules. Rats which died of fulminant hepatitis showed submassive necrosis. Regeneration of hepatocytes was observed in chronic hepatitis. Hyperplastic foci were composed of small hepatocytes with round nuclei and vacuolar or basophilic cytoplasm. These foci developed with age into hyperplastic nodules which were larger in size than hepatic lobules and which compressed the sur-

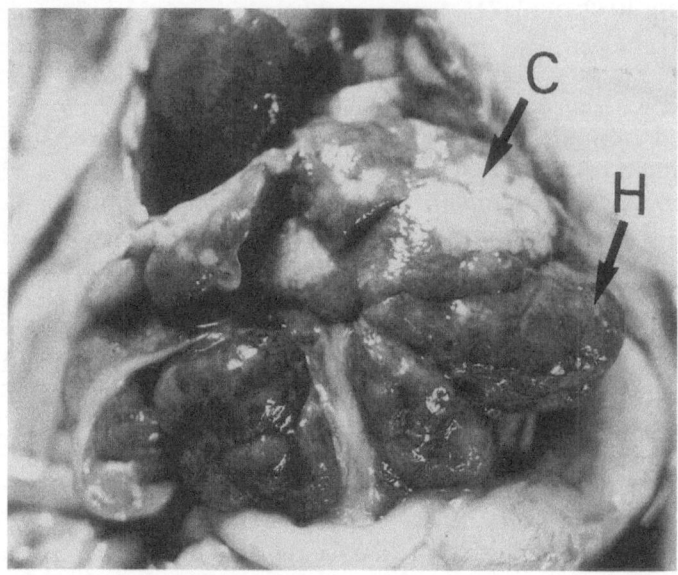

Fig. 1. Liver lesions of a 24-month-old female LEC rat. *H* Hepatoma with a reddish smooth surface, *C* Cholangiofibrosis with a white rough surface. (From [9])

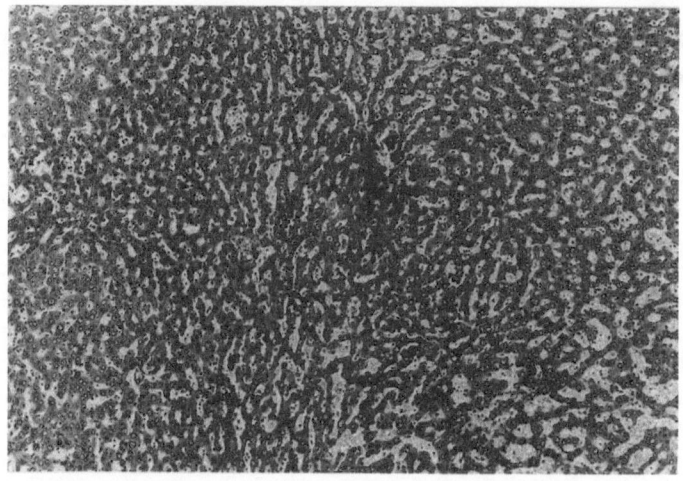

Fig. 2. Section of a well-differentiated hepatoma with a reddish smooth surface. These hepatocytes have round nuclei containing large nucleoli. Many erythrocytes are observed in wide sinusoids. H and E staining, × 100

rounding hepatocytes. These nodules became much larger and developed into hepatomas. Hepatomas were of a well-differentiated type with a trabecular structure of tumorous hepatocytes containing round nuclei with large nucleoli (Figs. 2, 3a). Tumorous hepatocytes had a more basophilic

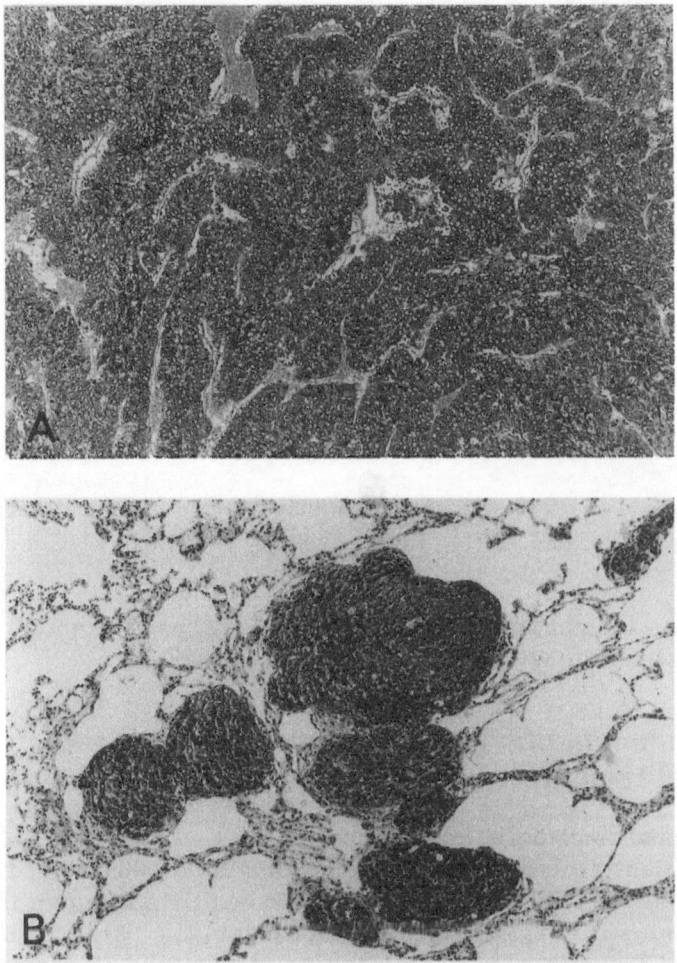

Fig. 3. **A** Section of a well-differentiated hepatoma with a whitish smooth surface and a trabecular structure of tumorous hepatocytes. H and E staining, ×100. **B** Metastatic lesions of hepatoma observed in the lung. H and E staining, × 100. (From [9])

cytoplasm than surrounding apparently normal hepatocytes. Metastatic specimens from lung tissues showed histological characteristics similar to the primary hepatoma (Fig. 3b). Cholangiofibrosis had various glandular structures surrounded by connective tissues (Fig. 4). Liver cirrhosis was not observed in any cases examined thus far. Leukemic cells were observed in the liver, spleen, kidney, lung, and lymph nodes of three of the rats described above. Although the bone marrow was not examined in this study, pleomorphism and infiltration of leukemic cells suggested a myeloid origin of the leukemia. Six LEA rats (3:3), as controls which survived for

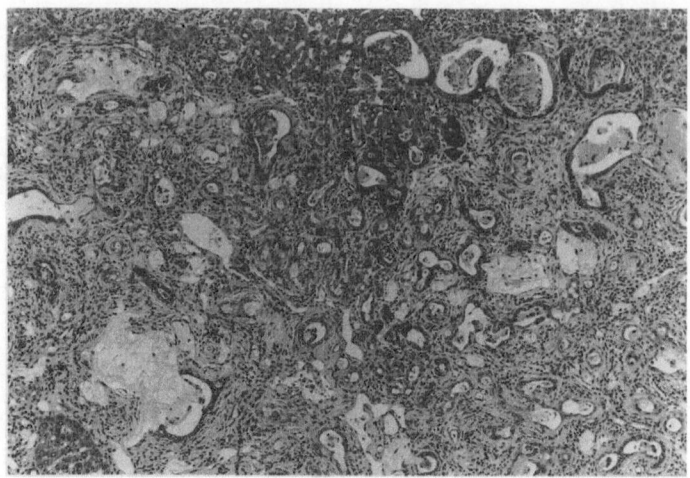

Fig. 4. Section of cholangiofibrosis showing various glandular structures surrounded by connective tissues. H and E staining, × 100. (From [9])

12 months, did not have either hepatitis or any hepatic tumor in gross and histological examinations.

Establishment of a Transplantable Cell Line From LEC Rat Hepatoma

Spontaneous hepatomas from 18 older than 12-month-old LEC rats were used for transplantation [10]. Each hepatoma tissue was minced into small pieces and then inoculated subcutaneously or intraperitoneally into 1-month-old LEC rats (recipients). Recipient rats were sacrificed and examined 1 month after transplantation. Among the 18 hepatomas, only one tumor from a male was successively transplanted in the recipients. The primary hepatoma of this particular case had multiple tumors of whitish and reddish nodules (about 5 × 5 × 5 mm) with metastatic lesions in the lung. One month after transplantation, tumors developed in two out of four recipients into which whitish nodules of this primary hepatoma were inoculated. Of the two recipients with transplanted tumors, one developed several small tumors surrounding the uterus. The other showed a widely spread growth of small nodules of tumors (about 1 × 1 × 1 mm) over the diaphragm. The small tumors in the latter case were transplanted into four recipients. On the other hand, no transplantable tumors were found when reddish nodules of the primary hepatoma were injected into four young LEC rats. The liver of the original male rat with the primary hepatoma weighed 28 g when the animal was sacrificed at 506 days of age, while the average weight of livers of 18 rats was 26 g (range: 16–52 g) with an average age when sacrificed of 550 days (range: 434–788 days).

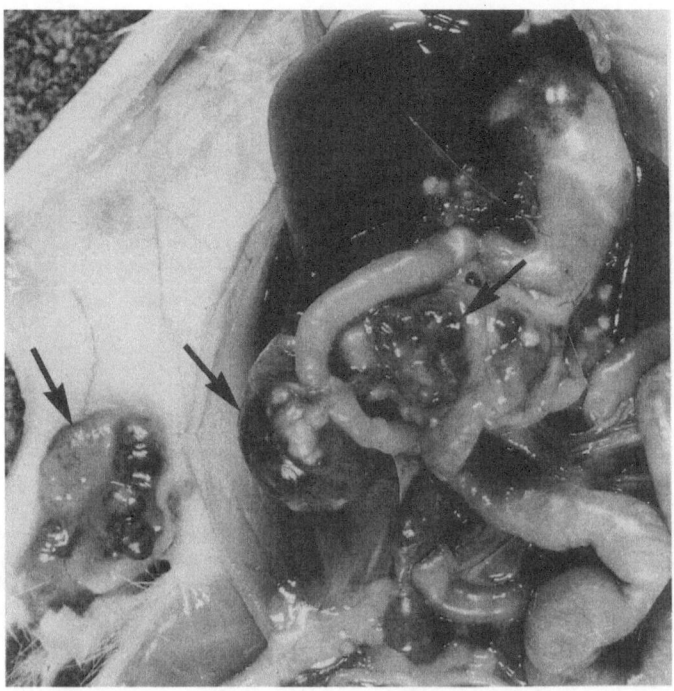

Fig. 5. Gross appearance of the abdominal cavity of a recipient rat 24 days after the fifth passage of LSH206G. Transplanted tumors with the various size are seen in subcutaneous tissues and the mesentery (*arrows*). (From [10])

In the second passage of transplanted hepatoma cells in LEC rats, all of the four recipients developed tumors in subcutaneous tissues or on the mesentery, spreading over the liver, kidney, uterus, or diaphragm. Within 1 month after transplantation, the development of tumors in recipients was detected by enlargement of the abdomen and subcutaneous tissues. Recipients which were not sacrificed died of large tumors (about 15 × 15 × 15 mm) within 2 months after transplantation. These large tumors were often hemorrhagic. To date, the seventh-passage tumors have been maintained in serial transplantation and were named LSH206G [10] (Fig. 5).

Histologically, the transplanted tumor LSH206G was similar to the primary hepatoma, showing a well-differentiated type with a trabecular structure of tumorous hepatocytes [10] (Fig. 6). The cells in both the primary hepatoma and LSH206G showed basophilic cytoplasm and round nuclei with clear nucleoli. The remaining 17 primary hepatomas which were not transplantable also appeared as a well-differentiated type of tumor. However, tumorous cells of whitish nodules in the above-mentioned male rat had more basophilic cytoplasm, higher nucleus-cytoplasm ratio, and more mitoses than those of reddish nodules in the same case and in 17 other hepatomas.

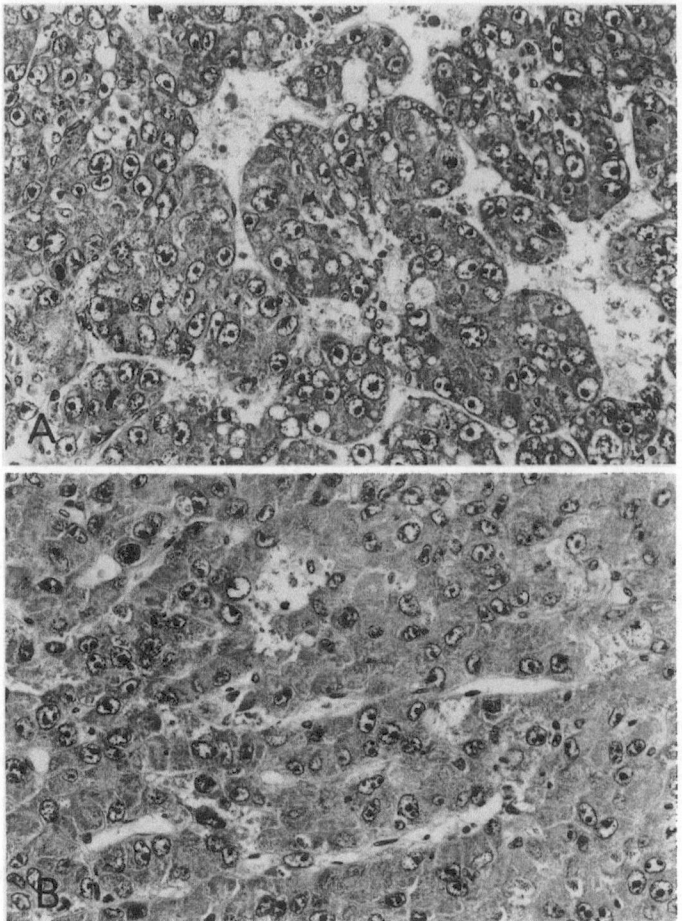

Fig. 6. A Section of a well-differentiated primary hepatoma with a trabecular structure of tumorous hepatocytes. H and E staining, × 340. **B** Section of LSH206G at the fifth passage, exhibiting histologically similar features to the primary hepatoma. H and E staining, × 340. (From [10])

Intracellular albumin was clearly detected as a fluorescent substance in the cytoplasm of LSH206G using fluorescein isothiocyanate-conjugated IgG fraction of goat anti-rat albumin serum [10] (Fig. 7). Such a positive immunofluorescence was observed in normal hepatocytes of a young LEC rat, while the spleen cells exhibited a negative reaction.

LSH206G is the first transplantable cell line of spontaneous hepatoma reported in the literature, although a number of liver tumor cell lines have previously been established from chemically induced hepatomas of laboratory animals. Among animal hepatomas related to viral hepatitis, only those in woodchuck cell lines have been reported [11–14]. LSH206G pro-

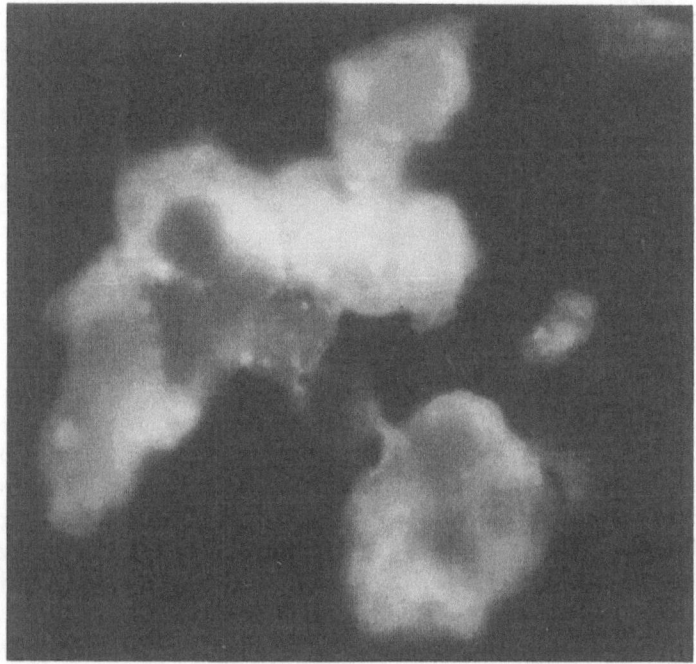

Fig. 7. Immunofluorescent staining of albumin of LSH206G cells from the fifth passage, showing a positive reaction in the cytoplasm. (From [10])

vides a novel material for further analysis of hepatocarcinogenesis of LEC rats and a control of chemically induced cell lines.

Time Course of Spontaneous Hepatocarcinogenesis of LEC Rats and Its Comparison With Other Hepatic Diseases

This study clarified that LEC rats have a remarkably high incidence of spontaneous liver neoplasia. As summarized in Fig. 8, all LEC rats developed hepatitis, often with severe jaundice, at about 4 months after birth, and 30% died of submassive necrosis of hepatocytes. The remaining 70% survived with residual chronic hepatitis which was caused by remission or recurrence of necrosis of the hepatocytes, and they expired from the development of hyperplastic foci, nodules, and hepatomas together with cholangiofibrosis.

Development of liver tumors in LEC rats is an age-associated phenomenon with serial hepatic alterations. A high incidence of hyperplastic foci and nodules was observed in LEC rats examined between 8 and 12 months of age, and hepatomas developed in older rats. A much higher incidence, possibly 100%, of preneoplastic and neoplastic lesions, might be expectd in

64   R. Masuda et al.

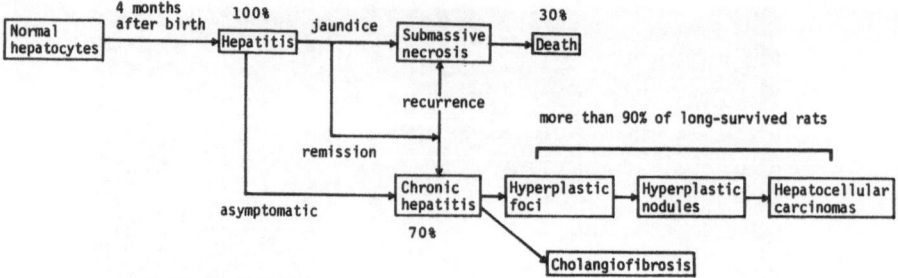

Fig. 8. Transition from normal hepatocytes to hepatitis and subsequent liver lesions in LEC rats. (From [9] with a slight modification)

fully aged LEC rats, since in this study, some younger animals were sacrificed for histological examinations before the development of liver tumors. In fact, hepatomas were observed in all of the rats examined when they were over 18 months of age. Therefore, development of hepatomas appears to be strongly correlated with these precancerous lesions in the liver in LEC rats which also had chronic hepatitis.

Stepwise transition from normal hepatocytes to precancerous lesions and to overt hepatomas is well investigated in chemical hepatocarcinogenesis [15]. It has been reported that hepatomas develop in human carriers of viral hepatitis [4,5] as well as in some animals [6–8], possibly through a course similar to chemical hepatocarcinogenesis. Although the cause of hepatitis in these animals may not be similar to that in LEC rats, each of their hepatocarcinogenesis seems to be promoted by regeneration stimuli caused by hepatitis. There were only a few reports of the occurrence of spontaneous liver tumors in laboratory rats and the incidence was very low in each case [16–18], except for the report of aged (older than 30 months) germ-free Wistar rats, but these rats did not develope hepatitis [19]. In long-surviving C3H-A^{vy} strain mice, a high incidence of spontaneous hepatomas was noted without causing hepatitis [20,21]. Therefore, the present LEC strain is unique and provides an excellent animal model of liver tumors associated with spontaneous hepatitis.

It is also interesting that a higher incidence of hepatomas of a relatively larger size was observed in males (97%) than in females (58%) (Table 3). It has been reported that more preneoplastic foci appeared in livers of male LEC rats than in those of females [22]. These findings correspond with other reports that the progressive growth of chemically induced hepatomas was influenced by sex hormones of the hosts, probably testosterone in the rat [23], and that the number of enzyme-altered foci was greater in male rats than in females [24]. By contrast, in most cases of this study, cholangiofibrosis was considerably more extensive in females than in males. All of the four rats which developed only cholangiofibrosis without hepatomas were females. Since there was an extensive degradation of hepatocytes by more severe chronic hepatitis in the females, it seems that preneoplastic lesions were replaced by cholangiofibrosis. A more severer degradation of hepatocytes and progressive growth of cholangiofibrosis may also be somehow affected by sex hormones.

Acknowledgments. We thank Mrs. Kazuko Kagami and Mr. Eikichi Kamimura from the Center for Experimental Plants and Animals of Hokkaido University for their assistance. R.M. was a recipient of a Fellowship for Japanese Junior Scientists from the Japan Society for the Promotion of Science. This work was supported in part by Grants-in-Aid for Scientific Research from the Ministry of Education, Science and Culture of Japan.

References

1. Sasaki M, Yoshida MC, Kagami K, Takeichi N, Kobayashi H, Dempo K, Mori M (1985) Spontaneous hepatitis in an inbred strain of Long-Evans rats. Rat News Lett 14:4–6
2. Yoshida MC, Masuda R, Sasaki M, Takeichi N, Kobayashi H, Dempo K, Mori M (1987) New mutation causing hereditary hepatitis in the laboratory rat. J Hered 78:361–365
3. Masuda R, Yoshida MC, Sasaki M, Dempo K, Mori M (1988) Hereditary hepatitis of LEC rats is controlled by a single autosomal recessive gene. Lab Anim 22:166–169
4. Popper H, Gerber MA, Thung SN (1982) The relation of hepatocellular carcinoma to infection with hepatitis B and related viruses in man and animals. Hepatology (Suppl) 2:1S–9S
5. Thiollais P, Pourcel C, Dejean A (1985) The hepatitis B virus. Nature 317:489–495
6. Summers J, Smolec MJ, Snyder R (1978) A virus similar to human hepatitis B virus associated with hepatitis and hepatoma in woodchucks. Proc Natl Acad Sci USA 75:4533–4537
7. Marion PL, Davelaar MJV, Knight SS, Salazar FH, Garcia G, Popper H, Robinson WS (1986) Hepatocellular carcinoma in ground squirrels persistently infected with ground squirrel hepatitis virus. Proc Natl Acad Sci USA 83:4543–4546
8. Omata M, Uchiumi K, Ito Y, Yokosuka O, Mori J, Terao K, Wei-Fa Y, O'Connell AP, London WT, Okuda K (1983) Duck hepatitis B virus and liver diseases. Gastroenterology 85:260–267
9. Masuda R, Yoshida MC, Sasaki M, Dempo K, Mori M (1988) High susceptibility to hepatocellular carcinoma development in LEC rats with hereditary hepatitis. Jpn J Cancer Res 79:828–835
10. Masuda R, Yoshida MC, Sasaki M, Dempo K, Mori M (1988) A transplantable cell line derived from spontaneous hepatocellular carcinoma of the hereditary hepatitis LEC rat. Jpn J Cancer Res 79:250–254
11. Kobayashi K, Fukuoka K, Matsushita F, Morimoto H, Hinoue Y, Honjo H, Tanaka N, Sugimoto T, Kato Y, Hattori N, Ueda S, Kato S (1983) Transplan-

tation of woodchuck hepatocellular carcinoma in nude mice. Hepatology 3: 663–666

12. Unoura M, Kobayashi K, Fukuoka K, Matsushita F, Morimoto H, Oshima T, Kaneko S, Hattori N, Murakami S, Yoshikawa H (1985) Establishment of a cell line from a woodchuck hepatocellular carcinoma. Hepatology 5:1106–1111

13. Abe K, Kurata T, Yamada K, Okumura H, Shikata T (1988) Establishment and characterization of a woodchuck hepatocellular carcinoma cell line (WH44KA). Jpn J Cancer Res 79:342–349

14. Ohnishi S, Aoyama H, Shiga J, Itai Y, Moriyama T, Ishikawa T, Sasaki N, Yamamoto K, Koshimizu K, Kaneko S, Murakami S, Hattori N, Imawari M (1988) Establishment of a new cell line from a woodchuck hepatocellular carcinoma. Hepatology 8:104–107

15. Squire RA, Levitt MH (1975) Report of a workshop on classification of specific hepatocellular lesions in rats. Cancer Res 35:3214–3223

16. Ward JM (1981) Morphology of foci of altered hepatocytes and naturally-occurring hepatocellular tumors in F344 rats. Virchows Arch [A] 390:339–345

17. Maekawa A, Kurokawa Y, Takahashi M, Kokubo T, Ogiu T, Onodera H, Tanigawa H, Ohno Y, Furukawa F, Hayashi Y (1983) Spontaneous tumors in F-344/DuCrj rats. Jpn J Cancer Res 74:365–372

18. Solleveld HA, Haseman JK, McConnell EE (1984) Natural history of body weight gain, survival, and neoplasia in the F344 rat. J Natl Cancer Inst 72: 929–940

19. Pollard M, Luckert PH (1979) Spontaneous liver tumors in aged germfree Wistar rats. Lab Anim Sci 29:74–77

20. Heston WE, Vlahakis G (1968) C3H-A^{vy} — A high hepatoma and high mammary tumor strain of mice. J Natl Cancer Inst 40:1161–1166

21. Ward JM, Vlahakis G (1978) Evaluation of hepatocellular neoplasms in mice. J Natl Cancer Inst 61:807–811

22. Oyamada M, Dempo K, Fujimoto Y, Takahashi H, Satoh MI, Mori M, Masuda R, Yoshida MC, Satoh K, Sato K (1988) Spontaneous occurrence of placental glutathione S-transferase-positive foci in the livers of LEC rats. Jpn J Cancer Res 79:5–8

23. Reuber MD (1969) Influence of hormones on N-2-fluorenyldiacetamide-induced hyperplastic hepatic nodules in rats. J Natl Cancer Inst 43:445–451

24. Mitaka T, Tsukada H (1987) Sexual difference in the histochemical characteristics of "altered cell foci" in the liver of aged Fischer 344 rats. Jpn J Cancer Res 78:785–790

PART II Hepatitis

1. Pathology

7 — Investigation of Infectious Agents Causing Spontaneous Hepatitis in LEC Rats

Tsutomu Namieno[1,2], Noritoshi Takeichi[1], Motomichi Sasaki[3], Kimimaro Dempo[4], Michio Mori[4], Jun-ichi Uchino[2], and Hiroshi Kobayashi[1]

Introduction

Two strains of Long-Evans rats, LEC and LEA were separated according to their coat colors. Acute hepatitis tends to occur spontaneously in the LEC rats after the 24th generation. As has been previously reported [1–3], the clinical course of the disease and the histopathological features closely resemble human fulminant hepatitis.

The characteristic features of this disease are a sudden onset of severe jaundice at 4–5 months after birth, accompanied by body weight loss, oliguria, bilirubinuria with an elevation of the blood bilirubin, and serum glutamic-oxaloacetic transminase (SGOT) and serum glutamic-pyruvic transaminase (SGPT) values (SGOT predominance). The histopathological features show liver atrophy and focal necrosis, and, in the progressive stage, widespread and multiple spotty necroses are seen. In this paper, we focus our study on the possibility of hepatitis virus participation, hereditary factors, and immunological abnormalities (the IgG level and its correlation to the onset of hepatitis).

Materials and Methods

Rats

We used two inbred strains of rats, LEC and LEA, which were isolated according to coat colors from a closed colony of LE rats. We also used Wistar King Aptekman/Hok (WKA/H) rats obtained from the Experimental Animal Institute, Hokkaido University School of Medicine.

[1] Laboratory of Pathology, Cancer Institute, [2] First Department of Surgery, School of Medicine, Hokkaido University, Sapporo, 060 Japan
[3] Sasaki Cancer Institute, Chiyoda-ku, Tokyo, 101 Japan
[4] Department of Pathology, Sapporo Medical College, Sapporo, 060 Japan

Observation of Hepatitis Virus by Electron Microscopy

In order to determine whether hepatitis virus is involved in the pathogenesis of acute hepatitis in the LEC rats, we tried to identify the virus morphologically. For specimens, we used livers, spleens, and kidneys of LEC rats in the stages of pre-hepatitis ($n = 6$), active hepatitis ($n = 6$), and post-hepatitis ($n = 6$). Each of the specimens was fixed immediately after dissection in 6.25% glutaraldehyde (pH = 7.4, 0.1 M sodium cacodylate buffer solution). After being washed 3 times in a 0.1 M cacodylate buffer solution, they were fixed in a 1% osmium acid solution (Millonig's method). Dehydration in graded alcohols was followed by propyleneoxide permeation and embedding in Epon 812. Ultra-thin sections were cut with an ultra-microtome (Porter-Bhem, MT-1 model), and double staining was performed with uranyl acetate and lead citrate (Reynold's method). Screening of a hepatitis virus was performed with the Hitachi model HU12A electron microscope. Photographs were taken simultaneously for later examination.

Detection of Hepatitis Virus Antigen by Indirect Fluorescent Antibody Method

The liver cells used were from hepatitis-developing LEC rats ($n = 10$) and the non-hepatitis control group LEA rats ($n = 10$) and were cultured in a standard condition.

As primary anti-serum, 2 kinds of serum were produced: (1) serum from the LEC rats which recovered from acute hepatitis, and (2) serum from the LEA rats which were inoculated with plasma from the LEC rats with hepatitis. Each serum was diluted two-, four-, and eightfold. As the secondary antibody, a fivefold diluted fluorescence-conjugated goat anti-rat-IgG serum (Cappel Co., USA) was used.

Collagenase (0.05%) and enzymatic separation were used to prepare suspensions of LEC ar LEA rat liver cells in the usual manner. Since it is believed that enzymatic treatment affects the antigens on liver cell surface, these suspensions were cultured for 3 days in the complete medium in a 55 mm plastic flask (Corning, New York).

After the treatment, cell suspensions were adjusted to 5×10^6 cells/ml, and 100 μl of cell suspensions was added to 100 μl of the primary antibody. After the mixture was allowed to sit at 37°C for 60 min, the cells were washed 3 times, 100 μl of the secondary antibody was added, and the resultant mixture was allowed to sit at 37°C for 60 min. The cells were then washed again, and the product from the reaction in the mixture was bedded onto a glass slide, fixed with acetone, and immediately examined and photographed through a fluorescence microscope (Nikon Optiphot: Nippon Optics Co. model, Tokyo). Either presence or absence of viral antigens was determined according to the protocols established by Yoshida [4] or Nomoto [5].

Passive Induction of Hepatitis

In order to examine whether a hepatitis virus is participating in the pathogenesis of acute hepatitis in the LEC rats, we first prepared liver homogenates and plasma or serum obtained from pre-hepatitis, hepatitis-suffering
and post-hepatitis LEC rats, and administered them to new-born LEA and
WKA/H rats.

A 0.15 ml aliquot of the liver homogenate which was diluted to 20%,
and a 0.15 ml aliquot of the undiluted plasma or serum were administered
(i.p.) to newborn LEA and WKA/H rats. After the observation period of
8 months, the rats were sacrificed for study histopathological studies.

Induction Facilitation of Hepatitis under
Steroid-Immunosupression

Immunosuppression is believed to induce hepatitis in the LEC rats and the
LEA rats. For the examination of a possible latent infection with hepatitis
virus in the LEC and LEA rats, the animals were immunosuppressed by the
administration of a high dose of a steroid hormone: administration (i.p.) of
triamcinolone acetonide (Kenacort-A) to 4- and 8-week-old LEC rats (0.4 or
0.8 mg/rat) and to 8-week-old LEA rats (1.2 mg/rat). Each rat was observed
for 8 months; jaundice was considered as the major clinical sign of
hepatitis development, and the diagnosis of hepatitis was confirmed by
histopathological studies. At the end of the observation period, the rats
with no hepatitis were sacrificed, and the histopathological abnormalities
in their livers and other organs were examined. During these experiments,
all of the immunosuppressed rats were raised in isolation.

Hereditary Factors of Hepatitis

For the study of influential hereditary foctors on the pathogenesis of
hepatitis in the LEC rats, a crossbreed was made by a hepatitis-developing
group of LEC rats and a non-hepatitis group of LEA rats. F_1s, F_2s and
backcrosses (hybrids [(LEC × LEA) × LEC]) were established, and we
studied the inheritance pattern by the incidence of acute hepatitis in these
rats.

A further crossbreed was also made by LEC and WKA/H rats and their
inheritance pattern was studied as well.

Correlation Between IgG-level and Hepatitis

Our study of the serum fractions from 6- and 12-week-old LEC rats by
cellulose acetate membrane electrophoresis revealed that the concentra-

tion of γ-globulin was so low that the densitometer could not detect it [3]. Another study of the correlation between the IgG level and the development of hepatitis was performed in parallel with the above-mentioned study of hereditary factors.

The test serum obtained from the LEC and the LEA rats, from the crossbreeds between the two strains, F_1s and F_2s, and from backcrosses between the F_2s and LEC rats. IgG was measured according to Mancini's method, a single radial immunodiffusion assay. In the preliminary experiments using anti-rat IgG (Cosmo-Bio KK, Tokyo), the antibody concentration in the agarose gel was set at 6%. In the agaroseplate, holes of 3 mm in diameter were made, and 5 μl of a standard solution with an established concentration and 5 μl of the test serum were pipetted into them independently. The plate was incubated for 3 h in a humidified 37°C environment. A calibration curve was drawn using the sedimentation rings of the standard solution, and the IgG concentration was calculated according to the test serum sedimentaion ring diameter at the time when equilibrium of the ring expansion was reached.

Statistical Analysis

The results were expressed as mean values ± standard deviation, and Student's t-test was applied as a test of significant differences between the groups.

Results

Screening Hepatitis Virus by Electron Microscopy

Specimens were prepared, as described in Materials and Methods, from livers, spleens, and kidneys of pre-hepatitis, hepatitis-suffering, and posthepatitis LEC rats for the morphological screening of hepatitis virus. No viral particles were detected in any of the numerous repetitions of the screening.

Detection of Hepatitis Virus Antigen by the Indirect Fluorescent Antibody Method

In order to define hepatitis virus antigen in the liver cells obtained from hepatitis-developing LEC rats and non-hepatitis LEA rats, we used the primary and secondary antibodies following the indirect fluorescent method..

The results revealed no evidence of hepatitis virus antigen in the liver cells of either the LEC or the LEA rats. Similar results were obtained from

Table 1. A trial of hepatitis induction in newborn LEA and WKA/H rats by the administration of serum and liver homogenates of LEC rats with acute hepatitis.

Strain	Injection with[a]	Age at injection	No. of rats with hepatitis/ no. of rats injected[b]
LEA	Serum	Newborn	0/8
	Liver homogenates	Newborn	0/13
WKA/H	Serum	Newborn	0/10
	Liver homogenates	Newborn	0/18

[a] Recipient rats were injected (ip) with 0.15 ml serum or 0.15 ml 20% liver homogenates
[b] All rats were observed for 8 months

all of the other organs as well. From the results of repeated experiments, we concluded that hepatitis virus antigen is not expressed in these liver cells.

Passive Induction of Hepatitis

Liver homogenates, plasma, or serum obtained from pre-hepatitis, hepatitis-suffering and post-hepatitis LEC rats were administered (i.p.) to newborn LEA and WKA/H rats. Among the LEA rats, 8 were administered serum and 13 were administered liver homogenates; among the WKA/H rats, 10 were administered serum and 18 were administered liver homogenates. All of the animals were kept under observation for 8 months with no occurrence of hepatitis. At the end of the observation period, liver tissue sections were prepared and stained with H and E for the study of pathological changes in the liver. In comparison to an untreated group of the same age, no abnormal findings were detected (Table 1). The animals which had been administered plasma or serum presented similar results.

Induction or Facilitation of Hepatitis under Steroid-Immunosuppression

Hepatitis developed in 100% ($n = 4$) of the 4-week-old LEC rats which received triamcinolone acetonide, 0.4 mg/rat, by im. injection. The average survival period of this group was 136 ± 18 days. There were no significant differences, however, in the hepatitis occurrence rate or in the average survival period in comparison to a control group of LEC rats of the same age which had not been given the steroid hormone ($n = 4$). Likewise, no significant differences were observed in the incidence of hepatitis, average survival days, and the onset time of hepatitis between the steroid hormone-administered cases ($n = 5$) and non-administered cases ($n = 4$) of 8-week-old LEC rats.

Table 2. Effects of immunosuppression induced by the administration of a steroid hormone on the induction of hepatitis in LEC and LEA rats.

Strain	Age at injection (Weeks)	Dose of steroid hormone[a] (mg/rat)	Incidence of hepatitis (Mean survival days)
LEC	4	0.4	4/4 (136 ± 18)
	4	none	4/4 (138 ± 27)
LEC	8	0.8	5/5 (142 ± 21)
	8	none	4/4 (135 ± 19)
LEA	8	1.2	0/8

[a] Recipient rats were injected (im.) with 0.5 ~ 0.11 mg triamcinolone acetonide (Kenacort-A)

A high dose of steroid hormone was administered to 8-week-old LEA rats in order to induce immunosuppression, but failed to induce hepatitis in these rats. The treated LEA rats were sacrificed after 8 months, and histopathological examinations revealed no abnormal findings (Table 2). During the experiments, all of the immunosuppressed rats were maintained in isolation, and no complication with newly occurring infectious diseases were observed in any of the cases.

Inheritance Background of Hepatitis

Among the 57 LEC rats used for the experiment, hepatitis developed in 50 (female 26, male 24), an occurrence rate of 88%. No male/female difference was detected regarding the onset of hepatitis. Hepatitis did not occur in any of the 34 LEA rats. In the F_1s, there were LEC (♀) × LEA (♂) = 38 subjects and LEA (♀) × LEC (♂) = 13 subjects; however, as in the

Table 3. Hereditary background of spontaneous hepatitis in LEC, LEA, F_1, F_2, and backcross rats.

Generation[b]	No. of rats examined (♀:♂)			
	Total No.	Jaundice (+)	Jaundice (−)	Hepatitis (%)
LEC	57	50 (26:24)	7 (3:4)	88
LEA	34	0	34 (18:16)	0
(LEC × LEA) F_1	38	0	38 (21:17)	0 ⎤ 0
(LEA × LEC) F_1	13	0	13 (6:7)	0 ⎦
(LEC × LEA) × (LEC × LEA) F_2	45	14 (5:9)	31 (15:16)	31 ⎤ 30
(LEA × LEC) × (LEA × LEC) F_2	38	11 (5:6)	27 (11:16)	29 ⎦
(LEC × LEA) × LEC	30	12 (6:6)	18 (7:11)	40 ⎤ 40
(LEA × LEC) × LEC	40	16 (10:6)	24 (10:14)	40 ⎦

[a] Hepatitis was diagnosed by histopathological investigation
[b] All rats were observed for more than 8 months

LEA rat group, no hepatitis developed in any of them. In the F_2s there were [LEC (♀) × LEA (♂)] × [LEC (♂) × LEA (♀)] = 47 subjects, and hepatitis developed in 14 of them, an occurrence rate of 31%. There were also [LEA (♀) × LEC (♂)] × [LEA (♀) × LEC (♂)] = 38 subjects, and hepatitis developed in 11 of these subjects, an occurrence rate of 29%. The overall hepatitis occurrence rate in the F_2s was 30% (25/83), with no significant difference between the sexes.

The hepatitis occurrence rate in the backcrosses was as follows: among 30 [LEC (♀) × LEA (♂)] × LEC rats, hepatitis occurred in 12 subjects (40%), and among 40 [LEA (♀) × LEC (♂)] × LEC rats, hepatitis developed in 16 subjects (40%). The overall hepatitis occurrence rate in the backcrosses was 40% (28/70), and the rate was higher in females than in males (Table 3). We also found that no hepatitis occurred in the F_1s between the LEC and the WKA/H rats, and that the hepatitis occurrence rates in the F_2s and the backcrosses were similar to those between the LEC and the LEA rats.

Inheritance Pattern of Hepatitis-Occurrence Indicated by IgG-level

In comparison to the IgG level of 15.7 ± 7.8 mg/ml in the non-hepatitis group (8-week-old) LEA rats ($n = 19$), the IgG level of 0.45 ± 0.2 mg/ml in the hepatitis-developing group LEC rats ($n = 16$) was markedly suppressed. The IgG level in the non-hepatitis F_1s ($n = 10$) was 9.3 ± 1.0 mg/ml, 2.8 ± 1.9 mg/ml in the hepatitis developing F_2s ($n = 23$), and 2.5 ± 2.0 mg/ml in the hepatitis-developing backcrosses ($n = 20$). It appears that in the groups with a greater genetic background of hepatitis, the IgG level was more suppressed in LEC rats (Fig. 1).

Discussion

It is incumbent upon us to answer whether the hepatitis virus is involved in the pathogenesis of spontaneous hepatitis in the LEC rats. If we assume that it is, the virus should be detected in the liver not only during the period of hepatitis, but before or/and after the duration of the disease, and not only in the liver, but also in other organs. In the study of infectious agents causing hepatitis, we divided the animals into clearly delineated groups of non-hepatitis, hepatitis in-progress, and survivors which recovered from the hepatitis 4 months after the spontaneous onset of the disease. Using a transmission electron microscope, we examined the livers, spleens, and kidneys in every group of the animals to verify the presence of hepatitis virus and failed to find any signs of it.

Since we suspected that we might still find virus antigen in the cytoplasm or on the membrane surface of liver cells from the animals infected with the hepatitis virus, an attempt was made to verify any

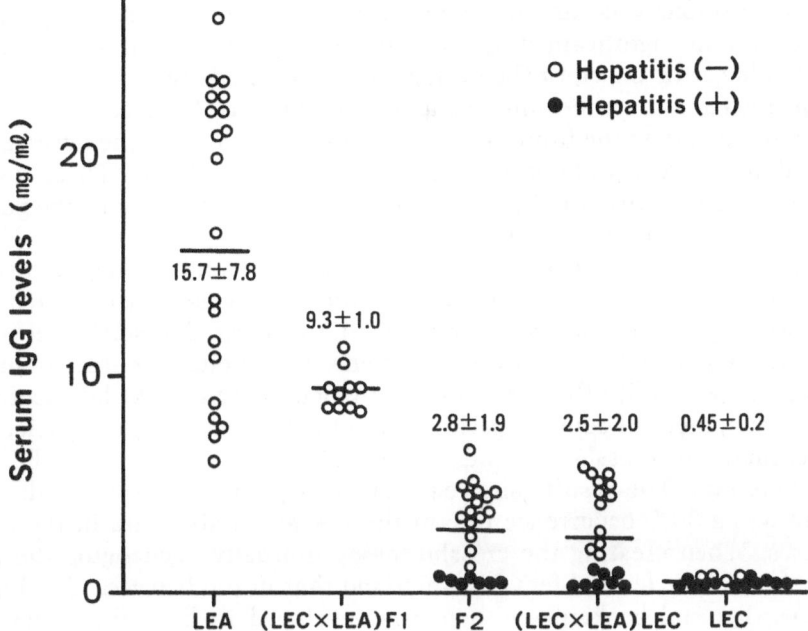

Fig. 1. Connection between serum IgG levels and hepatitis occurrence in LEC, LEA, F_1, F_2, and backcross rats

participation of hepatitis virus by localizing hepatitis virus antigens by the indirect fluorescent antibody method. However, no virus antigen was found.

Our next step was to study the participation of the hepatitis virus by an in vivo method. Since newborn rats have a weak immune system and are very susceptible to infection, putative inoculation with hepatitis virus was performed by administering liver homogenates, plasma, or serum taken from LEC rats to newborn LEA and WKA/H rats. The LEA and the WKA/H rats did not develop hepatitis during the 8-month observation period, and no pathological abnormalities were found in the liver tissue of these rats.

Several papers have reported that immuno-deficient animals, such as thymectomized mice, congenitally athymic nude mice, or the mice administered with anti-lymph ocyte serum or steroid hormones, are liable to present extensive changes in liver pathology after inoculation with a mouse hepatitis virus [6–11].

We speculate that if the LEC and the LEA rats were latently infected with the hepatitis virus, the LEC rats would show facilitated hepatitis development and the LEA rats would develop hepatitis upon induction of immunosuppression or immunodeficiency. The dose of the administered steroid hormone was sufficient enough to induce immunosuppression, but there were no significant differences in the hepatitis occurrence rate, the time of hepatitis onset, or the average survival time between the immuno-suppressed and the non-immunosuppressed LEC rats. No cases of hepatitis were found among the immunosuppressed LEA rats during the observation period, nor were any abnormalities in the liver tissue found. These results seem to confirm that the hepatitis virus does not participate in the patho-genesis of hepatitis in the LEC rats.

In a rat strain (Gunn rat) in which hereditary jaundice was discovered in 1938 [12], nuclear icterus developed immediately after birth which was followed by death; its cause was found to be an autosomal recessive genetic enzyme (UDP-glucuronyl transferase) deficiency. In order to inves-tigate the possibility that such an inheritance pattern might be a factor in the development of acute hepatitis in the LEC rats as well, we carried out experiments in crossbreeds and a backcross group between the LEC and the LEA rats. The results showed that no hepatitis occurred in the F_1s, there was a 30% occurrence rate in the F_2s, and a 40% rate in the back-crosses. When creating the crossbreeds by mutually exchanging the LEC and the LEA males and females, we found that in the hepatitis-developing groups, F_2s and backcrosses, hepatitis developed in both the males and females. These facts indicate the existence of a hereditary factor in the pathogenesis of hepatitis in the LEC rats. Thus, it appears that the develop-ment of hepatitis in the LEC rats is controlled by an autosomal recessive gene, in accordance with Mendel's classical laws of heredity.

It was difficult to detect γ-globulin in the tests of serum protein concen-tration in 6- and 12-week-old LEC rats, [3]. Since the main component of γ-globulin is IgG, the question arose as to whether there was a correlation between the IgG level and the development of hepatitis, and whether the hereditary pattern discussed above had any effect on the IgG level. It was found that the IgG level was relatively higher in the LEA rats and relatively lower in the LEC rats, and decreased gradually in the F_1s, F_2s, and the backcrosses, respectively. Therefore, it appears that in the groups with a greater contribution of LEC genetic factor(s), the IgG level is more sup-pressed. Moreover, in the hepatitis-developing F_2s, backcrosses, and LEC rats, the lower that the IgG level was, the higher was the hepatitis occur-rance rate. From these facts, it seems that there is a strong possibility that there is a close connection between the development of hepatitis in the LEC rats and an abnormality (mutation) in the gene which controls the production of IgG, and that the suppressed production of IgG leads to the development of hepatitis.

Based on the fact that hepatitis development in the LEC rats is attribu-table to an autosomal recessive gene, further research on the pathogenesis of hepatitis in the LEC rats should be carried out with emphasis upon enzyme abnormality as is seen in Gunn rats, as well as upon immune abnormality as is recognized in the correlation between lowered IgG levels and increased incidences of hepatitis.

Conclusions

In order to elucidate the pathogenesis of hepatitis in LEC rats, we investigated a possible involvement of a hepatitis virus, the presence of hereditary factors, and the correlation of the incidence of hepatitis with IgG levels. The following are our findings:

1. No hepatitis viruses were identified morphologically by electron microscopy or immunologically by the indirect fluorescent antibody method.
2. Newborn LEA and WAK/H rats were inoculated with a plasma/serum/liver homogenate from LEC rats with pre-/min-/post-hepatitis, but hepatitis could not be induced.
3. In order to find out whether or not immunosuppression facilitates the onset of hepatitis, a steroid hormone was administered to pre-hepatitis LEC and LEA rats. The results showed that the time before the onset was not shortened in the LEC rats, and hepatitis could not be induced in the LEA rats.
4. A crossbreed was developed between the hepatitis-developing group LEC rats and the non-hepatitis group LEA rats. No hepatitis was observed in the progeny of F_1, but hepatitis occurred in 30% of the progeny of F_2, and in 40% of the progeny of the backcross hybrid [(LEC × LEA) × LEC], with no differences between the sexes.
5. The average serum IgG levels showed a gradual decrease from the LEA to F_1s, F_2s, backcrosses, and the LEC rats, respectively, with a higher rate of the onset of hepatitis correlating with decreased IgG values.

From the above results, it appears that there is no participation of a hepatitis virus in the pathogenesis of hepatitis in the LEC rats, and that the appearance of hepatitis follows the pattern of an inherited autosomal recessive trait. Additionally, the suppressed IgG level, which also seems to follow the same hereditary pattern, correlates with the onset of hepatitis.

Acknowledgment. This work was supported in part by grants from the Ministry of Education, Science and Culture of Japan.

References

1. Sasaki M, Yoshida MC, Kagami K, Takeichi N, Kobayashi H, Dempo K, Mori M (1985) Spontaneous hepatitis in an inbred strain of Long-Evans rats. Rat News Lett 14:4–6
2. Yoshida MC, Masuda R, Sasaki M, Takeichi N, Kobayshi H, Dempo K, Mori M (1987) New mutation causing hereditary hepatitis in the laboratory rat. J Hered 78:361–365
3. Namieno T, Takeichi N, Sasaki M, Dempo K, Mori M, Uchino J, Kobayashi H in press. Clinical and pathological characteristics in Long-Evans Cinnamon (LEC) rats with spontaneous development of hepatitis. Gastroenterology

4. Yoshida T (1971) Membrane immunofluorescence method. In: Migita S (ed) Experimental immunology method and procedure I. Jpn Soc Immunol (Kanazawa) 243–245
5. Nomoto K (1971) Detection of cell membrane antigen using immuno-fluorescence method. In: Migita S (ed) Experimental immunology method and procedure I. Jpn Soc Immunol (Kanazawa) 239–241
6. Nelson JB (1952) Acute hepatitis associated with mouse leukemia. I. Pathological features and transmission of the disease. J Exp Med 96:293–302
7. Gledhill AW (1955) The nature of mouse hepatitis virus in weanling mice. J Exp Med 69:311
8. East J (1963) The appearance of a hepatotrophic virus in mice thymectomized at birth. J Exp Med 118:1069–1082
9. Gallily R (1964) Effect of cortisone on genetic resistance to mouse hepatitis virus in vivo and in vitro. Proc Natl Acad Sci USA 51:1158–1164
10. Pantelouris EM (1968) Absence of thymus in nude mouse mutant. Nature 217:370–371
11. Allison AC (1970) Effects of antilymphocytic serum on bacterial and viral infections and virus oncogenesis: Fed Proc 29:167–168
12. Gunn CK (1938) Hereditary acholuric jaundice in a new mutant strain of rats. J Hered 29:137–141

8 — Possible Involvement of Abnormal Cytokinesis and Karyokinesis in the Manifestation of Hepatitis in LEC Rats

YOSHINORI FUJIMOTO[1,2,3], MICHIO MORI[1], and MINAKO NAGAO[2]

Introduction

In jaundiced LEC rats, the histopathological characteristics of the liver include markedly enlarged hepatocytes with huge nuclei whose DNA content appears to be more than octaploid. At the age of 14 weeks, immediately prior to the onset of hepatitis, the nuclei of hepatocytes often vary in size, and their enlarged nuclei frequently possess several nucleoli. Based upon these observations, we have analyzed nuclei ploidy, the percentage of binucleated cells, and DNA synthesis in the hepatocytes of LEC rats at various ages in order to determine whether abnormal cytokinesis and karyokinesis occur in LEC rats [1,2].

Materials and Methods

Animals

The inbred rat strains LEC and LEA were established at Hokkaido University and maintained and raised at the Sapporo Medical College [3,4].

Isolation of Hepatocytes

Cells were isolated from the liver by digestion with collagenase [5], and, during perfusion, the lateral lobe was sectioned for light microscopic study.

[1] Department of Pathology, Sapporo Medical College, Sapporo, 060 Japan
[2] Carcinogenesis Division, National Cancer Center Research Institute, Chuo-Ku, Tokyo, 104 Japan
[3] Laboratory of Experimental Carcinogenesis, National Cancer Institute, National Institutes of Health, Bethesda, MD 20892, USA

Preparation of Nuclei for Flow Cytometry

Nuclei for flow cytometric analysis were prepared by the detergent-trypsin method [6]. After successive treatment with trypsin and RNase A, the cells were suspended in a citrate buffer, incubated on ice with propidium iodide, and then subjected to flow cytometer analysis using an EPICS C flow cytometer (Coulter Electronics, Inc., Hialeah, Fla., USA) at intervals between 15 min and 3 h after the addition of propidium iodide solution. A sample of 10^4 nuclei was utilized for each assay.

Labeling Index

BrdU (5-bromo-2'-deoxyuridine, 100 mg/kg body weight) in 1 ml buffered saline solution was injected intraperitoneally into the animals, and the livers were removed 1 h later and fixed in Carnoy's solution. After incubation of the liver sections with mouse anti-BrdU monoclonal antibody, BrdU incorporation was localized with an avidin-biotin-peroxidase complex, with color development of 3,3'-diaminobenzidine tetrahydrochloride. Liver sections were counterstained with hematoxylin. The labeling index was measured in three fields including the portal and central area in each slide. At least 5,000 nuclei per rat were counted.

Results

DNA Content of Hepatocyte Nuclei

Figure 1 shows the histogram of the DNA content of hepatocyte nuclei of a 20-week-old LEC rat with jaundice. The nuclei consisted of several different classes, all of which were found to be euploid. The dominant peak was that of diploid nuclei (2n) with additional peaks representing 4n, 8n, 16n, 32n, and 64n nuclei, respectively. Table 1 shows the frequency of polyploid nuclei in hepatocytes from LEC and LEA rats of various ages. The ratios of 4n ($P < 0.01$) at week 4, 4n ($P < 0.01$) and 8n ($P < 0.01$) at week 12, and 4n

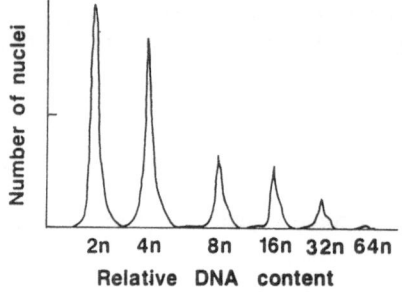

Fig. 1. Histogram of DNA contents of hepatocyte and oval cell nuclei of a 20-week-old LEC rat by a flow cytometer. (Adapted with permission from [1])

Table 1. Frequency (%) of polyploid nuclei in hepatocytes of LEC and LEA rats at various ages. (Adapted from [1]).

LEC	Weeks	2n	4n	8n	16n	>16n
	2	92	8	ND	ND	ND
	4	68	30	2	ND	ND
	6	51	33	6	ND	ND
	8	45	49	6	ND	ND
	12	35	56	9	ND	ND
	16	53	27	13	6	1
	20	50	32	13	3	2
	28	42	28	20	8	2
LEA	Weeks	2n	4n	8n	16n	>16n
	2	90	10	ND	ND	ND
	4	83	14	3	ND	ND
	6	59	37	4	ND	ND
	8	43	52	5	ND	ND
	12	44	51	5	ND	ND
	16	34	61	5	ND	ND

ND, not detected

($P < 0.01$), 8n ($P < 0.01$), and 16n ($P < 0.001$) at week 16 in the LEC rats were significantly higher than those observed in the LEA hepatocytes. The ploidy pattern of LEA rats was similar to that of other strains of rats, as reported previously [7].

Multinucleated Cells

The percent of binucleated hepatocytes of LEC and LEA rats were both about 7% at 2 weeks after birth, but at week 4 marked differences were observed. In LEA rats, approximately 25% of the hepatocytes were binucleated, while 50% of the hepatocytes were binucleated in the LEC animals. After week 6, the frequency of binucleated nuclei was 45% for both LEC and LEA rats, and no further significant differences were observed until week 16. Tri- and tetranucleated hepatocytes, which previously have not been observed in normal rats, were revealed in jaundiced LEC rats. The size of the nuclei within each multinucleated cell of LEC hepatocyte differed (Fig. 2). The percentage of trinucleated hepatocytes at week 16 and week 28 were 0.53% and 1.07%, respectively.

DNA Synthesis of Hepatocytes

After treatment with BrdU, approximately 10% of the hepatocytes were labeled and randomly distributed in the hepatic lobules of both LEC and

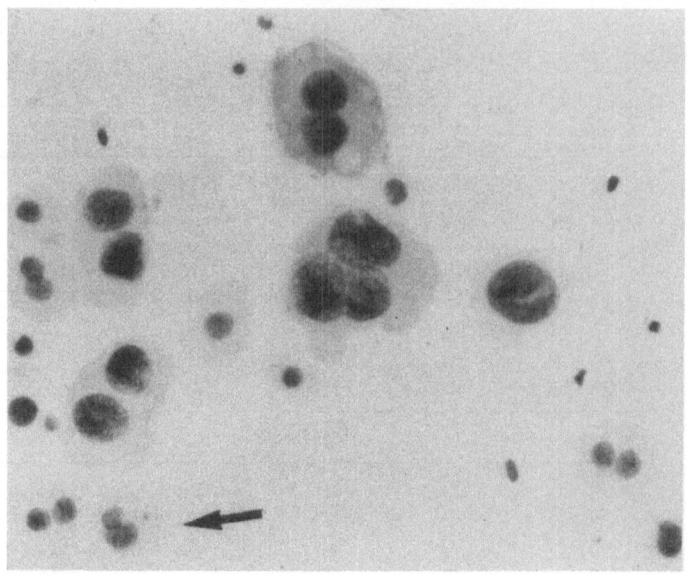

Fig. 2. Smear preparation of hepatocytes of a 20-week-old LEC rat with jaundice (Giemsa staining, × 340). Large trinucleated hepatocytes and binucleated hepatocytes whose nuclei differ in size (*arrow*) are observed. (Adapted with permission from [1])

LEA rats at day 1 after birth. The labeling indexes in both animals rapidly decreased during the first 2 weeks, continued to increase at week 4, and then exhibited a gradual decrease beginning at week 6 and continuing until week 14. Labeling indexes in LEC rats were significantly higher than those of LEA rats, except at week 6. At week 16, when hepatitis became manifest in LEC rats, the labeling index markedly increased to greater than 4%, and both large and small nuclei were labeled. An elevated labeling index persisted until at least week 28, at which time the LEC rats were in a chronic phase of hepatitis. The majority of the labeled cells were "oval cells" and small hepatocytes in the periportal area of the hepatic lobule, although a few large nuclei of hepatocytes were also labeled after the onset of hepatitis.

Discussion

Polyploidy is generally observed in the livers of older animals and in the regenerating liver following either partial hepatectomy or treatment with various chemicals. High polyploidy such as 64n has not been observed in rats, except in cases following treatment by carcinogens [8]. Three mechanisms, i.e., mitotic polyploidization [9], block in cell cycle at G2, and cell fusion [10], have been proposed for this polyploidization. In the first case, mitosis stops at the cytokinesis step, resulting in the formation of binucleated cells. If normal mitosis occurs at the next mitosis, then two tetraploid cells are produced. In the second case, if a block at G2 occurs with endoreduplication, then no mitotic figures should be observed. Alternatively, any anomalous cell fusion would result in the production of aneuploidy. Since both binucleated hepatocytes and mitotic figures of hepatocytes were detected, mitotic polyploidization appears to be the mechanism responsible for the formation of polyploidy in LEC rats. The presence of tri- and tetranucleated cells, and unequal-sized nuclei in bi- and trinucleated cells in hepatocytes of jaundiced LEC rats also suggest abnormality in cytokinesis or in karyokinesis, although it is unknown whether this abnormality is a cause or a result of hepatitis in LEC rats.

Conclusions

The histopathological characteristics of the liver in LEC rats suffering from hepatitis include enlarged hepatocytes with huge nuclei. Flow cytometric analysis of the DNA content of nuclei from jaundiced LEC rats revealed the presence of very high polyploids, such as 32n and 64n; however, no aneuploidy was detected. At the age of 12 weeks, shortly before the onset of hepatitis, 8 n polyploid nuclei were more frequent in LEC rats than in LEA rats. Binucleated hepatocytes were also more frequent in LEC rats than in LEA rats at the age of 4 and 8 weeks. Bi-, tri- and tetranucleated cells, whose nuclei occasionally differed in size, were observed after the manifestation of hepatitis. The number of proliferating liver cells, as determined by pulse labeling with 5-bromo-2'-deoxyuridine (BrdU), was higher in LEC rats prior to the development of hepatitis than in LEA rats. A remarkable increase of BrdU uptake was observed when jaundice developed. The possible involvement of abnormal cytokinesis and karyokinesis in the manifestation of hepatitis was suggested.

References

1. Fujimoto Y, Oyamada M, Hattori A, Takahashi H, Sawaki M, Dempo K, Mori M, Nagao M (1989) Accumulation of abnormally high ploid nuclei in the liver of LEC rats developing spontaneous hepatitis. Jpn J Cancer Res 80:45–50
2. Fujimoto Y, Takahashi H, Dempo K, Mori M, Wirth PJ, Nagao M, Sugimura T (1989) Hereditary hepatitis in LEC rats: Accumulation of abnormally high ploid nuclei. Cancer Detect Prev 14:235–237
3. Sasaki M, Yoshida MC, Kagami K, Takeichi N, Kobayashi H, Dempo K, Mori M (1985) Spontaneous hepatitis in an inbred strain of Long-Evans rats. Rat News Lett 14:4–6

4. Yoshida MC, Masuda R, Sasaki M, Takeichi N, Kobayashi H, Dempo K, Mori M (1987) New mutation causing hereditary hepatitis in the laboratory rat. J. Hered 78:828–835
5. Berry MN, Friend DS (1969) High-yield preparation of isolated rat liver parenchymal cells. J Cell Biol 43:506–520
6. Vindelof LL, Christensen IJ, Nissen NI (1983) A detergent-trypsin method for the preparation of nuclei for flow cytometric DNA analysis. Cytometry 3: 323–327
7. Roszell JA, Fredi JL, Irving CC (1978) The development of polyploidy in two classes of rat liver nuclei. Biochim Biophys Acta 519:306–316
8. Wiest L (1972) The effect of diethylnitrosamine on the distribution of cell classes in the parenchyma of the liver of newborn rats. Eur J Cancer 8:121–125
9. Brodsky WY, Uryvaeva IV (1977) Cell polyploidy: Its relation to tissue growth and function. Int Rev Cytol 50:275–332
10. LeBouton AV (1976) DNA synthesis and cell proliferation in the simple liver acinus of 10- to 20-day-old rats: Evidence for cell fusion. Anat Rec 184: 679–688

9 — Sensitivity of LEC Rats to the Hepatotoxic Effects of D-Galactosamine

HIDETOSHI TAKAHASHI, KATSUHIKO ENOMOTO, HIROFUMI SAKAMOTO, HIROTOSHI TOBIOKA, KIMIMARO DEMPO, and MICHIO MORI[1]

Introduction

Spontaneous hepatitis in the LEC rat is characterized by hyperbilirubinemia, increased levels of serum glutamic-oxaloacetic transaminase (GOT) and glutamic pyruvic transaminase (GPT) in laboratory examination and spotty coagulative necrosis of single hepatocyte without inflammatory cell response [1,2]. Although a single autosomal recessive gene (hts) has been shown to be responsible for the hepatitis, the mechanism(s) of hepatocyte necrosis in the LEC rat remains obscure. The histological features of the liver reveal a certain resemblance between the hepatitis of LEC rats and the liver necrosis induced by the administration of D-galactosamine (GalN).

Therefore, in this paper, we examined the hepatotoxic effects of GalN on the liver of the LEC rat before the onset of "spontaneous hepatitis", in order to obtain some clues for understanding the mechanisms of liver injury in the LEC rat. Several chemicals which are known to affect the liver through different mechanisms were also given to the animals to compare the sensitivity of LEC rats to each chemical.

Sensitivity of LEC Rats to D-Galactosamine

Eight-week-old male and female LEC rats (LEC/smc, F_{11}) were used in this study. LEA rats, which are also derived from the Long-Evans strain but do not show any hepatic disorder, were used as control. D(+)-GalN hydrochloride (Tokyo Kasei Chemicals) was administered intraperitonealy (i.p.) to the rats at dosages of 200, 400, or 800 mg/kg body weight. The rats were sacrificed with ether anesthesia at 24 h after injection, and blood samples were collected.

---

[1] Department of Pathology, Sapporo Medical College, Sapporo, 060 Japan

Table 1. Serum GOT and GPT after administration of GalN.

	Dose (mg/kg)	Strain	GOT (U)	GPT (U)
Male				
	200	LEC	143.4 ± 89.6	88.0 ± 70.5
		LEA	103.0 ± 50.1	51.5 ± 5.3
	400	LEC	459.3 ± 70.6	412.0 ± 79.2
		LEA	152.5 ± 80.4	85.5 ± 55.5
	800	LEC	874.5 ± 125.9	976.0 ± 149.7
		LEA	329.5 ± 146.4	253.3 ± 131.4
Female				
	200	LEC	142.0 ± 79.9	73.0 ± 59.2
		LEA	132.7 ± 11.7	53.0 ± 4.7
	400	LEC	162.5 ± 15.2	88.5 ± 9.6
		LEA	152.5 ± 3.9	60.0 ± 4.1
	800	LEC	325.3 ± 75.3	242.7 ± 47.8
		LEA	250.3 ± 12.4	135.7 ± 9.2

Values represent means ± SD

Levels of serum GOT and GPT in male LEC rats administered with GalN were significantly higher than those in male LEA rats, and increased in a dose-dependent manner (Table 1). Female rats were less sensitive to GalN than the male in both strains, and showed a significantly higher level of serum GPT only with a higher dose of GalN treatment.

Corresponding to the increase in the level of serum GOT and GPT, damaging histological changes to the liver, such as coagulative necrosis of hepatocytes and microgranulations, were seen in every male LEC rat treated with GalN, whereas in female LEC rats these changes appeared only at the higher doses of GalN treatment.

These results clearly showed that LEC rats are sensitive to the hepato-toxic effects of GalN. Liver injury by GalN is considered to be caused by the metabololite of the chemical. Decker and Keppler [3] reported that the mechanisms of liver damages by GalN are as follows. In i.p.-injected rats, GalN is taken up predominantly by the liver and phosphatized by the enzymes of the galactose pathway (galactokinase). Since GalN-1-phosphatase synthesis from GalN by galactokinase competes with glucose-1-phosphatase synthesis in the galactose pathway, this phosphatizing reaction inhibits the UDGP-pyrophosphorylase reaction which forms UDP-hexose from glucose, and subsequently inhibits RNA synthesis. The nucleolar segregation frequently observed electron microscopically in the nuclei of hepatocytes after GalN is thought to be a morphological counterpart of impaired RNA synthesis [4]. The appreciable reduction of glucoprotein synthesis causes necrosis of hepatocytes. It is interesting to note that identical nucleolar segregation and an increase in the number of interchromatin granules were frequently seen in the hepatocytes of 2-month-old LEC rats

Table 2. Sequential changes of serum GOT and GPT after administration of 800 mg/kg GalN.

Strain	Days after administration	GOT (U)	GPT (U)
LEC	0	96.0 ± 15.3	43.7 ± 3.9
	0.5	91.8 ± 4.1	38.5 ± 2.5
	1	874.5 ± 125.9	976.0 ± 149.7
	2	988.0 ± 46.0	989.5 ± 0.5
	4	222.0 ± 114.0	155.5 ± 85.5
	7	143.5 ± 11.5	115.0 ± 13.0
LEA	0	121.5 ± 15.5	56.0 ± 24.0
	0.5	509.0 ± 71.0	390.0 ± 64.0
	1	329.5 ± 146.4	253.3 ± 131.4
	2	270.0 ± 69.0	170.5 ± 0.5
	4	130.0 ± 5.0	57.0 ± 2.0
	7	148.0 ± 1.2	67.0 ± 13.0

Values represent means ±SD

before the onset of hepatitis without GalN treatment [5]. The sex difference in the response to GalN toxicity was not clarified. It may be related to the phenomenon of early occurrence of hereditary hepatitis in male LEC rats (male, 18.1-weeks-old; female, 18.8-weeks-old; average of F_1-F_7 generation; Division of Animal Experimentation in Sapporo Medical College, unpublished data).

In order to investigate sequential changes of the liver after GalN treatment, male LEC rats before the onset of hepatitis and age-matched LEA rats were injected i.p. with 800 mg/kg GalN and sacrificed at 12 h and 1, 2, 4, and 7 days thereafter. Serum GOT and GPT, and the histology of livers were examined as described above. Levels of serum GOT and GPT in LEA rats displayed a peak at 12 h after injection, whereas those in LEC rats reached a higher peak at 2 days after administration (Table 2). A large number of foci of coagulative necrosis of hepatocytes (Fig. 1a) were seen in the liver of LEC rats at 2 days after GalN injection. The appearance of megalocytic changes of hepatocytes with huge nuclei, as seen in the liver of LEC rats with hereditary hepatitis, was also observed. Single-cell necrosis of hepatocytes was still observed at 7 days after injection. Small regenerative hepatocytes intermingled with proliferated oval cells were seen in the periportal areas (Fig. 1b). On the other hand, the coagulative necrosis of hepatocytes was seen in LEA rats until 2 days after injection, and the lesions were completely recovered by 7 days after GalN administration. It was shown that the liver injury of LEC rats with GalN occurs slowly, but becomes more severe than that of LEA rats.

It was recently reported that cell death by GalN treatment is mediated by the activated complement system stimulated by endotoxin [6,7]. Levels of serum endotoxin in male LEC and LEA rats at 6 h and 1, 2, and 3 days

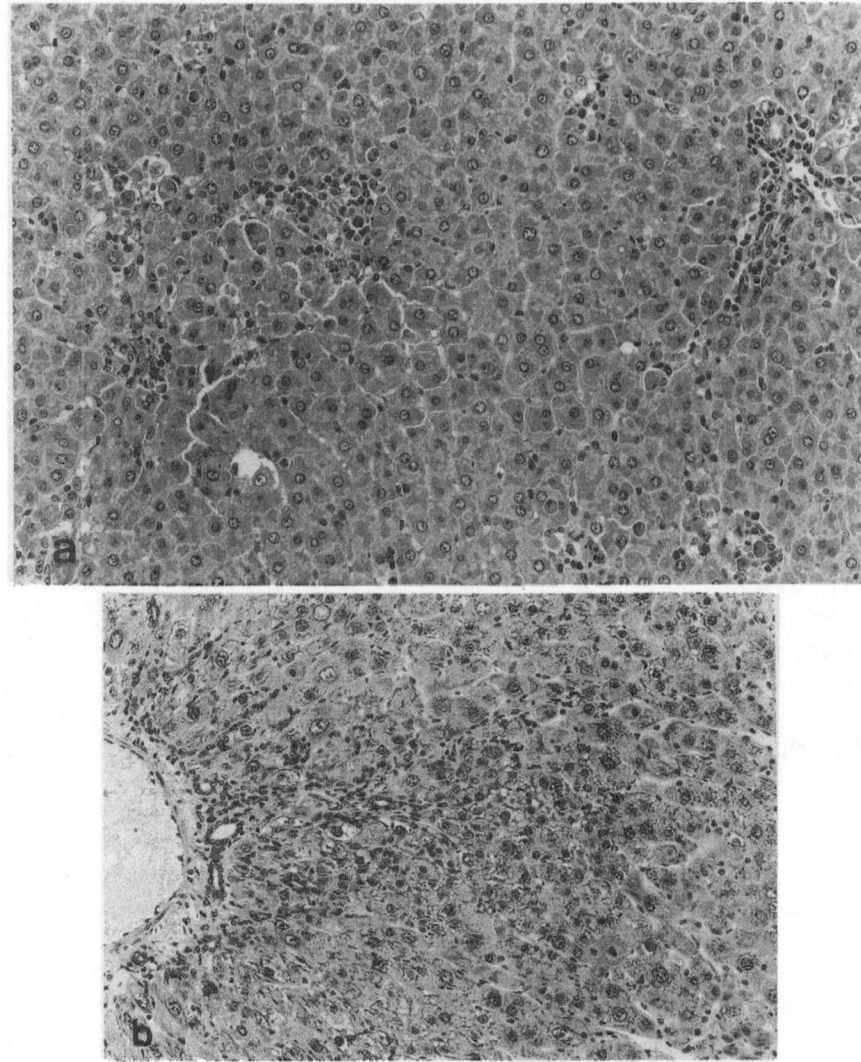

Fig. 1. Histological changes of the liver of LEC rats **a** 2 days and **b** 7 days after i.p. injection of 800 mg/kg D-galactosamine. H and E staining, × 235

after i.p. administration of 800 mg/kg GalN are shown in Table 3. LEC rats treated with GalN showed higher serum endotoxin than LEA rats. In LEC rats, serum endotoxin reached the highest level at 3 days after administration of GalN, whereas the endotoxin level in LEA rats reached a peak at 12 h and decreased thereafter. Thus, it is clear that the level of serum endotoxin fluctuated roughly in parallel with liver injury due to GalN, and rose in advance of the appearance of tissue damage. Therefore, serum lipopolysaccharide (endotoxin) may play a role in the GalN-induced liver

Table 3. Changes of serum endotoxin levels after administration of 800 mg/kg GalN.

Time (h)	LEC	LEA
0	15.33 ± 11.47	23.97 ± 9.64
6	28.30 ± 16.85	173.40 ± 78.45
12	89.72 ± 25.76	178.78 ± 79.39
24	160.82 ± 62.71	162.30 ± 59.28
48	144.14 ± 56.06	27.32 ± 12.66
72	212.20 ± 96.50	14.34 ± 5.40

Values represent mean (pg/ml) ±SD

necrosis of LEC rats, in addition to the direct effects of GalN. This suggests a possible relevance of lipopolysaccharides to the occurrence of fulminant hepatitis in LEC rats.

The mechanism(s) of such a high sensitivity to the hepatotoxic effects of GalN in the LEC rats is not known. However, it was recently shown that the LEC rat liver is already low in the activities of alpha- and beta-forms of S-adenosylmethionine synthetase at birth [8]. The activities were shown to decrease with age to one-half the level at the time of the manifestation of hepatitis, whereas the activity of glycine- and tRNA-methyltransferases in the liver remains normal. Since the decrease in hypomethylation of ribosomal RNA is followed by defects in protein synthesis, it seems reasonable to consider that the hypomethylation of ribosomal RNA is responsible for both the development of "spontaneous hepatitis" in LEC rats and for the high sensitivity of the rat to GalN, which induces further hypomethylation of ribosomal RNA.

Effects of Diethylnitrosamine, Carbon Tetrachloride, and Allyl Alcohol on the Development of Liver Necrosis in LEC Rats

LEC and LEA rats were administered i.p. diethylnitrosamine (DEN, Sigma, 25 or 100 mg/kg), or carbon tetrachloride (CCl$_4$, Kishida Chemical, 1 or 2 ml/kg), after which the rats were sacrificed with ether anesthesia at 24 h after injection. In the case of allyl alcohol administration (AA, Tokyo Kasei Chemicals, 0.5 or 1.0 mmol/kg), rats were sacrificed at 3 h after injection. Metabolic activation of these toxins has been known to depend upon P-450 activity [9,10]. Blood samples were collected from each rat at the time of sacrifice. The serum was separated and the activities of GOT and GPT were measured. The liver sections obtained from rats were fixed with Carnoy's solution for staining with hematoxylin and eosin (H and E).

Serum GOT and GPT levels of LEC rats administered with either 25 or 100 mg/kg DEN were slightly higher than those of LEA rats of either sex

Table 4. Serum GOT and GPT after administration of DEN.

Dose (mg/kg)	Strain	GOT (U)	GPT (U)
Male			
25	LEC	125.0 ± 24.6	81.0 ± 20.7
	LEA	131.3 ± 11.1	68.3 ± 2.9
100	LEC	184.0 ± 24.8	162.5 ± 54.0
	LEA	153.0 ± 9.0	102.0 ± 2.0
Female			
25	LEC	167.0 ± 25.1	195.0 ± 34.9
	LEA	102.7 ± 4.0	48.7 ± 4.6
100	LEC	134.7 ± 10.2	109.0 ± 14.2
	LEA	113.5 ± 3.5	71.5 ± 5.5

Values represent means ±SD

Table 5. Serum GOT and GPT after administration of CCl$_4$.

Dose (ml/kg)	Strain	GOT (U)	GPT (U)
Male			
1	LEC	362.7 ± 86.0	658.3 ± 222.3
	LEA	717.8 ± 162.1	520.5 ± 438.2
2	LEC	319.7 ± 66.3	449.5 ± 146.6
	LEA	720.0 ± 177.5	465.0 ± 238.6
Female			
1	LEC	375.0 ± 46.4	602.3 ± 165.8
	LEA	642.7 ± 171.4	283.7 ± 77.5
2	LEC	363.5 ± 106.6	465.0 ± 238.6
	LEA	795.0 ± 199.0	412.0 ± 135.0

Values represent means ±SD

Table 6. Serum GOT and GPT after administration of allyl alcohol.

Dose (mmol/kg)	Strain	GOT (U)	GPT (U)
Male			
0.5	LEC	152.7 ± 11.3	39.7 ± 2.9
	LEA	136.5 ± 5.5	29.5 ± 2.5
1	LEC	415.5 ± 128.2	154.5 ± 35.2
	LEA	1035.3 ± 110.3	607.7 ± 177.4
Female			
0.5	LEC	120.3 ± 12.8	39.6 ± 2.9
	LEA	136.5 ± 5.5	36.0 ± 2.2
1	LEC	671.0 ± 214.5	213.7 ± 191.0
	LEA	1043.0 ± 36.0	679.0 ± 121.0

Values represent means ±SD

(Table 4). Histologically, microgranulation was seen in the livers of both LEC and LEA rats, but no differences between the two strains were revealed.

Serum GOT levels in the CCl_4-administered LEA rats were significantly higher than those in LEC rats, but serum GPT did not show a constant value in either strain (Table 5). Histologically, central necroses in the livers of LEC rats were clearly stronger than those of LEA rats caused by CCl_4.

Serum GOT and GPT levels of LEA rats administered AA, either 0.5 or 1 mmol/kg, were significantly higher than those of LEC rats (Table 6). Histologically, damage to periportal hepatocytes was more prominent in LEA rats than in LEC rats.

In this study, we found that LEC rats were less sensitive to CCl_4 and AA compared to LEA rats. An extreme decrease of cytochrome P-450 content was reported in the LEC rat liver before the onset of hepatitis [11]. Our data, showing a decreased sensitivity of LEC rats to CCl_4 and AA, may be due to the low cytochrome P-450 content.

Although the pathogenesis of hereditary hepatitis is still not clear, the LEC rat strain is a useful model for the study of liver injury. Therefore, it is necessary to clarify the characteristics of the animals' drug sensitivity to understand the mechanisms of liver injury.

Acknowledgements. The authors are grateful to Ms. K. Kagami and Ms. N. Kawano for their careful breeding of the rats, and to Ms. T. Matsui, Ms. M. Kamada, and Ms. M. Kinoshita for technical assistance. This work was supported in part by a Grant-in Aid for Scientific Research (63480145) from the Ministry of Education, Science and Culture, Japan, and grants from the Princess Takamatsu Cancer Research Fund and the Uehara Memorial Foundation, Japan.

References

1. Yoshida MC, Masuda R, Sasaki M, Takeichi N, Kobayashi H, Dempo K, Mori M (1987) New mutation causing hereditary hepatitis in the laboratory rat. J Hered 78:361–365
2. Dempo K, Oyamada M, Fujimoto Y, Takahashi H, Satoh M, Hattori A, Mori M, Masuda R, Yoshida MC (1988) Pathological changes of the liver in LEC rats with hereditary hepatitis. J Toxicol Pathol 1:53–60
3. Decker K, Keppler D (1974) Galactosamine hepatitis: Key role for the nucleotide deficiency period in the pathogenesis of cell injury and cell death. Rev Physiol Biochem Pharmacol 71:77–106
4. Shinozuka H, Martin JT, Farber JL (1973) The induction of fibrillar nucleoli in rat liver cells by D-galactosamine and their subsequent re-formation into normal nucleoli. J Ultrastruct Mol Struct Res 44:279–292

5. Minase T, Piao Z, Takahashi H, Hattori A, Mori M, Yokoyama S (1989) Ultrastructural changes of the liver in LEC rats with hereditary hepatitis. J Clin Electron Microscopy 22:5–6
6. Liehr H, Grun M, Seelig HP, Seelig R, Reutter W, Heine WD (1978) On the pathogenesis of galactosamine hepatitis. Indication of extrahepatocellular mechanisms responsible for liver cell death. Virchows Arch [B] 26:331–344
7. Freudenberg MA, Keppler D, Galanos C (1986) Requirement for lipopolysac-charide-resposive macrophages in galactosamine-induced sensitization to endotoxin. Infect Immun 51:891–895
8. Shimizu K, Abe M, Yokoyama S, Takahashi H, Sawada N, Mori M, Tsukada K (1990) Decreased activities of S-adenosylmethionine synthetase isozymes in hereditary hepatitis in Long-Evans rats. Life Sci 46:1837–1842
9. Zimmerman HJ (1978) Indirect hepatotoxins. In: Hepatotoxicity, the adverse effects of drugs and other chemicals on the liver. Appleton-Century-Crofts, New York
10. Rees KR, Tarlow MJ (1967) The hepatotoxic action of allyl formate. Biochem J 104:757–761
11. Sugiyama T, Takeichi N, Kobayashi H, Yoshida MC, Sasaki M, Taniguchi N (1988) Metabolic predisposition of a novel mutant (LEC rats) to hereditary hepatitis and hepatoma: Alterations of the drug metabolizing enzymes. Carcinogenesis 9:1569–1572

10 — Consecutive Follow-up Study of the Liver of LEC Rats Before the Onset of Spontaneous Hepatitis

HIROFUMI SAKAMOTO, YASUHIRO KAMIMURA, TAKASHI MINASE,
SHIGEAKI YOKOYAMA, MASAAKI SATOH, and MICHIO MORI[1]

Introduction

Although the pathological changes in the liver of LEC rats after the onset of hepatitis are well established, the natural history of LEC rats before the manifestation of jaundice remains unresolved. Before the onset of hepatitis, the LEC rat is normal, at least as far as liver function tests are concerned. However, there are some reports that describe the presence of pathological changes in the liver of LEC rats before the onset of hepatitis, i.e., the appearance of abnormally high ploidy nuclei [1] and nuclear enlargement [2] in hepatocytes. Since these findings from different individual rats tend to be somewhat fragmentary, it seems worthy to assess whether such pathological findings are observed consistently in the liver of the same LEC rat throughout its life course before the onset of hepatitis. Therefore in this study, we designed a prospective follow-up study of the liver of LEC rats using consecutive needle biopsies. Much attention was placed on the ultrastructural changes in the nuclei in light of the abnormalities in the ploidy and nuclear size which have previously been reported.

Pathological Findings of Liver of LEC Rats Before the Onset of Hepatitis

Histological examination of liver specimens obtained by needle biopsies revealed no abnormalities at 5 weeks after birth (Fig. 1). On the other hand, at 9 weeks after birth, a few hepatocytes were necrotic and small areas of microgranulation were recognized (Fig. 2). At 19 weeks after birth, just before the manifestation of jaundice, the variation in the size of the nuclei of hepatocytes was remarkable (Fig. 3).

Electron microscopy, in contrast, already recognized vague abnormalities in the liver of LEC rats at 5 weeks after birth. Some nuclei of the LEC rat

---

[1] Department of Pathology, Sapporo Medical College, Sapporo, 060 Japan

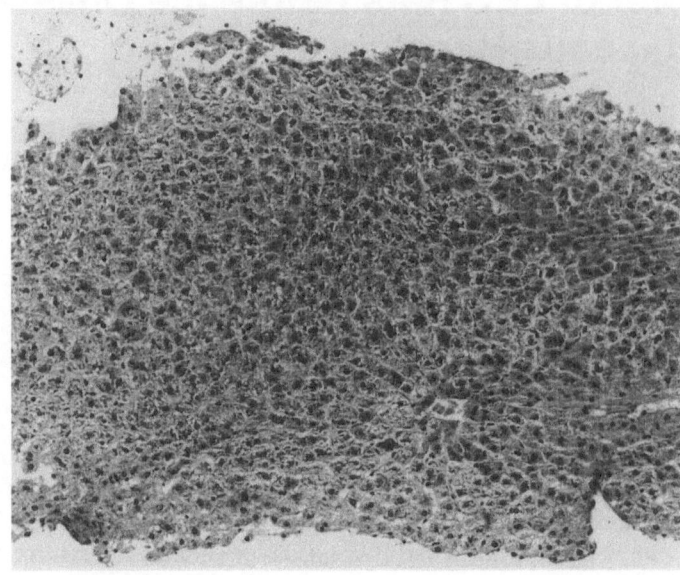

Fig. 1. A liver biopsy specimen from an LEC rat at 5 weeks of age. No abnormal findings are observed, H and E stain, × 100

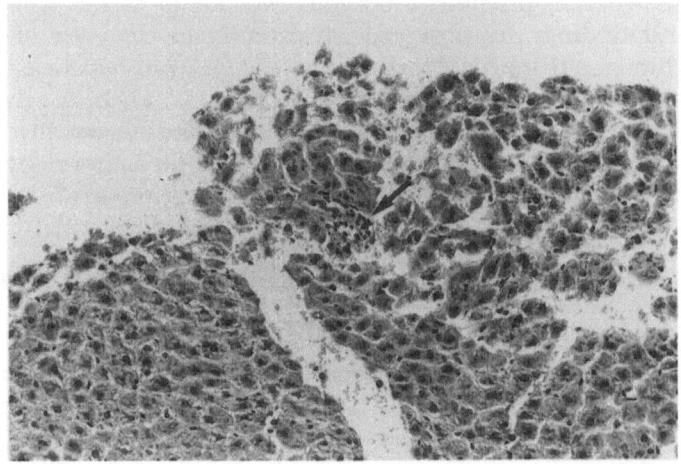

Fig. 2. A liver biopsy specimen from an LEC rat at 9 weeks of age. The *arrow* shows microgranulation, H and E stain, × 200

hepatocyte at this age showed scattered and decreased heterochromatin granules with nucleolar segregation. The segregated nucleoli were small in size because the granular component of the nucleoli was obscured and reduced in size. Contrarily, the fibrillar component was aggregated and

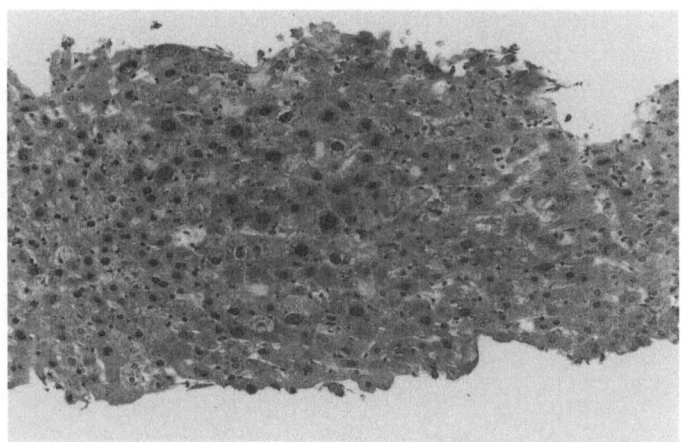

Fig. 3. A liver biopsy specimen from an LEC rat at 19 weeks of age. The variety of size of the nuclei is remarkable, H and E stain, × 200

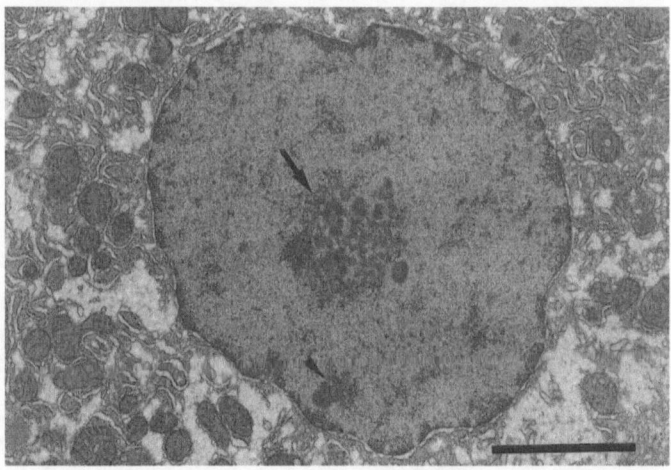

Fig. 4. A hepatocyte nucleus of the LEC rat at 5 weeks of age, before the onset of hepatitis. The nucleus is irregular in shape with scattered and decreased hetero-chromatin granules. The nucleolus near the nuclear envelope shows nucleolar segregation (*arrowhead*), but the one in the middle shows normal architecture (*arrow*). *Bar*, 3 μm

compact [3] (Figs. 4, 5). Such a segregation of the nucleoli, called "macro-segregation" [4], was consistently observed in the liver of the same LEC rat by consecutive biopsies before the onset of hepatitis, although the degree of segregation varied from cell to cell (Figs. 6–8). Segregation of the nucleoli is shown to occur in rat hepatocytes in a variety of conditions, such as (1) the administration of certain antibiotics, such as actinomycin D [5] and

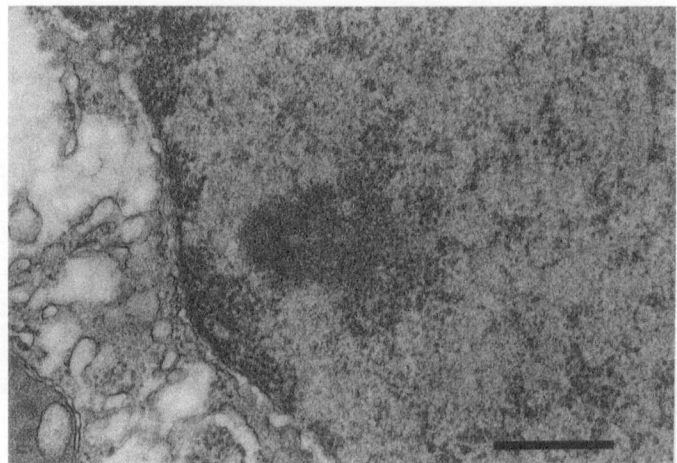

Fig. 5. A higher magnification of the nucleolus shown in Fig. 4, revealing nucleolar segregation. *Bar*, 0.5 μm

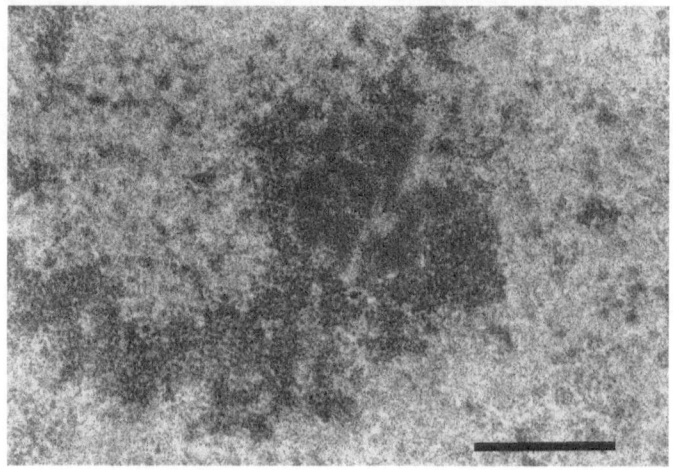

Fig. 6. A portion of hepatocyte nucleus of the LEC rat at 9 weeks of age. Aggregation of the fibrillar components of the nucleoli is prominent. *Bar*, 0.5 μm

adriamycin [6], which are known to impair the synthesis of ribosomal RNA, (2) the administration of alkilating agents [7], which are also known to inhibit ribosomal RNA synthesis, (3) infection with herpes viruses [8], and (4) neoplasia. However, thus far, viral infection and chemical administration were absent in these LEC rats, suggesting that the impairment of ribosomal RNA occurs constantly in the hepatocytes of LEC rats long before the onset of hepatitis. Recently, the activities of *S*-

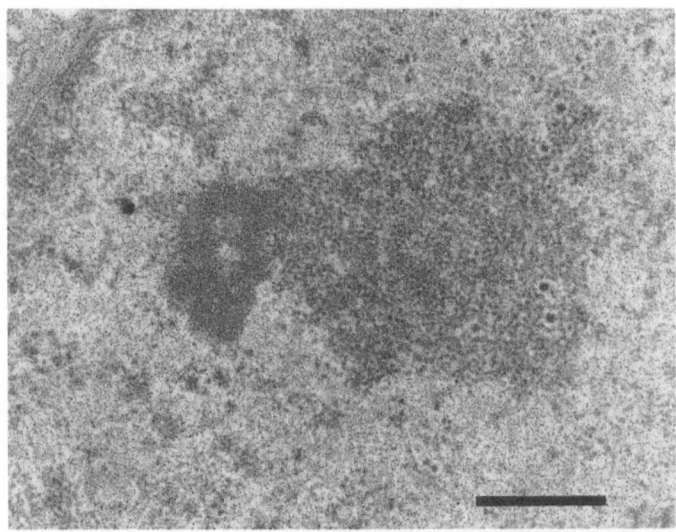

Fig. 7. A portion of hepatocyte nucleus of the LEC rat at 13 weeks of age. Aggregation of the fibrillar components of the nucleolus is dominant. *Bar*, 0.5 µm

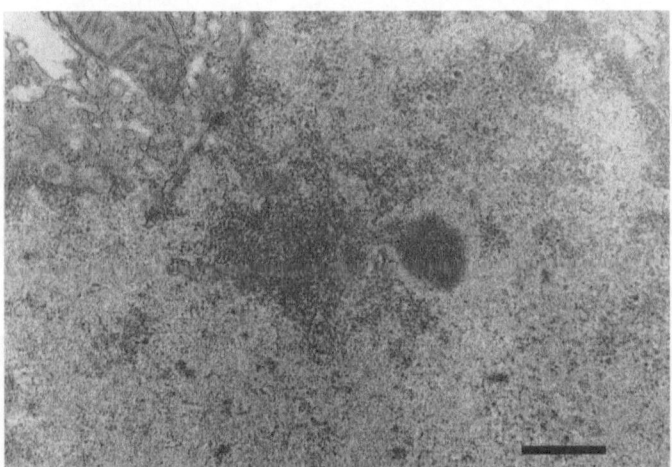

Fig. 8. A portion of hepatocyte nucleus of the LEC rat at 17 weeks of age. Separation of the fibrillar components of the nucleolus from granular components is seen. *Bar*, 0.5 µm

adenosylmethionine (AdoMet) synthetase isoforms in the LEC rat liver were shown to be low at birth. The activity of AdoMet synthetase progressively decreased with time to the level of one-half at the onset of hepatitis [9]. Since segregation of the nucleoli was induced in hepatocytes by the administration of D-galactosamine [10] which is known to cause

100   H. Sakamoto et al.

hypomethylation of ribosomal RNA [11], it seems reasonable to consider that the disturbance in methylation of ribosomal RNA due to decreased activities of AdoMet synthetase isoforms might be responsible for the development of nucleolar segregation in the LEC rat.

On the other hand, argyrophilic nucleolar organizer regions (AgNOR) are ribosomal DNA loops which have recently been shown to correlate with the transcriptional activity of the ribosomal RNA gene [12]. The number of AgNOR per hepatocyte nucleus measured in the biopsy specimens of the liver of our subjects revealed significant increases of these regions in the hepatocytes of the LEC rat before the onset of hepatitis. The increase in the number of AgNOR corresponded well to the development of nucleolar segregation. Taken together, these findings suggest the possibility that the synthesis of ribosomal RNA is impaired, whereas the transcription of ribosomal DNA is increased in the nucleoli of LEC rat hepatocytes.

In addition to the changes in the organization of the nucleoli, irregularity of the shape of the nuclei, appearance of nuclear pseudoinclusions, and an increase in the number of interchromatin granules were observed in the hepatocytes of the LEC rat before the manifestation of hepatitis [13], although the significance of these findings was not elucidated.

In the cytoplasm, proliferation of the smooth endoplasmic reticulum (SER) around the bile canaliculi was noted [13] (Fig. 9). Proliferation of the SER is a morphologic clue to a toxic reaction [14]. Administration of certain hepatotoxic chemicals, such as carcinogenic 3'-methyl-4-dimethylaminoazobenzen, aflatoxin B_1, and tannic acid, is known to induce both the nucleolar segregation and proliferation of the SER in hepatocytes [15]. Therefore, it is likely that LEC rats are already exposed to some hepatotoxic agents before the clinical and laboratory manifestation

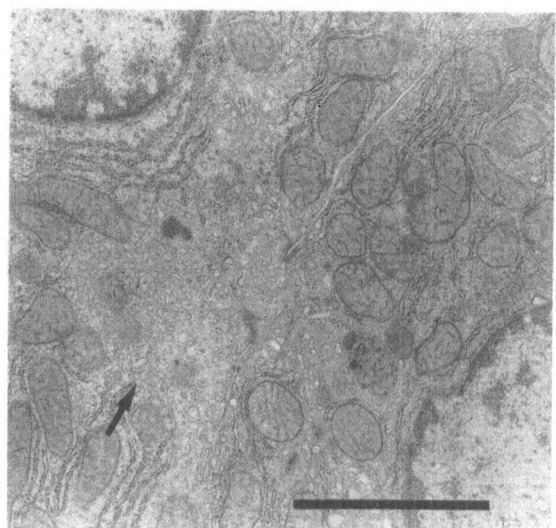

Fig. 9. Hepatocyte of the LEC rat at 15 weeks of age, before the onset of hepatitis. Significant proliferation of the SER (*arrow*) is observed around the bile canaliculus, whereas the rest of the ultrastructure is normal. *Bar*, 3 μm

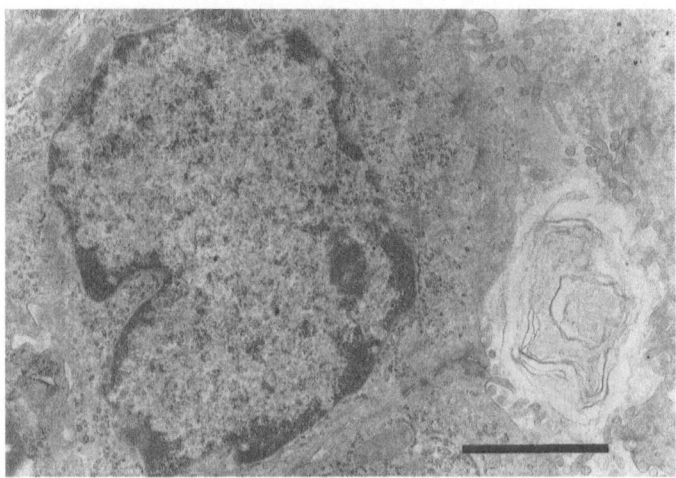

Fig. 10. Hepatocyte of the LEC rat at 23 weeks of age, the time of manifestation of jaundice. The nucleus is irregular in outline and the distended bile canalicular lumen is filled with a myelin-like substance. Cytoplasmic organelles are reduced in number and detachment of ribosomes from the ER is observed. *Bar*, 3 μm

of hepatitis. It was recently disclosed by Li et al. that an abnormal accumulation of copper takes place in the liver of LEC rats soon after birth [16]. The content of copper is reported to increase up to 40 times higher than normal levels at about 5 months of age, when the "spontaneous" hepatitis is manifested. It remains unresolved whether or not the changes in the nucleoli we observed in the livers of LEC rats directly reflect the accumulation of copper, but it was observed that the nuclear changes in the hepatocytes of LEC rats showed a tendency to increase with the development of manifested hepatitis (Fig. 10).

Conclusions

Sequential studies of the livers of LEC rats before the onset of hepatitis, using consecutive needle biopsies of the same animal with an average interval of 2 weeks revealed the following findings: (1) pathological changes of the liver at the ultrastructural level are already present at 5 weeks of age, suggesting that abnormalities in LEC rats begin before the onset of hepatitis, (2) segregation of the nucleoli is the most prominent pathological change in the hepatocytes of LEC rats before the onset of hepatitis, indicating that the impaired processing of ribosomal RNA in the nucleus may be responsible for the development of hepatitis, and (3) pathological changes of the liver progress with time toward the manifestation of hepatitis, suggesting that some hepatotoxic substance(s) may accumulate in the liver of LEC rats.

Acknowledgments. This work was supported in part by Grants-in-Aid from the Ministry of Education, Science and Culture, Japan, from Scientific Research (01304038), and by a Grant-in-Aid from the Ono Cancer Research Foundation.

References

1. Fujimoto Y, Oyamada M, Hattori A, Takahashi H, Satoh M, Dempo K, Mori M, Masuda R (1988) DNA analysis of megalocytic hepatocytes in LEC rats. Jpn Acta Hepatol 29:967–968
2. Dempo K, Oyamada M, Fujimoto Y, Takahashi H, Satoh M, Hattori A, Mori M (1988) Pathological changes of the liver in LEC rats with hereditary hepatitis. J Toxicol Pathol 1:53–60
3. Sakamoto H, Kamimura Y, Takahashi H, Nagai H, Yamaguchi T, Inaoka K, Minase T, Mori M (to be published) Sequential ultrastructural observations of the liver of LEC rats before the onset of hereditary hepatitis. J Clin Electron Microscopy 23
4. Zimmerman HJ (1978) Hepatotoxicity. In: Lesions seen by electron microscopy. Appleton-Century-Crofts, New York pp 80–84
5. De Man JCH, Noorduyn NJ (1967) Light and electron microscopic radioautography of hepatic cell nucleoli in mice treated with actinomycin D. J Cell Biol 33:489–496
6. Merski JA, Daskal I, Busch H (1976) Effects of adriamycin on ultrastructure of nucleoli in the heart and liver cells of rat. Cancer Res 36:1580–1584
7. Lantos PL (1971) The effect of a single dose of N-ethyl-N-nitrosourea in the fine structure of the brain of the rat. Experientia 27:1322–1321
8. Sirtori C, Bosisio M (1966) Oncolysis by Herpes simplex. Lancet I:96
9. Shimizu K, Abe M, Yokoyama S, Takahashi H, Sawada N, Mori M, Tsukada K (1990) Decreased activities of S-adenosylmethionine synthetase isozymes in hereditary hepatitis in Long-Evans rats. Life Sci 46:1837–1840
10. Dimova RN, Gajdardjieva KC, Dabeva MD, Hadjiolov AA (1979) Early effects of D-galactosamine on rat liver nucleolar structures. Biol Cell 35:1–10
11. Clawson GA, Sesno J, Milam K, Wang Y-F, Gabriel C (1990) The hepatocyte protein synthesis defect induced by galactosamine involves hypomethylation of ribosomal RNA. Hepatology 11:428–434
12. Howat AJ, Cotton DWK, Slater DN (1989) Nucleolar organizer regions in spitz nevi and malignant melanomas. Cancer 63:474–478
13. Minase T, Piao Zhe-Si, Takahashi H, Hattori A, Mori M, Yokoyama S (1989) Ultrastructural changes of the liver in LEC rats with hereditary hepatitis. J Clin Electron Microscopy 22:783–784
14. Schaffner F, Popper H (1975) Electron microscopy in the liver. In: Shiff L (ed) Diseases of the liver, 4th edn. Lippincott, Philadelphia, pp 51–86
15. Svoboda D, Higginson J (1968) A comparison of ultrastructural changes in rat liver due to chemical carcinogens. Cancer Res 28:1703–1733
16. Li Y, Togashi Y, Sato S, Emoto T, Kang J-H, Takeichi N, Kobayashi H, Kojima Y, Une Y, Uchino J (to be published) Spontaneous hepatic copper accumulation in LEC rats with hereditary hepatitis: A model of Wilson's disease. J Clin Invest

11 — Acute Tubular Necrosis in LEC Rats with Hereditary Hepatic Failure — A New Animal Model of Hepatorenal Syndrome

Hiroyuki Tochimaru, Yasushi Akutsu, Yasushi Nagata, Yasuo Takekoshi, Shuzo Matsumoto[1], and Noritoshi Takeichi[2]

Introduction

It has been reported that LEC rats are a useful animal model for spontaneous fulminant hepatitis [1] and liver cell carcinoma [2]. At 16–20 weeks of age, 80%–90% of LEC rats spontaneously develop severe hepatic disease, but its etiopathogenesis has not yet been clarified. The clinical features of these LEC rats are marked jaundice, ascitis, subcutaneous bleeding, and oliguria, and their low urinary output suggests the presence of an accompanying renal lesion. In this paper, we present the laboratory data and histopathological findings in the liver and kidney of LEC rats — hepatocellular lipid degeneration and acute renal failure due to acute tubular necrosis — and suggest that LEC rats can serve as an animal model for human hepatorenal syndrome.

Materials and Methods

Rats

Seven LEC rats, aged 16–20 weeks, were sacrificed 3–7 days after the onset of jaundice. Three 30-week-old LEC rats with no overt liver disorders were examined as controls. All the animals had been fed and kept in metabolic cages for 24-h urine collection for 3 days.

Biochemical Analysis

Serum bilirubin was measured using a Suntest Kit (Sanko Pharmaceutical Co., Japan). Serum levels of glutamic oxaloacetic transaminase (GOT), glutamic pyruvic transaminase (GPT), and serum lactic dehydrogenese

[1] Department of Pediatrics, and [2] Laboratory of Pathology, Cancer Institute, School of Medicine, Hokkaido University, Sapporo, 060 Japan

(LDH) levels were measured. Blood urea nitrogen (BUN) was determined by the urease-glutamic acid dehydrogense method. Serum and urinary potassium levels were measured by the Folin-Wu method. Serum and urinary sodium levels were measured by flame spectrophotometry. Urinary albumin levels were determined by means of ELISA. Urinary N-acetyl-β-D-glucosaminidase (NAG) levels were measured by spectrophotometry.

Histological Examination

Light microscopy.

Liver and kidney tissues were fixed in 10% buffered formalin for observation by light microscopy and were processed routinely. The paraffin-embedded sections were stained with hematoxilin-eosin and periodic acid-Schiff stain. Sections of freshly frozen liver and kidney tissues were stained with Sudan III.

Electron microscopy.

Liver and kidney tissues were fixed in 2% glutaraldehyde and processed routinely for observation by electron microscopy. Epok-812 embedded ultrathin sections were stained with uranyl-acetate and lead-citrate and examined with a Hitachi H-800 electron microscope.

Statistical Analysis

All biochemical data are expressed as means ±SD. Statistical analysis was performed by means of t test. Statistical significance level was defined as $P < 0.05$.

Results and Discussion

Biochemical data (Tables 1, 2)

Tables 1 and 2 show the results of the biochemical data. In LEC rats with jaundice, serum total bilirubin concentrations were elevated (24.7 ± 5.6 mg/dl). Liver function studies revealed marked elevation of serum GOT (790.8 ± 250.6 K.U/l), GPT (229.3 ± 103.3 K.U/l), and LDH (2354.3 ± 353.5 Wrob.U/l) levels. BUN levels were also elevated (89.9 ± 13.5 mg/dl). Serum creatinine levels were normal (0.5 ± 0.1 mg/dl) in 4 rats, but were slightly elevated in 3 (0.9 ± 0.5 mg/dl). Urinary sodium excretion was low (4–10 mEq/l) in 5 of the 7 LEC rats with jaundice. The urinary NAG concentration was elevated (30.4 ± 5.8 U/l) in all of the jaundiced rats. Urinary alubumin excretion of the jaundiced rats was slightly elevated (206.5 ± 60.8 mg/dl).

Table 1. Serum biochemical data of LEC rats.

	T.BIL. (mg/dl)	GOT (K.U./l)	GPT (K.U./l)	LDH (Wrob.U./l)	BUN (mg/dl)	Creatinine (mg/dl)
Jaundiced LEC rats (n = 7)	24.7 ± 5.6	790.8 ± 250.6	229.3 ± 103.3	2354.3 ± 353.5	89.9 ± 13.5	0.9 ± 0.5
Non-jaundiced LEC rats (n = 3)	0.2 ± 0.1	210.1 ± 56.5	110.5 ± 35.9	1962.5 ± 453.7	25.0 ± 9.2	0.5 ± 0.2
	P < 0.001	P < 0.05	N.S.	N.S.	P<0.01	N.S.

N.S., no signicant difference

Table 2. Urinary biochemical data of LEC rats.

	Protein (mg/dl)	Creatinine (mg/dl)	Na (mEq/lℓ)	FENa	NAG (U/l)
Jaundiced LEC rats (n = 7)	206.5 ± 60.8	24.8 ± 5.3	19.2 ± 10.8	2.21 ± 0.59	30.4 ± 5.8
Non-jaundiced LEC rats (n = 3)	106.5 ± 24.8	10.9 ± 1.9	77.7 ± 18.6	11.12 ± 5.83	4.5 ± 2.8
	N.S.	N.S.	$P < 0.05$	$P < 0.01$	$P < 0.001$

N.S., no significant difference

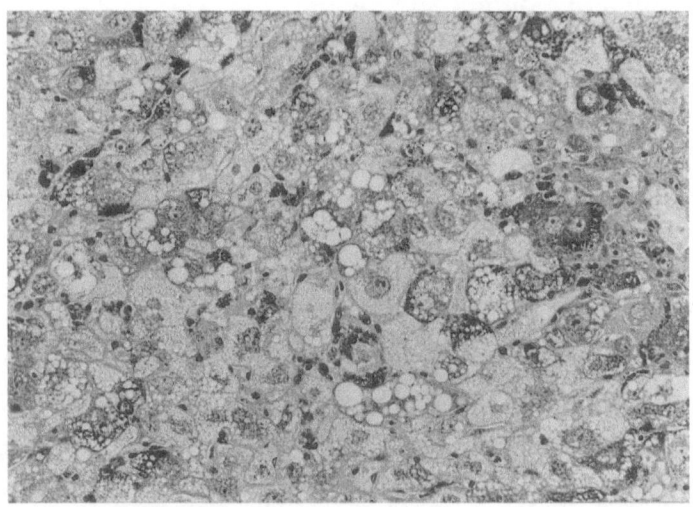

Fig. 1. Light micrograph of the liver of a 20-week-old LEC rat showing severe lipid degeneration of the heptocytes. PAS, × 200

These laboratory data show that LEC rats with jaundice developed severe renal failure as well as hepatic failure. The characteristic urinary finding was low sodium excretion, which has been reported to be one of the most important laboratory findings in patients with hepatorenal syndrome [3]. Elevated urinary NAG level is also a common laboratory finding among the jaundiced rats and patients with hepatoranal syndrome [3].

In contrast, although LEC rats without jaundice had elevated serum levels of GOT (210.1 ± 56.5 K.U/l) and LDH (1962.5 ± 245.8 Wrob.U/l), their renal function was within normal limits in terms of BUN (25.0 ± 3.8 mg/dl), serum creatinine (0.5 ± 0.3 mg/dl), and urinary concentration of NAG (4.5 ± 2.8 U/l). These data revealed that: (1) LEC rats without jaundice also exhibited hepatic dysfunction albeit milder than that seen in jaundiced LEC rats, but (2) they did not develop renal failure.

Histological Findings

Histological findings in the liver and kidney correlated well with the biochemical data. Light microscopy showed that one of the most characteristic features of the livers of LEC rats with jaundice was severe lipid degeneration of the hepatocytes with slight inflammatory cell infiltration (Fig. 1). Most of the hepatocytes were Sudan III-positive. Electron microscopy revealed the cytoplasma and nuclei of the hepatocytes to contain numerous small lipid droplets (Fig. 2). In LEC rats without jaundice, light micros-copy revealed the basic structure of liver to be well preserved, however, some hepatocytes had large nuclei (Fig. 3). Electron microscopy

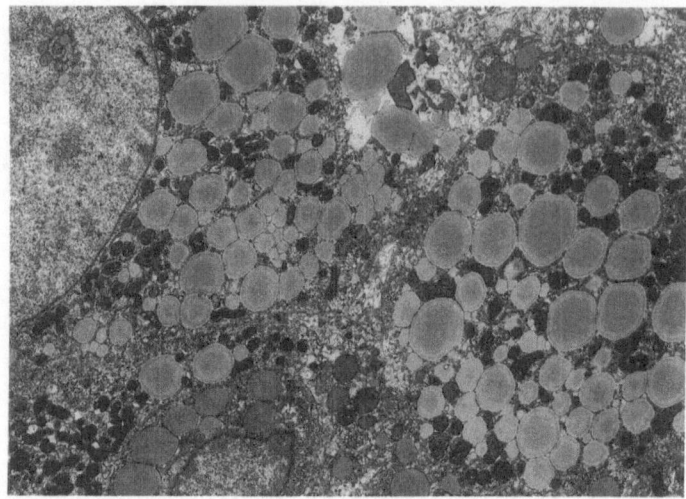

Fig. 2. Electron micrograph of the liver of a 20-week-old LEC rat showing numerous small lipid droplets in the cytoplasma as well as in the nuclei, ×3,000

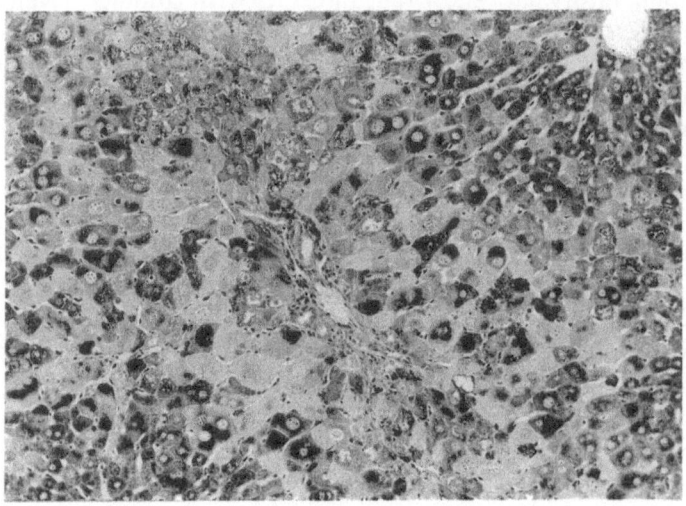

Fig. 3. Light micrograph of the liver of a 30-week-old LEC rat showing well-preserved hepatic acinar architecture. Some hepatocytes, however, have large nuclei with mild lipid degeneration. PAS, ×200

showed lipid degeneration of hepatocytes with mitochondrial vacuolization (Fig. 4).

We believe that the lipid degeneration seen in the liver is a finding closely associated with the pathogenesis of the liver disease observed in

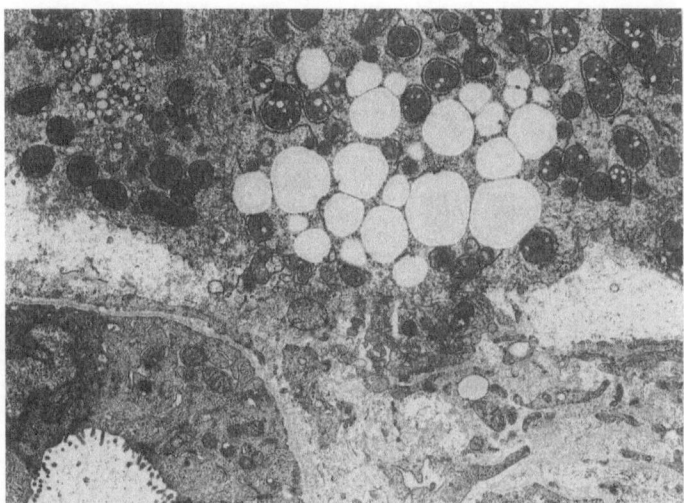

Fig. 4. Electron micrograph of the liver of a 30-week-old LEC rat showing hepatocytes with lipid droplets and vacuolated mitochondria, ×3,000

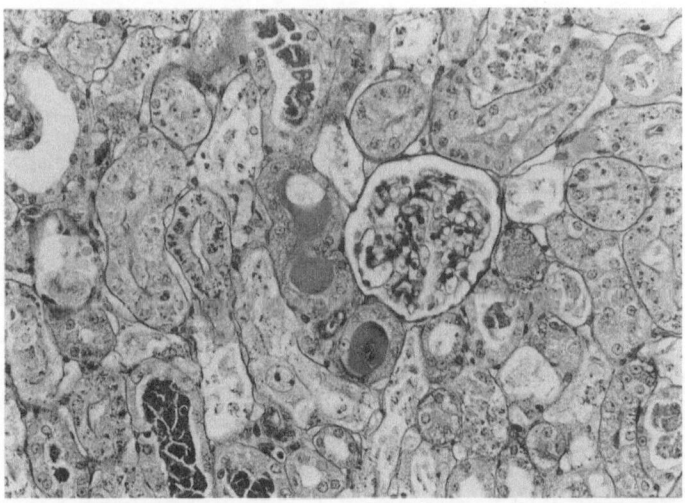

Fig. 5. Light micrograph of the kidney of a 20-week-old LEC rat showing acute tubular necrosis. In contrast, the glomerulus exhibits no proliferative changes nor capillary wall thickning. PAS, ×200

the LEC rat. In humans, certain metabolic disorders, such as tyrosinemia type I [4], lecithin-cholesterol acyltransferase deficiency [5], and Wilson's disease [6], are reported to involve the liver and kidney simultaneously. Masuda et al. [7] showed, on the basis of a crossbreeding study with other species, that development of liver disease is governed by a single gene and

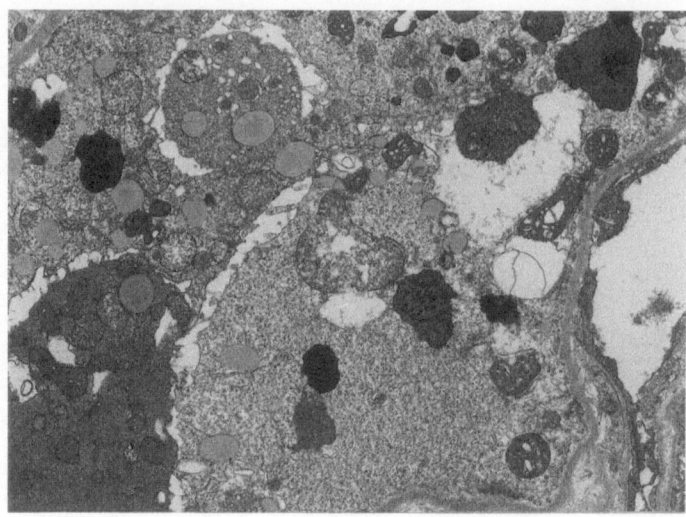

Fig. 6. Electron micrograph of the kidney of a 20-week-old LEC rat showing separation of a severely damaged tubular epithelial cell from tubular basement membrane, ×3,000

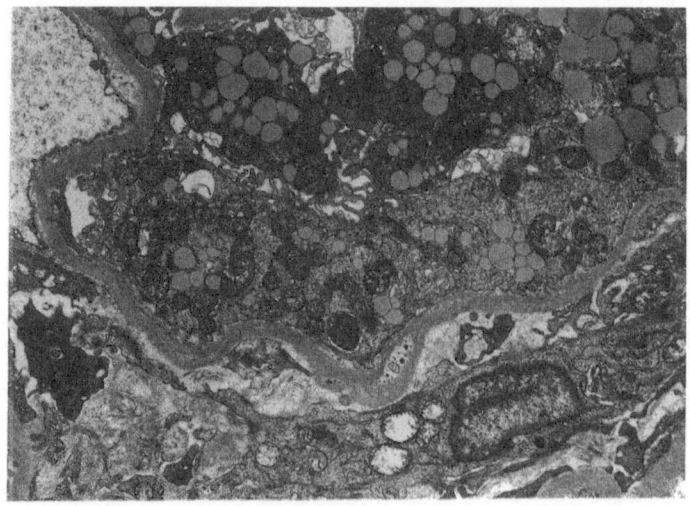

Fig. 7. Electron micrograph of the kidney of a 20-week-old LEC rat showing tubular epithelial cells containing lipid droplets similar to those seen in hepatocytes, ×3,000

is inherited as an autosomal recessive trait, suggesting that some metabolic disorders can cause liver disease in the LEC rat.

Severe tubular necrosis was observed in the kidney of LEC rats with jaundice (Fig. 5). Electron microscopy showed that tubular epithelial cells

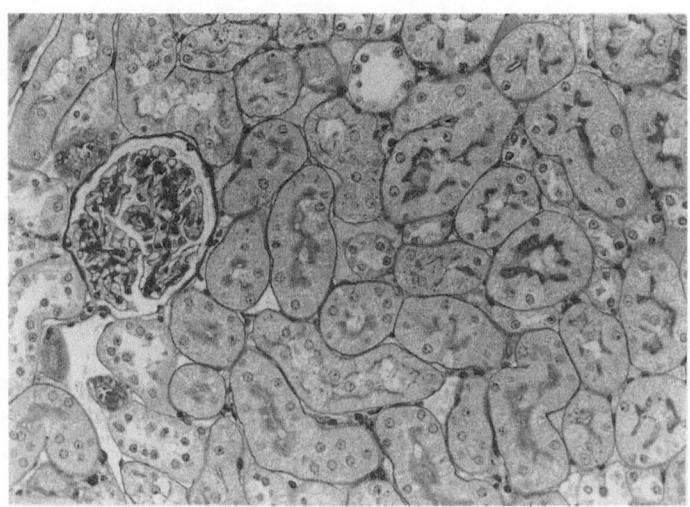

Fig. 8. Light micrograph of the kidney of a 30-week-old LEC rat showing no abnormal findings in the glomerulus or tubules. PAS, ×200

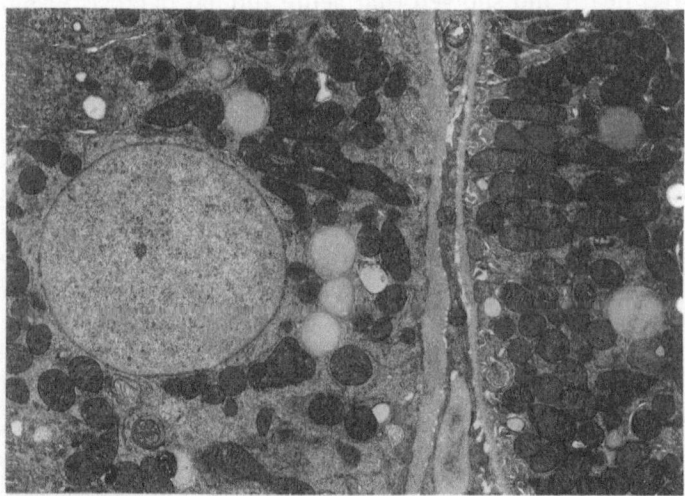

Fig. 9. Electron micrograph of the kidney of a 30-week-old LEC rata showing tubular epithelial cells containing fewer lipid droplets, ×3,000

were separated from the tubular basement membrane (Fig. 6). The remaining epithelial cells exhibited severe degenerative changes consisting of mitochondrial swelling, disorganization of their cristae, the appearance of dark bodies within the mitochondria, as well as the formation of segresomes. Lipid droplets similar to those seen in the hepatocytes were also observed (Fig. 7). In contrast, the glomerulus showed minor glomerular abnormalities (Fig. 5).

These histological findings are compatible with those of acute tubular necrosis (ATN), which we believe to be responsible for the acute renal failure in jaundiced LEC rats.

On the other hand, LEC rats without jaundice showed no abnormal findings in their glomeruli or tubules when examined by light microscopy (Fig. 8). Mild lipid degeneration in tubular epithelial cells, however, was observed by electron microscopy (Fig. 9).

It is well known that renal failure is often complicated by severe liver disease in humans as well. Unless the cause of the renal failure can be determined, e.g., sepsis, hypotension, radiographic contrast material, etc., the acute renal failure of these patients is diagnosed as hepatorenal syndrome [3]. Functional disturbances have been usually emphasized in the pathogenesis of hepatorenal syndrome, rather than morphological abnormalities [8]. The histopathology of the kidney of hepatorenal syndrome, however, has not been fully investigated, since it is often quite difficult to perform renal biopsies in patients with hepatorenal syndrome. Recently, several investigators have reported the histopathology of the kidney in patients with hepatorenal syndrome [9–12]. Mandel et al. [9] examined kidney tissue from five patients with typical hepatorenal syndrome within 2 hours after death and showed that acute tubular necrosis was uniformly present in these patients. They suggested that the acute tubular necrosis might be due to the reduced renal blood flow and intense cortical vasoconstriction which has been reported in patients with hepatorenal syndrome. Soletz et al. [10] reviewed the histopathological data of patients with hepatorenal syndrome and concluded that hepatorenal syndrome and acute tubular necrosis are not separate entities but are, in fact, interrelated.

The histopathological findings in the kidney reported in human hepatorenal syndrome by Mandel et al. [9] were quite similar to those observed in LEC rats, except for the presence of lipid degeneration. The low urinary sodium excretion, which is one of the most characteristic findings of hepatorenal syndrome, was detected in LEC rats as well. These histopathological and biochemical findings suggest that LEC rats can serve as an animal model of spontaneous hepatorenal syndrome.

References

1. Takeichi N, Kobayashi H, Yoshida MC, Sasaki M, Dempo K, Mori M (1988) Spontaneous hepatitis in Long-Evans rats. Acta Pathol Jpn 38:1369–1375
2. Masuda R, Yoshida MC, Sasaki M, Dempo K, Mori M (1988) A transplantable cell line derived from spontaneous hepatocellular carcinoma of the hereditary hepatitis LEC rat. Jpn J Cancer Res 79:250–254
3. Epstein M (1988) Hepatorenal syndrome. In: Epstein M (ed) The kidney in liver diseases. Williams and Wilkins, Baltimore p 89
4. Weinberg AG, Mize CE, Worthen HG (1976) The occurrence of hepatoma in the chronic form of hereditary tyrosinemia. J Pediatr 88:434–438

5. Hovig T, Blomhoff JP, Holme R, Flatmark A, Gjone E (1978) Plasma lipoprotein alerations and morphologic changes with lipid deposition in the kidney of patients with hepatorenal syndrome. Lab Invest 38:540–549
6. Elsas LJ, Hayslett JP, Spargo BH, Durant JL, Rosengerg LE (1971) Wilson's disease with reversible renal tubular dysfunction: Correlation with proximal tubular ultra structure. Ann Intern Med 75:427–435
7. Masuda R, Yoshida MC, Sasaki M, Dempo K, Mori M (1988) Hereditary hepatitis of LEC rats is controlled by autosomal recessive gene. Lab Anim 22:166–172
8. Koppel MH, Coburn JW, Mims MM, Goldstein H, Boyle JD, Rubini ME (1969) Transplantation of cadaveric kidneys from patients with advanced liver disease. N Engl J Med 280:1367–1371
9. Mandel AK, Lansig M, Fahmy A (1982) Acute tubular necrosis in hepatorenal syndrome: An electron microscopy study. Am J Kidney Dis 2:363–374
10. Solez K (1983) Pathogenesis of acute renal failure. Int Rev Exp Pathol 24: 277–333
11. Solez K, Racusen LC, Jewell LD (1988) Pathology of acute renal failure occurring in liver disease. In: Epstein M (ed) The Kidney in liver disease. Williams and Willkins, Baltimore, p 182
12. Wilkinson SP, Hirst D, Day DW, Wiliams R (1976) Spectrum of renal damage in renal failure secondary to cirrhosis and fulminant hepatic failure. J Clin Pathol 31:101–107

12 — Inhibitory and Intensifying Effects of Long-Term Exposure to Chemicals on Spontaneous Hepatic Injury in LEC Rats

Keisuke Izumi, Hisanori Uehara, Hisashi Otsuka[1], and Kozo Matsumoto[2]

Introduction

Liver disease, including the so-called hereditary hepatitis [1–4] and subsequent hepatocellular carcinoma [5,6], and hypoplasia of the thymus [7], are presently known as characteristic morphological abnormalities in LEC rats. Basically, the hepatic lesions of this mutant strain of rat are liver cell degeneration and necrosis, and accumulation of hepatocytes with polyploid huge nuclei [8]. The pathogenesis of hepatic injury has not yet been elucidated, but recently the possibility of the abnormality of methionine metabolism has been suggested from the results of DL-ethionine administration [9]. In examining the response to short-term administration of chemicals or to physical stimulation, the following results have been reported: (1) delay of the hepatic injury by daily intragastric administration of high doses of phenobarbital [10], (2) intensification of hepatic injury by a choline-deficient diet [11] or 0.1% DL-ethionine [9], (3) high susceptibility to initiation by diethylnitrosamine [12], and (4) inhibitory effect of a two-thirds partial hepatectomy on hepatic injury [13].

Induction of Hepatic Lesions Mimicking LEC Rat Liver

Histologically, the hepatic lesions in LEC rats resemble those induced by hepatocarcinogens or hepatotoxic agents in rats in terms of the presence of megalocytic degeneration and oval cell proliferation [14–16]. To induce hepatic lesions morphologically similar to LEC rat liver, we administered several chemicals to 6-week-old male F344/DuCrj rats (Charles River Japan Inc., Kanagawa) as follows: (1) 0.04 2-acetylaminofluorene in a powdered diet for 2 and 4 weeks, (2) 0.06% 3'-methyl-4-dimethylaminoazobenzene in

[1] Second Department of Pathology, and [2] Institute for Animal Experimentation, School of Medicine, University of Tokushima, Tokushima, 770 Japan

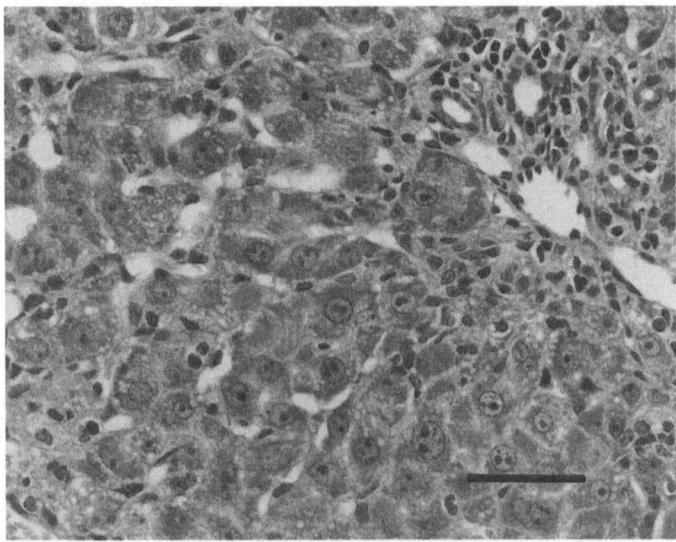

Fig. 1. The liver in a 6-week-old male F344 rat treated with a single sc. injection of 750 mg/kg D-galactosamine hydrochloride and sacrificed on day 3. H and E, *bar* = 50 μm

a powdered diet for 2, 4, and 8 weeks, (3) 0.1% α-naphthylisothiocyanate in a powdered diet for 1, 2, and 3 weeks, and (4) single or repeated sub-cutaneous (sc.) injection of 300 mg/kg or 750 mg/kg D-galactosamine hydro-chloride (GAL) dissolved in 0.9% NaCl. The lesion most similar to LEC rat liver was present on the liver of a rat treated with GAL (Fig. 1). Touch-smeared hepatocyte nuclei of LEC and GAL-treated Fischer rats were stained with 4′, 6-diaminido-2-phenylindole and the DNA content was measured with a Nikon microfluorometer. DNA content reached 32n to 64n maximally in LEC rats, but in GAL-treated F344 rats it was at most 16n and the hepatic lesions were reversible. The livers in transgenic mice expressing HBV genes [17,18] may be more similar to LEC rat liver.

Effects of Long-term Exposure to D-Galactosamine Hydrochloride, Dipyrone, Phenobarbital, and Clofibrate on Spontaneous Hepatic Injury

In order to investigate the inhibitory and intensifying effects of drugs and other chemicals on spontaneous hepatic injury in LEC rats, which is present with jaundice between 4 and 6 months of age, we treated 6-week-old female and male LEC rats for 30 weeks as follows: (1) weekly sc. injections of 300 mg/kg GAL dissolved in 0.9% NaCl, (2) weekly sc. injections of 0.9% NaCl (0.2 ml/100g body weight), (3) 0.3% dipyrone (DP) in

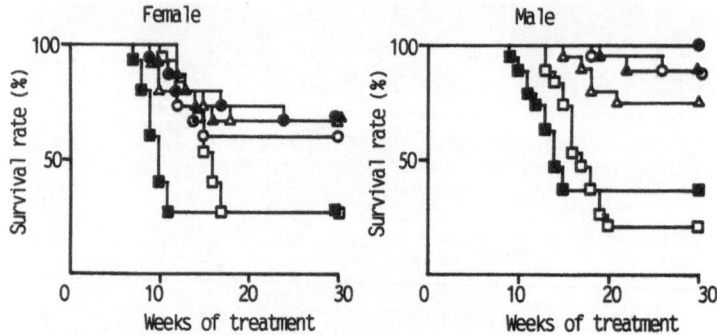

Fig. 2. Survival curves of the female and male LEC rats in each group. Six-week-old rats were treated for 30 weeks as follows: weekly sc. injections of 300 mg/kg GAL (● — ●); weekly sc. injections of 0.9% NaCl (○ — ○); 0.3% DP in drinking water (▲ — ▲); 0.05% phenobarbital in drinking water (■ — ■); 0.3% clofibrate in diet (□ — □); untreated control (△ — △). Many PB and CF treated female and male rats died of hepatic injury by 20 weeks while none of GAL-treated male rats died

drinking water, (4) 0.05% phenobarbital (PB) in drinking water, (5) 0.3% clofibrate (CF) with pellet diet, and (6) untreated control. The doses of these chemicals were chosen by referring to those which have been often used in two-stage carcinogenicity studies [19–21] or used in our own carcinogenicity studies of F344 rats. The doses, except in GAL, are not toxic, at least to F344 rats. In our previous experiment, when 300 mg/kg of GAL was injected sc. to male F344 rats, on day 3 the bromodeoxyuridine-labeled hepatocytes rose to about 3%, which was 5 times or more higher than in the vehicle control. In this study, we used GAL to accelerate the cell renewal of hepatocytes of LEC rats by repeated application.

Survival curves are shown in Fig. 2. The earliest death occurred in week 7 in a 0.05% PB-treated female rat. Death occurred mostly by the end of 20 weeks from the start of treatment. Survival rates at 30 weeks and incidences of the development of jaundice are shown in Table 1. Survival rates in PB- and CF-treated groups were significantly lower than in other groups, and none of the GAL-treated males died. The incidences of jaundice in GAL- and DP-treated males were lower than in corresponding controls. In this study, we found that: (1) long-term administration of low doses of PB and CF intensified the hepatic injury of LEC rats, (2) GAL, weekly injected sc., and DP inhibited the hepatic injury, and (3) weekly sc. injection of 0.9% NaCl delayed the development of jaundice.

These data suggest that: (1) the amount of metabolizing enzymes of PB and CF, such as cytochrome P-450, which is markedly decreased in LEC rats [22], may be reduced during the treatment, and (2) GAL treatment may prevent the development of jaundice by the increase of cell renewal. Histologically, livers of animals which died or were sacrificed in each group showed a similar severe hepatic injury pattern (Fig. 3).

Table 1. Survival rates and incidences of the development of jaundice in LEC rats treated with chemicals.

Treatment	Route	Female		Male	
		Survival rate[a]	Development of jaundice	Survival rate	Development of jaundice
D-galactosamine, 300 mg/kg	SC.[b]	10/15 (67%)	11/15 (73%)	20/20 (100%)	2/20 (10%)[e]
0.9% NaCl	SC.	9/15 (60%)	10/15 (67%)	17/19 (89%)	15/19 (79%)
0.3% dipyrone	W[c]	10/15 (67%)	11/15 (73%)	17/19 (89%)	6/19 (32%)
0.05% phenobarbital	W	4/15 (27%)[g]	12/15 (80%)	7/19 (37%)[g]	14/19 (74%)
0.3% clofibrate	D[d]	4/15 (27%)[g]	12/15 (80%)	4/19 (21%)[f]	16/19 (84%)
Control		10/15 (67%)	11/15 (73%)	15/20 (75%)	11/20 (55%)

[a] At 30 weeks from the start of the treatment
[b] Weekly subcutaneous injection
[c] W, in drinking water
[d] D, with pellet diet
[e,f,g] Significantly different by Fisher's exact probability test: [e]$P < 0.001$ (vs 0.9% NaCl); [f]$P < 0.005$ (vs untreated control), [g]$P < 0.05$ (vs untreated control)

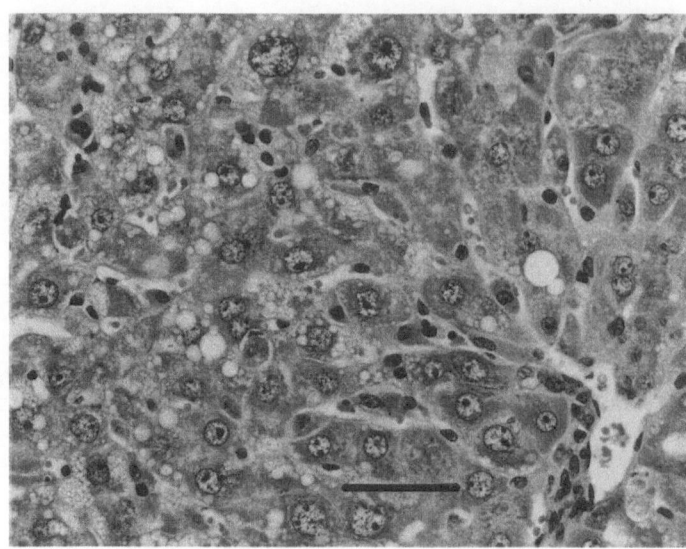

Fig. 3. The liver in a PB-treated female LEC rat which died 8 weeks from the start of treatment. H and E, *bar* = 50 μm

References

1. Sasaki M, Yoshida MC, Kagami K, Takeichi N, Kobayashi H, Dempo K, Mori M (1985) Spontaneous hepatitis in an inbred strain of Long-Evans rats. Rat News Lett 14:4–6
2. Yoshida MC, Masuda R, Sasaki M, Takeichi N, Kobayashi H, Dempo K, Mori M (1987) New mutation causing hereditary hepatitis in the laboratory rat. J Hered 78:361–365
3. Takeichi N, Kobayashi H, Yoshida MC, Sasaki M, Dempo K, Mori M (1988) Spontaneous hepatitis in Long-Evans rats. A potential animal model for fulminant hepatitis in man. Acta Pathol Jpn 38:1369–1375
4. Matsumoto K, Ono E, Izumi K, Otsuka H, Yoshida MC, Sasaki M, Takeichi N, Kobayashi H (1987) Expression of new esterases and pathologic profiles in LEC rats with spontaneous fulminant hepatitis. Transplant Proc 19:3207–3211
5. Masuda R, Yoshida MC, Sasaki M, Dempo K, Mori M (1988) High susceptibility to hepatocellular carcinoma development in LEC rats with hereditary hepatitis. Jpn J Cancer Res 79:828–835
6. Sawaki M, Enomoto K, Takahashi H, Nakajima Y, Mori M (1990) Phenotype of preneoplastic and neoplastic liver lesions during spontaneous liver carcinogenesis of LEC rats. Carcinogenesis 11:1857–1861
7. Agui T, Oka M, Tamada T, Sakai T, Izumi K, Ishida Y, Himeno K, Matsumoto K (1990) Maturational arrest from CD4$^+$8$^+$ to CD4$^+$8$^-$ thymocytes in a mutant strain (LEC) of rat. J Exp Med 172:1615–1624
8. Fujimoto Y, Oyamada M, Hattori A, Takahashi H, Sawaki M, Dempo K, Mori M, Nagao M (1989) Accumulation of abnormally high ploid nuclei in the liver of LEC rats developing spontaneous hepatitis. Jpn J Cancer Res 80:45–50

9. Matsunaga M, Ikeda Y, Sugiyama T, Taniguchi N (1990) Correlation between the methionine metabolism and the expression of the drug metabolizing enzymes in spontaneous hepatitis and hepatoma LEC rats. Proc Jpn Cancer Assoc (49th annual meeting) p 90
10. Togashi Y, Konaka S, Namieno T, Li Y, Kang J, Takeichi N, Kobayashi H (1990) Effects of phenobarbital on spontaneously developed hepatic injury and carcinoma in LEC rats. Proc Jpn Cancer Assoc (49th annual meeting) p 79
11. Sugiyama T, Ookawara T, Kinoshita N, Suzuki K, Taniguchi N (1989) Effect of choline deficient diet on the hepatic drug metabolizing enzymes in spontaneous hepatitis and hepatoma LEC rats. Proc Jpn Cancer Assoc (48th annual meeting) p 256
12. Takahashi H, Enomoto K, Nakajima Y, Mori M (1990) High sensitivity of the LEC rat liver to the carcinogenic effect of diethylnitrosamine. Cancer Lett 51:247–250
13. Takahashi H, Sawada N, Isomura H, Enomoto K, Mori M (1990) Supression of hepatitis in LEC rats by partial hepatectomy. Proc Jpn Cancer Assoc (49th annual meeting) p 66
14. Dempo K, Chisaka N, Yoshida Y, Kaneko A, Onoe T (1975) Immunofluorescent study on α-fetoprotein-producing cells in the early stage of 3'-methyl-4-dimethylaminoazobenzene carcinogenesis. Cancer Res 35:1282–1287
15. Shinozuka H, Lombardi B, Sell S, Iammarino, RM (1978) Early histological and functional alterations of ethionine liver carcinogenesis in rats fed a choline-deficient diet. Cancer Res 38:1092–1098
16. Keppler D, Lesch R, Reutter W, Decker K (1968) Experimental hepatitis induced by D-galactosamine. Exp Mol Pathol 9:279–290
17. Chisari FV, Filippi P, Buras J, McLachlan A, Popper H, Pinkert CA, Palmiter RD, Brinster RL (1987) Structural and pathological effects of synthesis of hepatitis B virus large envelope polypeptide in transgenic mice. Proc Natl Acad Sci USA 84:6909–6913
18. Dunsfold HA, Sell S, Chisari FV (1990) Hepatocarcinogenesis due to chronic liver cell injury in hepatitis B virus transgenic mice. Cancer Res 50:3400–3407
19. Peraino C, Michael Fry RJ, Staffeldt E (1971) Reduction and enhancement by phenobarbital of hepatocarcinogenesis induced in the rat by 2-acetylaminofluorene. Cancer Res 31:1506–1512
20. Weisburger JH, Madison RM, Ward JM, Viguera C, Weisburger EK (1975) Modification of diethylnitrosamine liver carcinogenesis with phenobarbital but not with immunosuppression. J Natl Cancer Inst 54:1185–1188
21. Hosokawa S, Tatematsu M, Aoki T, Nakanowatari J, Igarashi T, Ito N (1989) Modulation of diethylnitrosamine-initiated placental glutathione S-transferase positive preneoplastic and neoplastic lesions by clofibrate, a hepatic peroxisome proliferator. Carcinogenesis 10:2237–2241
22. Sugiyama T, Takeichi N, Kobayashi M, Yoshida MC, Sasaki M, Taniguchi N (1988) Metabolic predisposition of a novel mutant (LEC rats) to hereditary hepatitis and hepatoma: Alterations of the drug metabolizing enzymes. Carcinogenesis 9:1569–1572

2. Biochemistry

13 — Abnormal Copper Accumulation in the Liver of LEC Rats: A Rat Form of Wilson's Disease

Yu Li[1,2], Yuji Togashi, and Noritoshi Takeichi[1]

Introduction

Since the hepatitis in LEC rats is controlled by a single autosomal recessive gene [1], a genetic metabolic disorder is likely to be the cause of the hepatitis. Although interesting biochemical changes associated with the development of the hepatitis have been reported [2–4], they have been unable to provide any direct evidence about the pathogenesis of the rats.

Copper is a prosthetic element of several metalloenzymes which are essential for mammalian life. Excess copper in the liver caused by an autosomal recessive disorder is believed to lead to Wilson's disease, one of the hereditary human hepatic diseases [5]. Recently, we have found that LEC rats also have an abnormally high copper accumulation in the liver and show biochemical features which are very similar to those found in Wilson's disease [6]. In this paper we describe the copper profiles of LEC rats, and compare them with the same profiles in cases of Wilson's disease.

Excessive Copper Accumulation in the Liver of LEC Rats

The copper concentrations in the liver of 2-, 3- and 8-month-old LEC rats were more than 40 times higher than those of age- and sex-matched LEA rats (Fig. 1). The copper concentrations in LEC rats reached a toxic level at the age of 3 months, which suggests that the development of the hepatitis is closely related to the copper toxicity. The decrease of the copper level between the ages of 2 days and 1 month is comparable to that observed in age-matched LEA rats; this could be the consequence of a switch from a fetal to an adult mode of copper metabolism.

Histochemical rhodanine staining for copper and orcein staining for copper-associated protein failed to stain the hepatocytes of LEC rats. How-

[1] Laboratory of Pathology, Cancer Institute, and [2] First Department of Surgery, Hokkaido University School of Medicine, Sapporo, 060 Japan

Fig. 1. Copper concentration in the liver of LEC (□) and LEA (■) rats aged 2 days (D) and 1, 2, 3, 8 and 29 months (M). *$P < 0.001$, **$P < 0.05$, ***$P < 0.005$ vs age- and sex-matched LEA rats, #$P < 0.001$, ##$P < 0.05$, ND, not done

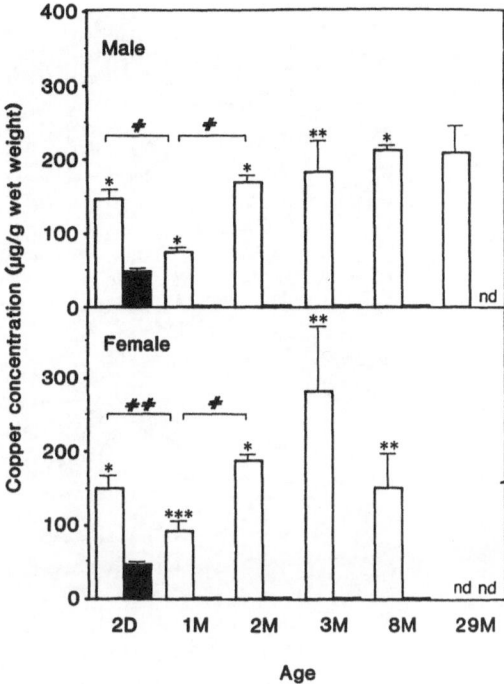

ever, modified Timm's method, a highly sensitive histochemical staining for copper [7], demonstrated copper accumulation in the centrilobular hepatocytes of LEC rats (Fig. 2).

Copper concentrations in the brain were low in 3-month-old LEC rats, but were high in 8-month-old LEC rats compared with those of age- and sex-matched LEA rats. Copper concentrations in the kidney of 8-month-old LEC rats were over 1.8-times higher than those of LEA rats (Table 1). We have observed tubular necrosis in the kidney of LEC rats with jaundice. Electron microscopy showed that tubular epithelial cells were separated from the basement membrane, and that the epithelial cells which were retained showed severe degenerative changes (H. Tochimaru et al., unpublished results). Recently, we have observed that some rats aged between 8 and 12 months have occasionally gone into convulsions. These findings, too, may possibly be associated with copper toxicosis in the kidney and brain.

Prevention of the Development of Hepatitis in LEC Rats by D-Penicillamine

An oral administration of d-penicillamine (100 mg/kg per day), a chelating agent known as an effective therapeutic measure for treatment of Wilson's disease, prevented the development of the hepatitis in LEC rats both

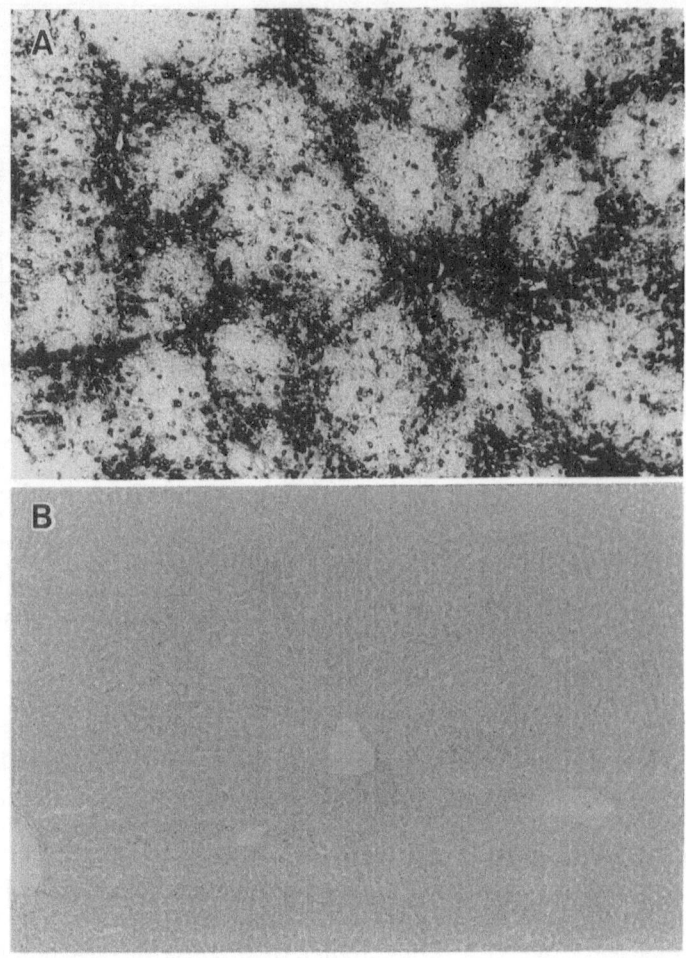

Fig. 2. A MDSD staining of liver of 8-month-old male LEC and **B** LEA rats. Centrilobular hepatocytes of LEC rats stain intensely, demonstrating excessive copper accumulation, × 25

Table 1. Copper concentration in the kidney and brain of LEC and LEA rats.

Sex	Age (months)	Kidney		Brain	
		LEC	LEA	LEC	LEA
Male	3	5.13 ± 0.24	7.08 ± 1.51	1.37 ± 0.07*	1.91 ± 0.03
	8	14.53 ± 3.27	5.37 ± 0.82	2.70 ± 0.04*	1.99 ± 0.09
Female	3	8.95 ± 3.13	6.35 ± 0.31	1.51 ± 0.07*	2.16 ± 0.04
	8	13.04 ± 4.02	6.96 ± 1.08	3.58 ± 0.96	2.30 ± 0.24

Copper concentration was determined by atomic absorption spectrophotometry. Data are means ± SE (µg/g wet weight; $n = 3$).
* $P < 0.005$ vs age- and sex-matched LEA rats

Table 2. Effect of d-penicillamine on the development of hepatitis in LEC rats.

Treatment	Jaundice		Lethality	
	Male	Female	Male	Female
None	3/5	5/5	2/5	4/5
D-penicillamine*	0/5	0/5	0/5	0/5

* Three-month-old LEC rats were given oral administration of d-penicillamine (100 mg/kg per day) for 12 weeks

clinically and biochemically. Over 90% of LEC rats develop acute hepatitis with severe jaundice about 4 months after birth [8], but those rats which had been treated with d-penicillamine, starting at the age of 3 months, did not show any clinical symptoms, at least not until the age of 6 months (Table 2). Although non-treated LEC rats, either jaundiced or asymptomatic, showed a remarkable elevation of serum glutamic-oxaloacetic transaminase (SGOT) and serum glutamate-pyruvate transaminase (SGPT) [8], the levels of these transaminases in the d-penicillamine-treated rats were almost the same as the levels in LEA rats (Fig. 3). These findings were confirmed by histological observation: the untreated LEC rats showed numerous enlarged hepatocytes with huge nuclei and spotty necrosis in the liver, whereas the treated rats did not (Fig. 4). The treated rats showed increased copper excretion into urine (Table 3) and a reduction of the copper level in the liver (Table 4); these resemble the biochemical changes in patients with Wilson's disease under chelation therapy [5,9]. Such findings clearly demonstrate that an abnormal copper metabolism that leads to an excess of hepatic copper causes hepatitis in LEC rats.

Comparison of Hepatitis in LEC Rats and Wilson's Disease in Humans

Ceruloplasmin is a glycoprotein containing 90%–95% of the copper in the serum [5]. In both 3- and 8-month-old LEC rats, the serum levels of ceruloplasmin and copper decreased markedly (Table 5). Since excess hepatic copper, ceruloplasmin deficiency, and hepatitis constitute the definition of Wilson's disease [5,9], the hepatitis in LEC rats can be considered to be a form of Wilson's disease in rats.

Several other important similarities exist between LEC hepatitis and Wilson's disease. Both diseases are inherited by autosomal recessive means, and both respond to d-penicillamine treatment. Histochemical Sudan III staining revealed steatosis in the hepatocytes of LEC rats (Fig. 5). Ultrastructural examination revealed lipid droplets in the cytoplasm of the hepatocytes, too, and showed a striking pleomorphism of mitochondria (Fig. 6); these features resemble histological features found in Wilson's

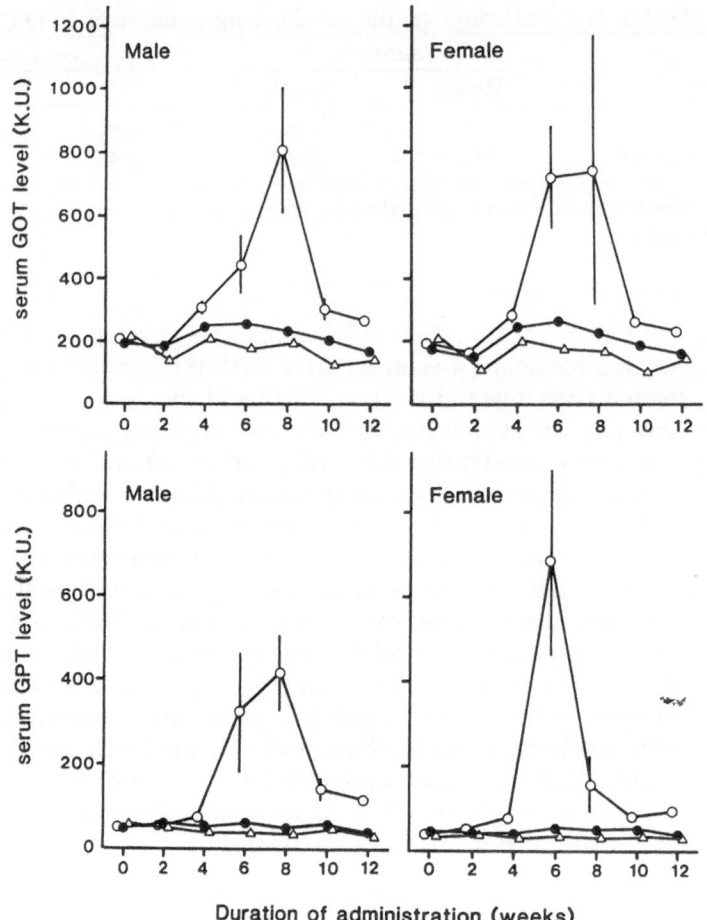

Fig. 3. Chronological changes in serum GOT and GPT levels in d-penicillamine-treated (100 mg/kg per day, p.o.) LEC rats (●), untreated LEC rats (○) and LEA rats (△)

disease [5,9]. Neither rhodanine nor orcein was able to stain the hepatocytes of LEC rats. However, such stainings do not show positive for hepatocytes in the majority of cases of Wilson's disease [5,9]; this failure to stain is thought to be because the copper is diffusely distributed in the cytosol [10].

Differences between the two diseases also exist, however. The huge nuclei of hepatocytes in LEC rats [11] differ from the ballooned glycogen nuclei of hepatocytes in Wilson's disease. The liver disorder in the rats with chronic hepatitis results in cholangiofibrosis [11], which is not the same as the liver cirrhosis found in Wilson's disease. The Kayser-Fleischer ring in the cornea, one of the characteristics of Wilson's disease [5,9], was not detected macroscopically in LEC rats until the age of 8 months. These

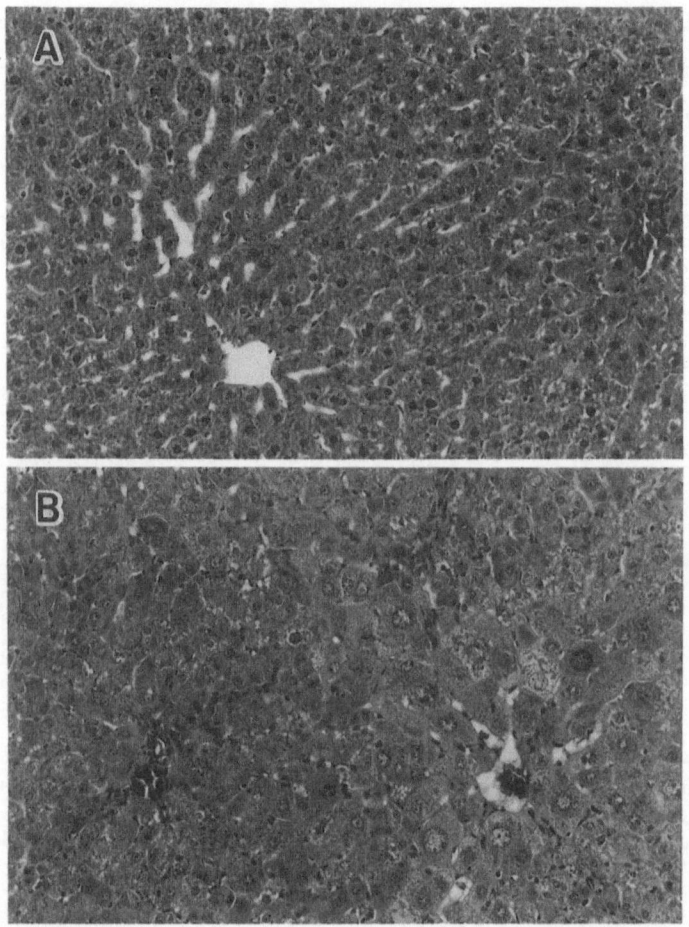

Fig. 4. A Histological examination of liver of d-penicillamine-treated and **B** untreated 6-month-old male LEC rats. H and E, × 50

Table 3. Effects of d-penicillamine on copper concentration in the urine of LEC rats.

Treatment	LEC		LEA	
	Male	Female	Male	Female
None	68.1 ± 7.4	64.1 ± 16.9	21.6 ± 1.2*	25.3 ± 1.8
D-penicillamine[a]	241.2 ± 34.5*	206.1 ± 15.0**	ND	ND

[a] Three-month-old LEC rats were given oral administration of d-penicillamine (100 mg/kg per day) for 1 week
* $P < 0.01$, ** $P < 0.001$ vs age- and sex-matched nontreated LEC rats, *ND*, not done. Data are means ± SE (μg/dl; LEC, $n = 5$; LEA, $n = 3$)

Table 4. Effects of d-penicillamine on copper concentration in the liver of LEC rats.

Treatment	LEC		LEA	
	Male	Female	Male	Female
None	213.3 ± 18.2	259.6 ± 19.6	3.8 ± 0.1*	4.3 ± 0.1
D-penicillamine[a]	110.8 ± 5.8**	154.0 ± 7.0**	ND	ND

[a] Three-month-old LEC rats were given oral administration of d-penicillamine (100 mg/kg per day) for 12 weeks
* $P < 0.01$, ** $P < 0.001$ vs age- and sex-matched untreated LEC rats, ND, not done. Data are means ± SE (µg/g wet weight; untreated, $n = 3$; d-penicillamine-treated, $n = 5$)

Table 5. Ceruloplasmin and copper concentrations in the serum of LEC and LEA rats.

Sex	Age	Ceruloplasmin concentration (unit/liter)		Copper concentration (µg/dl)	
		LEC	LEA	LEC	LEA
Male	2 Days	ND	ND	52.3 ± 11.0	57.0 ± 1.5
	3 Months	0.9 ± 0.5**	162.2 ± 7.2	38.0 ± 11.0*	135.7 ± 2.3
	8 Months	15.0 ± 9.5**	175.0 ± 4.1	52.7 ± 2.4*	137.3 ± 7.2
Female	2 Days	ND	ND	50.0 ± 12.0	68.7 ± 8.1
	3 Months	3.1 ± 0.8**	195.8 ± 7.5	31.3 ± 2.1*	158.0 ± 2.7
	8 Months	7.1 ± 0.2**	214.3 ± 19.9	47.3 ± 3.8*	161.3 ± 9.7

Ceruloplasmin concentration was determined by the method of Schosinski et al. [18]. Copper concentration was determined by atomic absorption spectrophotometry. Data are means ± SE with 3 rats. * $P < 0.001$, ** $P < 0.005$ vs age- and sex-matched LEA rats ND, not done

differences may be due to different repairing responses to copper toxicity between rats and humans.

Toxic milk mice and Bedlington terriers also develop genetically controlled hepatic copper toxicosis. Since, in the former, the pups fed with their mother's milk develop copper deficiency [12] while in the latter the dogs show normal or elevated serum ceruloplasmin levels [13], LEC rats seem likely to provide the closest animal model for the study of Wilson's disease.

Excessive Copper Accumulation in Spontaneously Developed Hepatocellular Carcinoma in LEC Rats

In three 29-month-old LEC rats, copper accumulated not only in non-cancerous liver tissues but also in spontaneously developed hepatocellular carcinoma (HCC) (Fig. 7). Thus, it seems that the abnormal copper metabolism may be maintained during the process of carcinogenesis. It has been reported that almost all of the LEC rats which have survived for more than 1

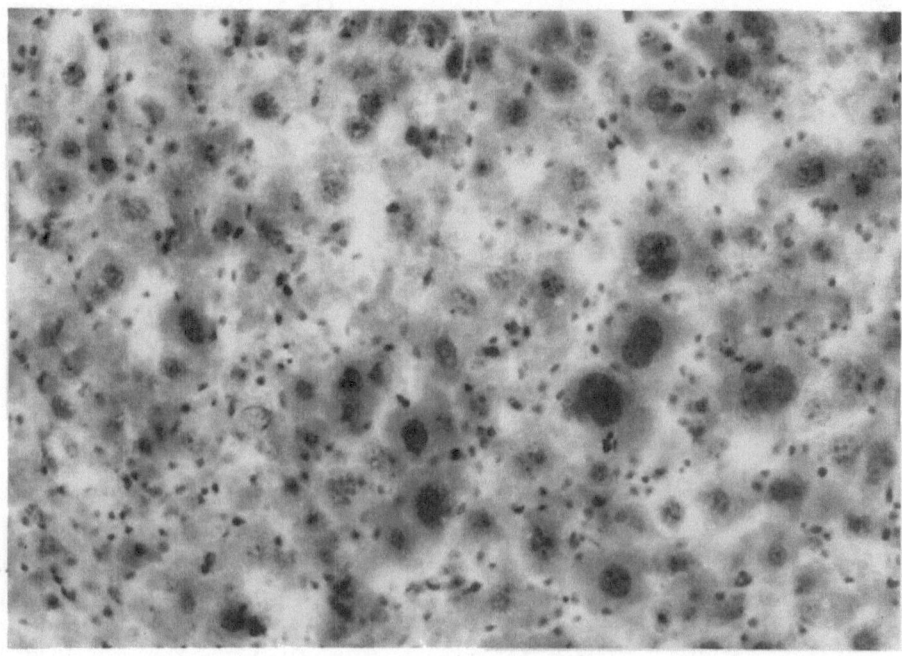

Fig. 5. Histochemical staining of liver of 5-month-old female LEC rats. Hepatocytes stain with Sudan III (orange) indicating an abundance of lipid droplets, × 200

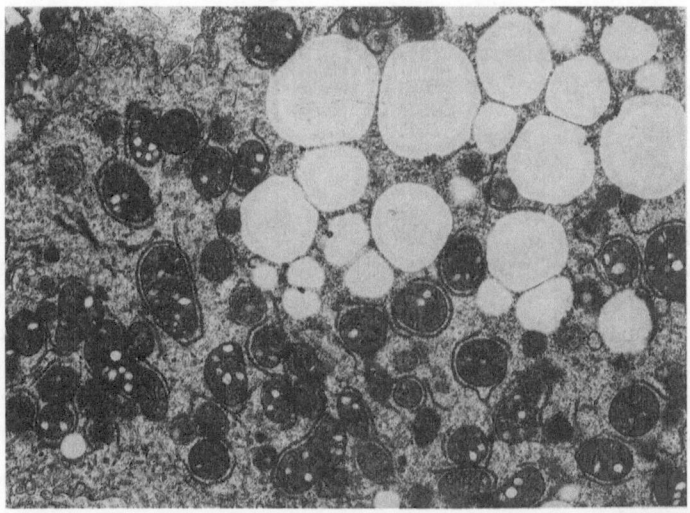

Fig. 6. Electron micrograph of liver of 7-month-old female LEC rats. The hepatocyte contains numerous lipid droplets in cytoplasm. Mitochondria show striking pleomorphism with electron-lucent vacuoles, × 3,000

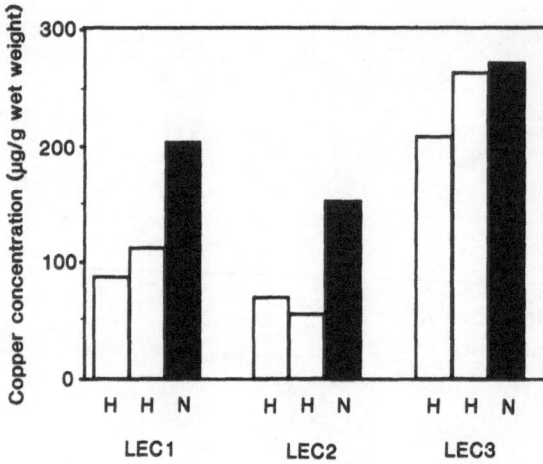

Fig. 7. Copper concentration in spontaneously developed hepatocellular carcinoma (□, *H*) and corresponding noncancerous liver tissues (■, *N*) of three 29-month-old male LEC rats, LEC1–LEC3

year develop HCC spontaneously [14], whereas only a dozen cases of Wilson's disease developed HCC [15]. It has been hypothesized that, as in the case of chemically induced hepatic carcinogenesis in copper-loading rats [16,17], copper may protect the liver against carcinogenesis in patients with Wilson's disease [5,15]. However, a more likely explanation is that the non-treated patients died before a malignant change could occur, while in medically well-treated patients the liver lesion becomes so quiescent that the stimulus to carcinogenesis is removed [9]. Although it is yet unknown whether copper itself acts as a hepatic carcinogen, the high incidence of HCC and the excessive copper accumulation in the liver of LEC rats suggest that an abnormal copper metabolism may be linked with hepatic carcinogenesis. LEC rats will provide us with a valuable opportunity to further study the role of copper in carcinogenesis.

Summary

The inheriting manner, clinical course, and copper profiles, including excessive copper accumulation in the liver and reductions of serum levels of copper and ceruloplasmin, in LEC rats strikingly resemble these features in patients with Wilson's disease. An oral administration of d-penicillamine, effective in the treatment of Wilson's disease, prevented the development of hepatitis in LEC rats completely. Such similarities suggest that hepatitis in LEC rats may be a form of Wilson's disease in rats.

References

1. Masuda R, Yoshida MC, Sasaki M, Dempo K, Mori M (1988) Hereditary hepatitis in LEC rats is controlled by a single autosomal recessive gene. Lab Anim 22:166–169

2. Sugiyama T, Suzuki K, Ookawara T, Kurosawa T, Taniguchi N (1989) Selective expression and induction of cytochrome $P450_{PB}$ and $P450_{MC}$ during the development of hereditary hepatitis and hepatoma of LEC rats. Carcinogenesis 10:2155–2159

3. Matsumoto K, Ono E, Izumi K, Otsuka H, Yoshida MC, Sasaki M, Takeichi N, Kobayashi H (1987) Expression of new esterases and pathologic profiles in LEC rats with spontaneous fulminant hepatitis. Transplant Proc 19:3207–3211

4. Wirth PJ, Fujimoto Y, Takahashi H, Mori M, Yoshida MC, Sugiyama T, Nagao M (1990) Two-dimensional electrophoretic analysis of hepatitis-associated polypeptides in liver of LEC rats developing spontaneous hepatitis. Jpn J Cancer Res 81:477–482

5. Gollan JL (1989) Copper metabolism, Wilson's disease, and hepatic copper toxicosis. In: Zakim D, Boyer TD (eds) Hepatology. WB Sauders, Philadelphia, p 1249

6. Li Y, Togashi Y, Sato S, Emoto T, Kang J-H, Takeichi N, Kobayashi H, Kojima Y, Une Y, Uchino J (to be published) Spontaneous hepatic copper accumulation in LEC rats with hereditary hepatitis: A model of Wilson's disease. J Clin Invest

7. Kozma M, Szerdahelyi P, Kása P (1981) Histochemical detection of zinc and copper in various neurons of the central nervous system. Acta Histochem 69:12–16

8. Sasaki M, Yoshida MC, Kagami K, Takeichi N, Kobayashi H, Dempo K, Mori M (1985) Spontaneous hepatitis in an inbred strain of Long-Evans rats. Rat News Lett 14:4–6

9. Walshe JM (1987) The liver in Wilson's disease (hepatolenticular degeneration). In: Shiff L, Shiff ER (eds) Diseases of the liver. JB Lippincott, Philadelphia, p 1037

10. Nartey NO, Frei JV, Cherian MG (1987) Hepatic copper and metallothionein distribution in Wilson's disease (hepatolenticular degeneration). Lab Invest 57:397–401

11. Yoshida MC, Masuda R, Sasaki M, Takeichi N, Kobayashi H, Dempo K, Mori M (1987) New mutation causing hereditary hepatitis in the laboratory rat. J Hered 78:361–365

12. Biempica L, Rauch H, Quintana N, Sternlieb I (1988) Morphologic and chemical studies on a murine mutation (toxic milk mice) resulting in hepatic copper toxicosis. Lab Invest 59:500–508

13. Su L-C, Ravanshad S, Owen CA Jr, McCall JT, Zollman PE, Hardy RM (1982) A comparison of copper-loading disease in Bedlington terriers and Wilson's disease in humans. Am J Physiol 243:G226–G230

14. Masuda R, Yoshida MC, Sasaki M, Dempo K, Mori M (1988) High susceptibility to hepatocellular carcinoma development in LEC rats with spontaneous hepatitis. Jpn J Cancer Res 79:828–835

15. Polio J, Enriquez RE, Chow A, Wood WM, Atterbury C (1989) Hepatocellular carcinoma in Wilson's disease. Case report and review of the literature. J Clin Gastroenterol 11:220–224

16. Kamamoto Y, Makiura S, Sugihara S, Hiasa Y, Arai M, Ito N (1973)The inhibitory effect of copper on DL-ethionine carcinogenesis in rats. Cancer Res 33:1129–1135

17. Yamane Y, Sakai K, Umeda T, Murata N, Ishizeki S, Ogihara I, Takahashi A, Iwasaki I, Ide G (1984) Suppressive effect of cupric acetate on DNA alkylation,

DNA synthesis and tumorigenesis in the liver of dimethylnitrosoamine-treated rats. Jpn J Cancer Res 75:1062–1069

18. Schosinski KH, Lehmann HP, Beeler MF (1974) Measurement of ceruloplasmin from its oxidase activity in serum by use of o-dianisidine dihydrochloride. Clin Chem 20:1556–1563

14—Hereditary Low Levels of Plasma Ceruloplasmin in LEC Rats

Takao Ono, Syuiti Abe, and Michihiro C. Yoshida[1]

Introduction

The LEC rats with hereditary hepatitis show an abnormal accumulation of copper in various organs such as liver, kidney, and brain, together with a marked decrease in the level of serum or plasma ceruloplasmin (Cp) [1]. Cp is a copper-binding protein primarily involved in the transport of copper from the liver [2]. The apoprotein is synthesized in the liver [3], and then binds from six to eight atoms of copper per Cp molecule [4,5]. Most of the copper in plasma is present as the Cp-bound form. Thus, impaired copper metabolism may bear an etiological significance for the hepatic lesions in LEC rats, although the basic defect involved in the occurrence of hepatitis still remains obscure.

In this study, we examined the level of Cp in LEC and other strains of rats and in their hybrids in order to ascertain whether low Cp level is heritable in LEC rats and if it is associated with the occurrence of hepatitis. In addition, plasma copper levels were examined for correlation with the Cp levels in these rats.

Materials and Methods

Animals

Three inbred LEC, LEA and BN (brown Norway) strain rats were used, all of which were maintained at the Center for Experimental Plants and Animals of Hokkaido University. As described in the previous chapters, LEC rats develop acute hepatitis with severe jaundice at about 4 months after birth. About one-third to one-fourth of the affected animals died of

---

[1] Chromosome Research Unit, Faculty of Science, Hokkaido University, Sapporo, 060 Japan

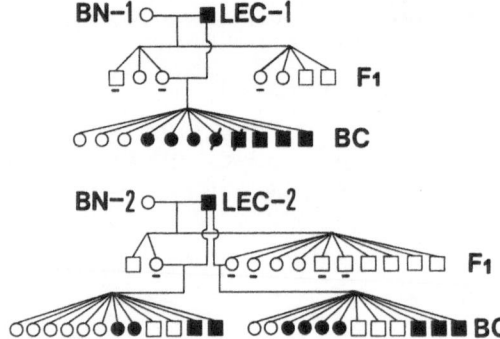

Fig. 1. The pedigree of F_1 and backcross rats (BC) used. All backcross rats were examined for the levels of plasma Cp and/or copper, whereas only F_1 rats (*underlined*) were used for these examinations

submassive necrosis in the liver within 1 week after the onset of jaundice. The remainder, which recovered from jaundice, developed chronic hepatitis terminating in hepatocellular carcinoma.

LEA and BN rats do not develop hepatitis, and both served as controls in the present study. As shown in Fig. 1, 5-month-old male LEC rats which had recovered from jaundice were mated with age-matched female BN rats. Backcross hybrid rats were obtained from matings with female F_1 rats.

Determination of Plasma Cp and Copper Levels

Cp in the plasma of blood collected from the animals at different ages was measured as ferroxidase activity [3,6] by using a commercially available Determiner Cp Kit (Kyowa Medics, Tokyo), as previously described [7]. Concentration of plasma copper was determined by using a Cu Neo Shino-Test Kit (Shino-Test, Tokyo), which is based on the chelation of copper ion with 2-(2-Thiazolylazo)-4-methyl-5-sulfomethylaminobenzoic acid (TAMSMB).

Histological Examination

Histological study on paraffin sections of liver tissue with hematoxylin-eosin (H and E) and dimethylaminobenzylidine rhodanine staining was made for confirmation of hepatic lesions and copper accumulation in the liver of the animals.

Cp Levels in LEC and Other Strains of Rats

LEC rats exhibited a markedly low level of Cp compared with LEA and BN rats (Table 1). Although the Cp ferroxidase activity tended to increase with age in all strains of examined rats, no statistically significant difference was observed in young and old rats except for the BN strain. The level of Cp in old BN and LEA rats was similar, whereas it remained low in old LEC

Table 1. Level of plasma ceruloplasmin (Cp) in three strains, F_1 and backcross rats.

Animal	No. and Sex of subjects ♀	No. and Sex of subjects ♂	Age (Weeks)	Cp Ferroxidase activity (mU/ml) Range	Cp Ferroxidase activity (mU/ml) Mean ± SE	Concentration of Cp (mg/dl)[a] Mean ± SE
LEC (young)	4	3	5	0.49– 5.64	2.58 ± 0.66[c]	3.43 ± 0.88
LEC (old)[b]	1	5	61–100	0.18–12.00	5.04 ± 1.59[c]	6.71 ± 2.11
BN (young)	3	4	7	11.01–20.98	15.75 ± 1.19	20.94 ± 1.59
BN (old)	4	0	56	21.86–25.16	23.33 ± 0.78[d]	31.03 ± 1.04
LEA (young)	3	3	7	15.21–24.34	19.15 ± 1.20	25.47 ± 1.60
LEA (old)	1	2	33	18.21–26.69	23.23 ± 2.57	30.90 ± 3.42
F_1 (BN × LEC)	5	3	54–63	12.81–24.30	20.79 ± 1.34	26.92 ± 1.92
BC (F_1 × LEC): With hepatitis	9	8	40–53	1.69–12.96	6.24 ± 0.61[c]	8.30 ± 0.81
Without hepatitis	11	5	40–53	16.57–33.69	22.60 ± 1.06	10.05 ± 1.41

[a] Concentration of Cp was given by the converting formula as follows: Cp (mg/dl) = Ferroxidase activity of Cp (mU/ml) × 1.33 (Manufacturer's instructions, Determiner Cp Kit)

[b] All rats developed hepatic lesions including chronic hepatitis or hepatoma and cholangiofibrosis. One female had sebacious carcinoma in the lower abdomen (data not shown)

[c] Statistically significant compared with each of young or old BN and LEA and F_1 rats ($P < 0.005$ in all cases, t-test)

[d] Statistically significant compared with young BN rats ($P < 0.005$)

rats, being nearly one-fifth of the two other strains' value (23 mU/ml vs 5 mU/ml).

Parallel histological study revealed no hepatic lesions in 5-week-old young LEC rats, whereas the old LEC rats (61–100 weeks) had hepatic lesions, including chronic hepatitis, cholangiofibrosis, and hepatocellular carcinoma. Although the levels of Cp ferroxidase activity ranged widely (from 0.18 to 12.0 mU/ml) in old LEC rats, they did not seem to correlate with the stage of hepatic lesions observed. These results indicate that both young and old LEC rats show a low level of Cp ferroxidase activity, irrespective of the occurrence of hepatic lesions.

Cp Levels in F_1 and Backcross Hybrid Rats

The (BN × LEC) F_1 hybrids at 54–63 weeks old showed a level of Cp similar to that of older BN and LEA rats (Table 1). Although F_1 rats never had any hepatic lesions, approximately 50% of (BN × LEC) × LEC backcross rats (19 out of 35 from three litters, as shown in Fig. 1) developed hepatic lesions such as those found in the parental LEC rats (Fig. 2). No backcross rats had hepatocellular carcinoma at the time of examination. Thus, the segregation rate of hepatitis in backcross rats followed a single autosomal recessive mode of inheritance, as previously described [8]. While the backcross rats without hepatitis showed a level of Cp ferroxidase activity similar to that of old BN, LEA, and F_1 rats, backcross rats with hepatitis exhibited a significantly decreased Cp level compared with BN and LEA rats at all ages and with F_1 hybrids ($P < 0.005$ in all cases). Although the backcross rats with hepatitis had a wide range of Cp levels (from 1.69 to 12.96 mU/ml), no relationship was found between the level of Cp and the stage of hepatic lesions as evidenced in old LEC rats. These results indicate that the low Cp level in LEC rats is heritable in a single autosomal recessive mode.

Copper Levels in Parental Strain and Hybrid Rats

Plasma copper concentrations in LEC and BN rats and in their F_1 and backcross progeny are summarized in Table 2. Young LEC rats exhibited the most decreased level of copper concentration among the groups of examined rats. Although the copper levels tended to increase with age in both strains of rats, copper concentration in old LEC rats was significantly low compared with old BN and F_1 rats. Levels of plasma copper concentration in F_1 and backcross rats without hepatitis were similar to that of aged BN rats, whereas the backcross rats with hepatitis showed a significantly low level of copper concentration compared with F_1 and backcross rats without hepatitis ($P < 0.05$). Thus, the plasma copper concentration in old LEC and backcross rats with hepatitis was similar, both showing a significantly decreased level compared with old BN, F_1, and backcross rats without hepatitis.

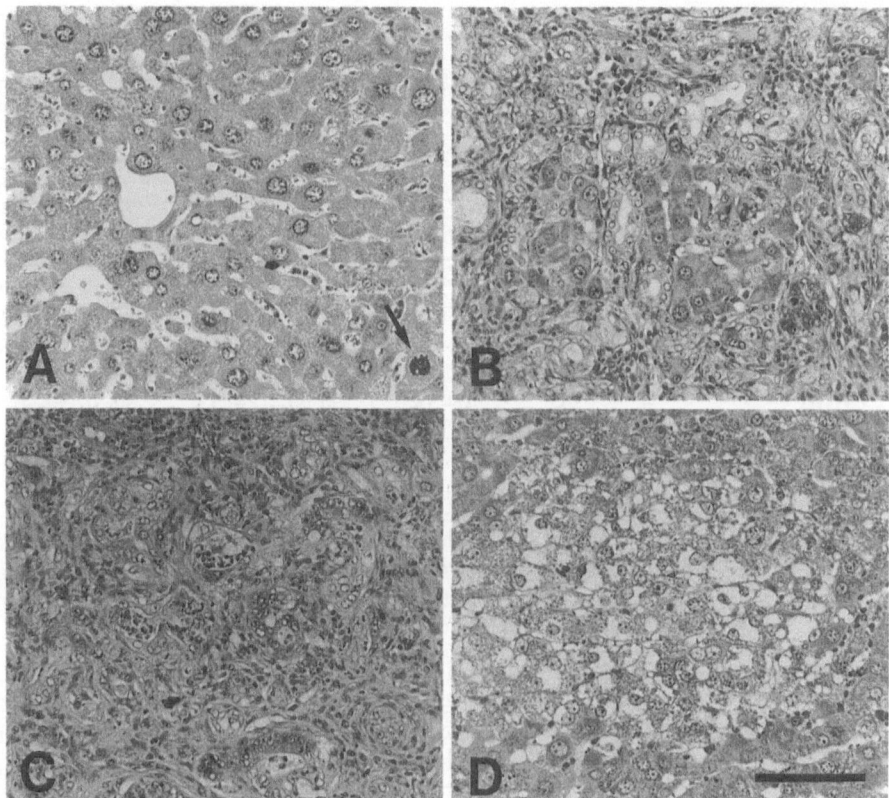

Fig. 2. Histological findings of livers in backcross rats [(BN × LEC) × LEC] with hepatitis (H and E staining). **A** Enlarged hepatocytes with large nuclei are observed (male, 45 weeks old). *Arrow* indicates a mitotic cell. **B** Hepatocytes are enclosed with cholangiofibrosis, looking like islands (female, 47 weeks old). **C** Well-developed cholangiofibrosis with various-sized glands (famale, 53 weeks old). **D** A focus of cells with light cytoplasm (male, 53 weeks old). **A–D** are same magnification and *bar* indicates 100 μm

Histological examination with rhodanine staining revealed copper accumulation in the liver of LEC and backcross rats with hepatitis (Fig. 3). The level of copper accumulation as detected by the histochemical staining was variable among the affected animals (data not shown), although the localization of copper was found in Kupffer's cells.

Association of Cp and Copper Levels with Hepatic Lesions in LEC Rats

The present study revealed apparently low Cp levels in LEC rats with hereditary hepatitis at all ages. Backcross rats with hepatitis also showed decreased Cp levels, whereas F_1 and backcross rats without hepatitis re-

Table 2. Plasma copper concentrations in LEC and BN strains, and F_1 and back-cross rats.

Animals	No. and Sex of Subjects ♀	No. and Sex of Subjects ♂	Age (Weeks)	Plasma coper (µg/dl) Range	Plasma coper (µg/dl) Mean ± SE
LEC (young)	1	2	5	14.00– 23.08	19.23 ± 2.67[a]
LEC (old)	0	3	61–73	39.74– 43.59	41.88 ± 1.13[b]
BN (young)	1	2	7	46.15– 75.64	58.12 ± 8.95[c]
BN (old)	3	0	56	61.54–114.10	88.89 ± 15.21
F_1 (BN × LEC)	2	2	54–63	76.92–126.93	97.12 ± 10.63
BC (F_1 × LEC):					
With hepatitis	4	3	40–53	34.62– 69.23	52.56 ± 4.29[d]
Without hepatitis	3	4	40–53	80.77–162.82	95.42 ± 17.54

[a] Statistically significant compared with each group ($P < 0.05$, t-test)
[b] Statistically significant compared with old BN and F_1 rats ($P < 0.01$)
[c] Statistically significant compared with F_1 rats ($P < 0.05$)
[d] Statistically significant compared with F_1 and BC without hepatitis ($P < 0.05$)

tained Cp levels similar to LEA and BN rats without hepatitis. These findings indicate a very close association of Cp levels with hepatitis in LEC and backcross rats, although the observed decrease in Cp levels may not be the primary cause of hepatitis in these rats.

The decreased Cp level is a neonatal feature of all mammalian species examined thus far [9–11], although this level increases with age, as seen in LEA and BN rats examined here. It has been reported that the Cp gene is

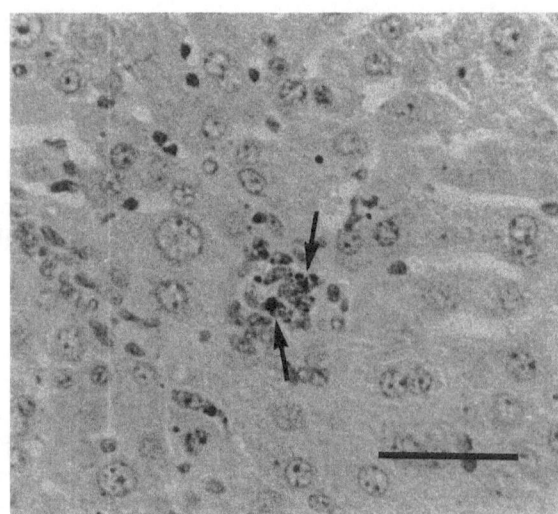

Fig. 3. Rhodanine stained liver section from a male backcross rat with hepatitis. Accumulated copper is observed as coarse granules (*arrows*) in Kupffer's cells but not in hepatocytes. *Bar* indicates 50 µm

Fig. 4. Levels of plasma Cp ferroxidase activity and plasma copper concentration in LEC, BN, F_1 (BN × LEC) and backcross (F_1 × LEC) rats at age 40–100 weeks. *BCh* and *BCn* indicate backcross rats with and without hepatitis, respectively. Range *bars* indicate standard error of the mean activity of Cp ferroxidase

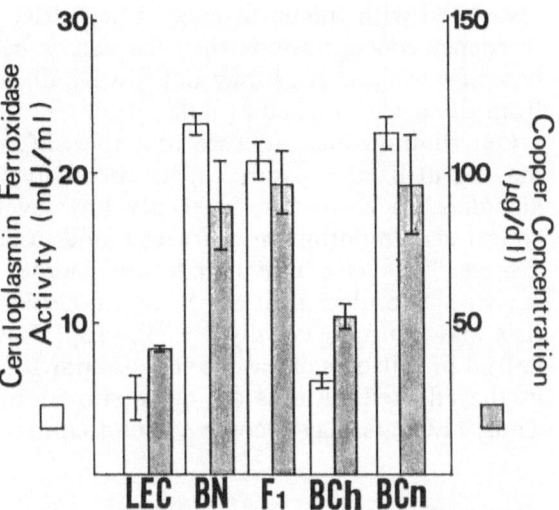

transcribed to a normal adult level of mRNA in the newborn Wistar strain of rats [10], suggesting a post-transcriptional regulation in neonatal low Cp production. If this is the case, a genetically altered translational process, rather than a defective Cp gene, may account for the observed low Cp levels in LEC rats. Another possibility not to be excluded, however, is an unknown intermediate(s), which is normally involved in the incorporation of copper into apoprotein, may be impaired genetically and modifies the copper-binding, particularly since a possible metabolic link has been recently suggested among apo-Cp, Cu(I)-thionein, and activated leucocytes in blood plasma [5]. These possibilities should be examined by further studies.

Plasma copper concentration mostly parallels Cp ferroxidase activity in the hybrids and their parental strain rats, thereby showing an association of copper levels with the occurrence of hepatitis (Fig. 4). The observed low copper concentration may be ascribed to a possible decrease in the copper transport from the liver by the lowered level of Cp in LEC and hepatitis-bearing backcross rats. It is thus conceivable that the observed hepatic copper accumulation is related to the decreased levels of plasma Cp and copper in these rats.

Conclusions

Our findings clearly demonstrate the heritable low levels of plasma Cp in LEC rats. Because of the very close association of Cp levels with the occurrence of hepatitis, the decreased Cp level may become a useful marker for detecting affected animals among F_2 and backcross rats derived from crossing LEC and other strains of rats. Plasma copper concentration is also associated with the occurrence of hepatitis. However, a smaller difference of copper concentrations than Cp values between rats with and without hepatitis (Tables 1, 2) may not always discriminate the affected animals from the backcross and F_2 rats.

Our findings also indicate that the LEC rats with hereditary hepatitis may be utilized to study copper metabolism and pathogenesis of related disorders. In particular, markedly low levels of plasma Cp and hepatic copper accumulation are features found in patients affected with Wilson's disease. This is a rare hereditary disorder with chronic and relentless copper accumulation in the liver and nervous system which causes hepatitis and neurological disease [12–16]. However, the primary defect involved in Wilson's disease is still unknown. The pathogenic features found in the affected patients are quite similar to those observed in LEC rats. Thus, LEC rats may become a useful animal model for Wilson's disease.

Acknowledgments. We thank Mr. E. Kamimura, the Center for Experimental Plants and Animals of Hokkaido University, for careful breeding of the rat strains used, and Dr. T. Nojima and Ms. Y. Fukushima, Department of Pathology, Hokkaido University School of Medicien, for histological preparations and pathological diagnosis of hepatic lesions in LEC rats. This work was supported in part by Grants-in-Aid for Cancer Research from the Ministry of Education, Science and Culture and from the Ministry of Health and Welfare, Japan.

References

1. Li Y, Togashi Y, Sato S, Emoto T, Kang, J-H, Takeichi N, Kobayashi H, Kojima Y, Une Y, Uchino J (1991) Spontaneous hepatic copper accumulation in Long-Evans Cinnamon rats with hereditary hepatitis: A model of Wilson's disease. J Clin Invest 87:1858–1861
2. Cousins RJ (1985) Absorption, transport, and hepatic metabolism of copper and zinc: Special reference to metallothionein and ceruloplasmin. Physiol Rev 65:238–309
3. Ryden L, Bjork I (1976) Reinvestigation of some physicochemical and chemical properties of human ceruloplasmin (ferroxidase). Biochemistry 15:3411–3417
4. Koschinsky ML, Funk WD, van Oost BA, MacGillivray RTA (1986) Complete cDNA sequence of human preceruloplasmin. Proc Natl Acad Sci USA 83: 5086–5090
5. Schechinger T, Hartmann H-J, Weser U (1986) Copper transport from Cu(I)-thionein into apo-ceruloplasmin mediated by activated leucocytes. Biochem J 240:281–283
6. Johnson DA, Osaki S, Frieden E (1967) A micromethod for the determination of ferroxidase (ceruloplasmin) in human serums. Clin Chem 13:142–150
7. Ono T, Abe S, Yoshida MC (1991) Hereditary low level of plasma ceruloplasmin in LEC rats associated with spontaneous development of hepatitis and liver cancer. Jpn J Cancer Res 82:486–489

8. Masuda R, Yoshida MC, Sasaki M, Dempo K, Mori M (1988) Hereditary hepatitis of LEC rats is controlled by a single autosomal recessive gene. Lab Anim 22:166–169
9. Srai SKS, Burroughs AK, Wood B, Epstein O (1986) The ontogeny of liver copper metabolism in the guinea pig: Clues to the etiology of Wilson's disease. Hepatology 6:427–432
10. Barrow L, Tanner MS, Critchley DR (1989) Expression of the caeruloplasmin gene in the adult and neonatal rat liver. Clin Sci 77:259–263
11. Shokeir MHK (1971) Investigations on the nature of ceruloplasmin deficiency in the newborn. Clin Genet 2:223–227
12. Scheinberg IH, Gitlin D (1952) Deficiency of ceruloplasmin in patients with hepatolenticular degeneration (Wilson's disease). Science 116:484–485
13. Czaja MJ, Weiner FR, Schwarzenberg SJ, Sternlieb I, Scheinberg IH, Van Thiel DH, LaRusso NF, Giambrone M-A, Krischner R, Koschinsky ML, MacGillivray RTA, Zern MA (1987) Molecular studies of ceruloplasmin deficiency in Wilson's disease. J Clin Invest 80:1200–1204
14. Walshe JM (1975) The liver in hepatolenticular degeneration. In: Schiff L (ed) Diseases of the liver. J B Lippincott, Philadelphia, pp 1000–1016
15. Nartey NO, Frei JV, Cherian MG (1978) Hepatic copper and metallothionein distribution in Wilson's disease (hepatolenticular degeneration). Lab Invest 57:397–401
16. Frydman M, Bonne-Tamir B, Farrer LA, Conneally PM, Magazanik A, Ashbel S, Goldwitch Z (1985) Assignment of the gene for Wilson's disease to chromosome 13: Linkage to the esterase D locus. Proc Natl Acad Sci USA 82:1819–1821

15 — Differential Expression of Mn- and Cu,Zn-Superoxide Dismutases in Various Tissues of LEC Rats

KEIICHIRO SUZUKI, TOSHIYUKI NAKATA, HAN GEUK SEO, NOBUKO MIYAZAWA, TOSHIHIRO SUGIYAMA, and NAOYUKI TANIGUCHI[1]

Introduction

Oxy-radicals are thought to play important roles in the course of multistep carcinogenesis [1–3]. Accurate detection of oxy-radicals is impossible, however, because of their instability and short half-life. Therefore, evaluation of the levels of enzymes involved in the metabolism of oxy-radicals appears to be the most reliable means of assessing oxy-radical metabolism in vivo.

Superoxide dismutase (SOD) is one of the most important enzymes in the anti-oxidant defense system. The enzyme scavenges superoxide anion (O_2^-), which is the first product of oxy-radicals. In mammalian tissues, there are three SOD isozymes designated Cu,Zn-SOD, Mn-SOD, and extracellular SOD (EC-SOD). The measurement of the activity of SOD, which is usually determined by the inhibition method, is both unreliable and complicated. Moreover, activities of different isozymes are difficult to discriminate, while the measurements of SOD protein levels are more accurate.

We previously developed a monoclonal antibody against human Mn-SOD [4] and reported that serum levels of Mn-SOD were elevated in several malignant diseases, such as ovarian carcinoma and primary hepatoma [5,6]. Oxy-radicals may also play an important role in the process of hepatitis and hepatoma in LEC rats.

In the present study, we developed an enzyme-linked immunosorbent assay (ELISA) for rat Cu,Zn-SOD and Mn-SOD using specific polyclonal antibodies, and determined the levels of immunoreactive SODs in the various organs of LEC rats. SOD levels in Wistar rats were also measured for comparison.

---

[1] Department of Biochemistry, Osaka University Medical School, Suita, Osaka, 565 Japan

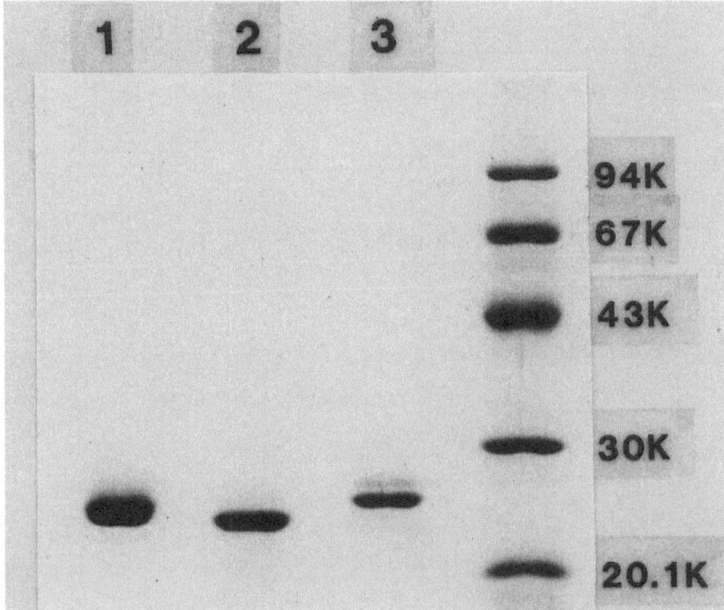

Fig. 1. Polyacrylamide gel electrophoresis of purified Mn-SOD. *Lanes 1, 2,* and *3* depict human, dog, and rat Mn-SOD, respectively. The *faint band* observed was SH-modified Mn-SOD as reported previously [1]

ELISA of SODs

Rat Mn-SOD was purified from livers (800 g) of male Wistar rats by the same procedure used for human Mn-SOD [7]. Polyacrylamide gel electro-phoresis of purified rat Mn-SODs is shown in Fig. 1. A polyclonal antibody against the purified rat Mn-SOD was raised in rabbits and purified by precipitation with 50% saturated ammonium sulfate, DEAE-cellulose chromatography, and immuno-affinity column chromatography using purified Mn-SOD as an adsorbent. Figure 2 shows the specificity of this antibody as judged by Western blotting analysis. An ELISA was developed with the polyclonal antibody using a sandwich method. The ELISA was able to measure 5–100 ng/ml Mn-SOD (Fig. 3)

An ELISA for Cu,Zn-SOD has been also established, and the range of measurement was found to be 0.1–2.0 ng/ml.

Tissue Distribution of Mn-SOD

Five LEC rats (male, 18-week-old) were sacrificed and ten tissues were obtained from each rat. Each tissue was homogenized and centrifuged at 900 × g, and the supernatant was sonicated. Protein levels of each sample were measured by the BCA method (Pierce), and Mn-SOD levels were

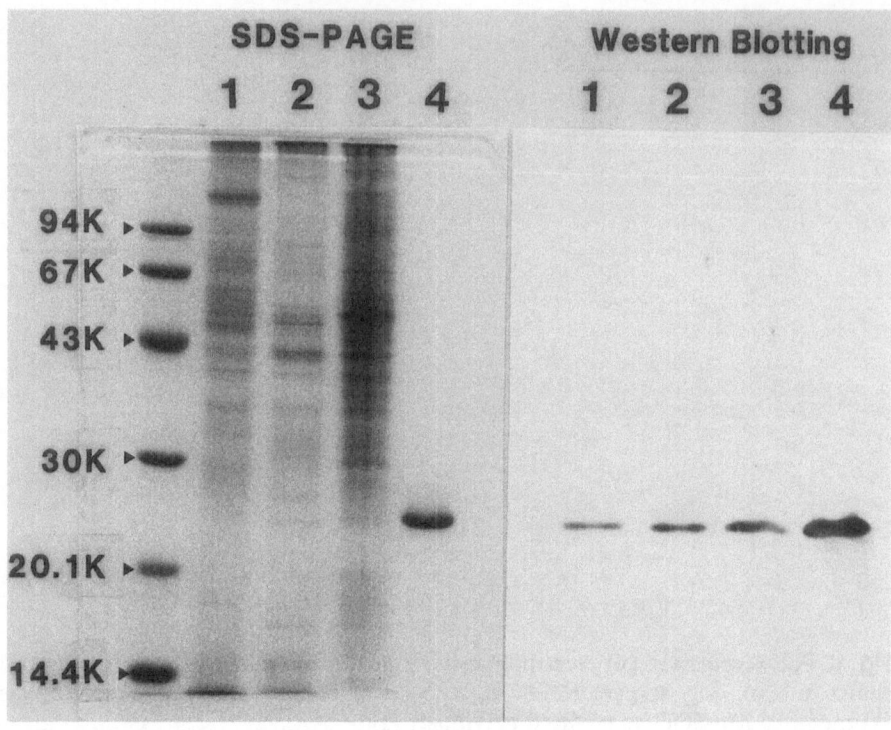

Fig. 2. Specificity of purified polyclonal antibody against rat Mn-SOD. *Left panel,* SDS-PAGE; *right panel,* Western blotting. *Lanes 1, 2, 3,* and *4* of both panels indicate the samples from liver, heart, and brain and purified Mn-SOD, respectively

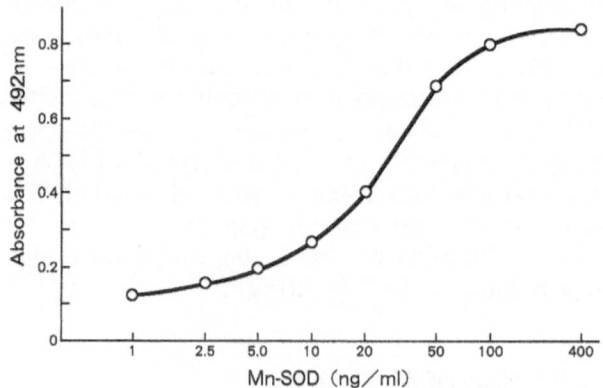

Fig. 3. Standard curve of ELISA for rat Mn-SOD

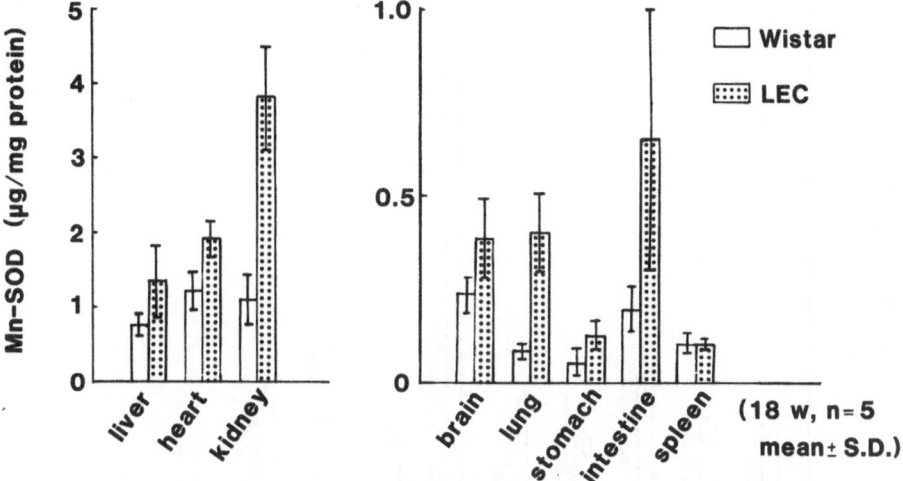

Fig. 4. Tissue distribution of Mn-SOD in LEC and Wistar rats

measured by ELISA. As a control, Mn-SOD levels were also determined for tissues of five Wistar rats (male, 11-week-old) which had about the same body weight as the LEC rats.

Mn-SOD concentrations were higher in LEC rats than in Wistar rats in almost all of the tissues except in the spleen (Fig. 4). Mn-SOD was abundant in liver, heart, and kidney of both Wistar and LEC rats.

Tissue Distribution of Cu,Zn-SOD

The distribution of Cu,Zn-SOD was also determined. Cu,Zn-SOD levels of liver, kidney, and intestine were lower in LEC rats than in Wistar rats (Fig. 5). In the other examined organs, Cu,Zn-SOD levels in LEC rats were almost the same as those in Wistar rats.

Discussion

It was recently found that copper ion accumulated in LEC rats and that the pathogenesis of hepatitis and hepatoma in LEC rats was similar to Wilson's disease [8]. However, LEC rats also display various abnormalities in the expression of drug-metabolizing enzymes [9–12] and maturation of T cells [13]. Therefore, the occurrence of hepatitis and hepatoma cannot be explained by a single mechanism. It is well known that copper ion enhances the generation of oxy-radicals in various tissues. It could be expected that an increase in oxy-radicals is associated with hepatitis and hepatocarcinogenesis in LEC rats. In fact, Mn-SOD levels were found to be much higher

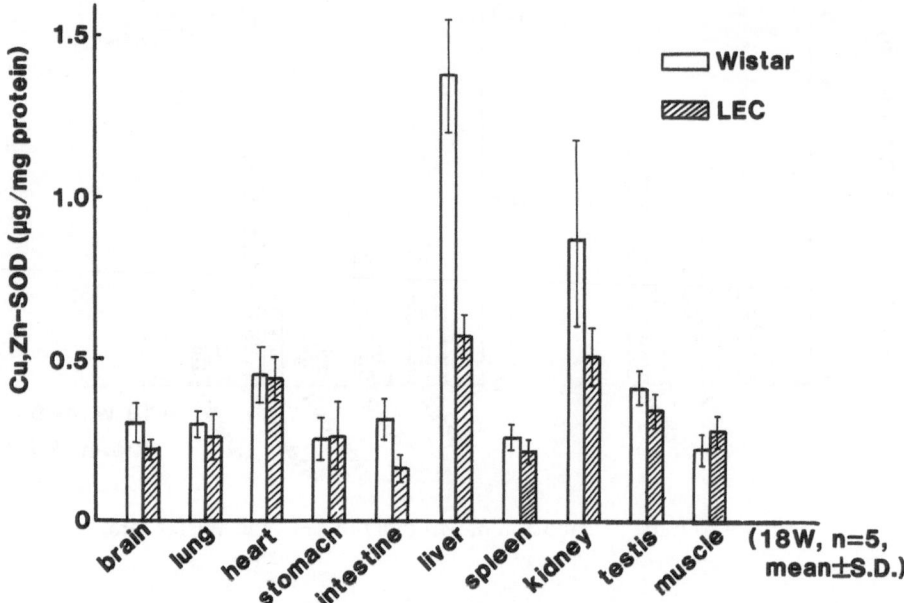

Fig. 5. Tissue distribution of Cu,Zn-SOD in LEC and Wistar rats

in LEC rats than in Wistar rats, whereas Cu,Zn-SOD levels were lower in the LEC rats. These facts suggested that the regulation of expression of each SOD in LEC rats is quite different, and that the SODs serve different roles in the tissues.

Cu,Zn-SOD is located in cytosol, while Mn-SOD is located in mitochondria. In human cell lines, the tumor necrosis factor (TNF) and Interleukin-1 (IL-1) increase both mRNA and protein levels of Mn-SOD, but Cu,Zn-SOD is insensitive to these cytokines [14–16]. Mn-SOD production in LEC rats may be also induced by TNF or IL-1 released from macrophages or neutrophiles during the process of hepatitis and hepatocarcinogenesis. A possible mechanism for Mn-SOD expression in the LEC rats is shown in Fig. 6.

The total activity and content of SODs in human liver seem to be kept at constant values [17]. In the liver of LEC rats, the Mn-SOD content is higher but Cu,Zn-SOD is lower than in Wistar rats. It appears that Cu,Zn-SOD production is suppressed in rat liver and kidney in which Mn-SOD production is increased, and that the total level of SOD in the liver and kidney seems to remain at a constant as it does in human tissues. The low level of Cu,Zn-SOD and the high level of Mn-SOD are probably adaptive responses to intrahepatic oxy-radical formation. Cu,Zn-SOD is considered to be labile to oxy-radicals, whereas Mn-SOD is resistant [18]. Therefore, a mechanism for preferential production of Mn-SOD may exist to optimize the defense of the tissues against oxy-radicals.

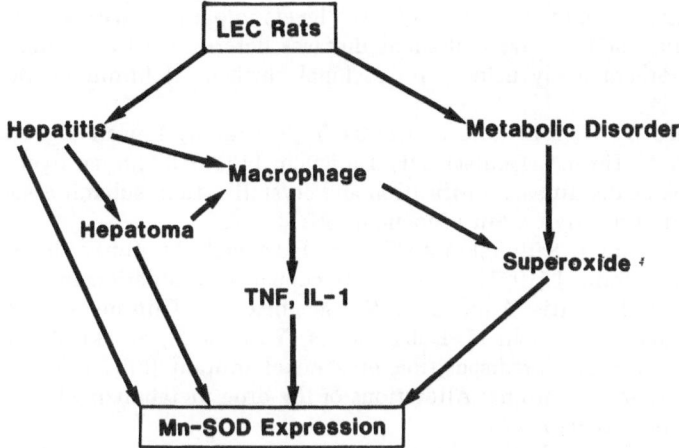

Fig. 6. A possible mechanism of Mn-SOD expression in LEC rats

Conclusions

High expressions of Mn-SOD and low expressions of Cu,Zn-SOD were found in LEC rats. These data suggest that oxy-radicals may play an important role in the process of hepatitis and hepatocarcinogenesis in LEC rats and that some system to regulate synthesis of SODs is active in these rats.

References

1. Oberley LW, Oberley TD (1986) Free radicals, cancer, and aging. In: Johnson JE Jr, Walford R, Harma D, Michel J (eds) Free radicals, aging and degenerative diseases. Alan R Liss, New York, pp 325–371
2. Cerutti PA (1985) Prooxidant states and tumor promotion. Science 227:375–381
3. Troll W, Fenke K, Teebor G (1984) Free oxygen radicals: Necessary contributions to tumor promotion and cocarcinogenesis. In: Fukiki H (ed) Cellular interactions by environmental tumor promoters. VUN Science, Utrecht, pp 207–210
4. Kawaguchi T, Noj, S, Uda T, Nakashima Y, Takeyasu A, Kawai Y, Takagi H, Tohyama M, Taniguchi N (1989) A monoclonal antibody agaist COOH-terminal peptide of human liver manganese superoxide dismutase. J Biol Chem 264:5762–5767
5. Ishikawa M, Yaginuma Y, Hayashi H, Shimizu T, Endo Y, Taniguchi N (1990) Reactivity of a monoclonal antibody to manganese superoxide dismutase with human ovarian carcinoma. Cancer Res 50:2538–2542
6. Kawaguchi T, Suzuki K, Matsuda Y, Nishiura T, Uda T, Ono M, Sekiya C, Ishikawa M, Iino S, Endo Y, Taniguchi N (1990) Serum Mn-superoxide dis-

mutase: Normal values and increased levels in patients with acute myocardial infarction and several malignant diseases determined by enzyme-linked immunosorbent assay using a monoclonal antibody. J Immunol Methods 127: 249–254

7. Matsuda Y, Higashiyama S, Kijima Y, Suzuki K, Kawano K, Akiyama M, Kawata S, Tarui S, Deutsch HF, Taniguchi N (1990) Human liver manganese superoxide dismutase: Purification and crystallization, subunit association and sulfhydryl reactivity. Eur J Biochem 194:713–720

8. Li Y, Togashi Y, Sato S, Emoto T, Kang J, Takeichi N, Kobayashi H, Kojima Y, Une Y, Uchino J (1991) Spontaneous copper accumulation in LEC rats with hereditary hepatitis: A model of Wilson's disease. J Clin Invest 87:1858–1861

9. Sugiyama T, Takeichi N, Kobayashi H, Yoshida M, Sasaki M, Taniguchi N (1988) Metabolic predisposition of a novel mutant (LEC rats) to hereditary hepatitis and hepatoma: Alterations of the drug metabolizing enzymes. Carcinogensis 9:1569–1572

10. Sugiyama T, Suzuki K, Ookawara T, Kurosawa T, Taniguchi N (1989) Selective expression and induction of cytochrome $P450_{PB}$ and $P450_{MC}$ during the development of hereditary hepatitis and hepatoma of LEC rats. Carcinogenesis 10:2155–2159

11. Suzuki K, Sugiyama T, Ookawara T, Kurosawa T, Taniguchi N (1991) High sensitivity to 5-azacytidine in LEC rats, a strain with a metabolic predisposition to hepatitis and hepatoma: Possible involvement of DNA methylation in the expression of cytochrome P-450 and γ-glutamyl transpeptisdase. Biochem Int 23:9–14

12. Sugiyama T, Matsunaga M, Jain SK, Jain S, Ikeda Y, Taniguchi N (1991) Enhancing effect of a choline-deficient diet on alterations of hepatic drug-metabolizing enzymes in hepatitis- and hepatoma-predisposed rats (LEC rats). Jpn J Cancer Res 82:390–396

13. Agui T, Oka M, Yamada T, Sakai T, Izumi K, Ishida Y, Himeno K, Matsumoto K (1990) Maturational arrest from $CD4^+8^+$ to $CD4^+8^-$ thymocytes in a mutant strain (LEC) of rat. J Exp Med 172:1615–1624

14. Wong GHW, Goeddel DV (1988) Induction of manganous superoxide dismutase by tumor necrosis factor: Possible protective mechanism. Science 242:941–944

15. Masuda A, Longo DL, Kobayashi Y, Appella E, Oppenheim JJ, Matsushima K (1988) Induction of mitochondrial manganese superoxide dismutase by interleuken 1. FASEB J 2:3087–3090

16. Kawaguchi T, Takeyasu A, Matsunobu K, Uda T, Ishizawa M, Suzuki K, Nishiura T, Ishikawa M, Taniguchi N (1990) Stimulation of Mn-superoxide dismutase expression by tumor necrosis factor-α: Quantitative determination of Mn-SOD protein levels in TNF-resistant and sensitive cells by ELISA. Biochem Biophys Res Commun 171:1378–1386

17. Deutsch HF, Hoshi S, Matsuda Y, Suzuki K, Kawano K, Kitagawa Y, Katsube Y, Taniguchi N (1991) Preparation of human manganese superoxide dismutase tri-phase-partitioning and preliminary crystallographic data. J Mol Biol 219: 103–108

18. Salo DC, Pacifici RE, LIn SW, Giulivi C, Davies KJA (1990) Superoxide dismutase undergoes proteolysis and fragmentation following oxidative modification and inactivation. J Biol Chem 265:11919–11927

16 — Decreased Activities of S-Adenosylmethionine Synthetase Isozymes in Hereditary Hepatitis in LEC Rats

KINJI TSUKADA[1] and MICHIO MORI[2]

Introduction

In mammalian livers, methionine is mostly degraded via a trans-sulphuration pathway in which S-adenosylmethionine (AdoMet) transfers methyl groups to other molecules.

Enzymatic synthesis of AdoMet is catalyzed by AdoMet synthetase (ATP: L-methionine S-adenosyltransferase, EC 2.5.1.6):

$$\text{Methionine} + \text{ATP} \rightarrow \text{AdoMet} + \text{PPi} + \text{Pi}$$

As reported by Cantoni and Durell [1,2], the three phosphates of ATP are cleaved. The 5'-deoxyadenosyl group of ATP is transferred to one free electron pair from the sulfur atom of L-methionine and tripolyphosphate is formed at the same time. This then generates pyrophosphate and inorganic phosphate; the former originates from α- and β-phosphate groups, and the latter from the γ-phosphate of ATP. The enzyme-bound intermediate, tripolyphosphate, is cleaved by a tripolyphosphatase that is associated with purified AdoMet synthetase from yeast [3], E. coli [4], and rat liver [5].

Three isozymes, termed α (or I), β (or III) and γ (or II), of AdoMet synthetase have been demonstrated in mammalian tissues [6–13]. These isozymes can be distinguished by their dependency on sulfhydryl reagents, sensitivity to dimethyl sulfoxide (Me$_2$SO), kinetic properties, and molecular weights. At least two isozymes, the α- and β-forms, are present in adult liver, and the γ-form is found in kidney, fetal liver [8,11], and every other tissue, except for adult liver [11]. The β-form was purified to homogeneity from rat liver cytosol [14,15], and antiserum against the β-form was shown to cross-react with the α-form and the β-form, but not with the γ-form [14]. The general properties of AdoMet synthetase isozymes are shown in Table 1.

[1] Department of Pathological Biochemistry, Medical Research Institute, Tokyo Medical and Dental University, Chiyoda-ku, Tokyo, 101 Japan
[2] Department of Pathology, Sapporo Medical College, Sapporo, 060 Japan

Table 1. Properties of AdoMet synthtetase isozymes.

Properties	Liver (α)	Liver (β)	Kidney (γ)
	Relative activity (% control)		
Control assay system	100	100	100
$-Mg^{2+}$	1	1	1
$-K^+$	1	1	1
−Dithiothreitol	33	27	97
−Dithiothreitol + p−mercurubenzoate	2	5	78
+Dimethylsulfoxide	135	1500	86
+Tripolyphosphate	20	175	32
Molecular mass (kd)	200	100	160−190
$s20,w$ (S)	8.0	5.5	7.5
Subunits (kd)	4 × 48	2 × 48	?
K_m for methionine (μM)	17	500	6
K_m for ATP (μM)	500	2000	70

The γ-form predominantly exists in fetal rat liver and gradually decreases along with appearance of the α- and β-forms during development [13]. When adult rats are treated with a hepatocarcinogen, N-2-fluorenylacetamide, the α- and β-forms are replaced by the γ-form according to the stages of carcinogenesis in the liver [16]. Recently Mato's groups have reported a marked decrease (around 50%) in the activity of AdoMet synthetase of human cirrhotic liver [17]. This decrease was due to a specific reduction in the higher molecular weight (α-form) of AdoMet synthetase in a group of cirrhotic patients We demonstrated a markedly decreased activity of AdoMet synthetase isozymes in LEC rat liver with hereditary hepatitis, and also in rat liver treated with CCl₄ [18].

Decreased Activities of AdoMet Synthetase from Livers of LEC Rats with Time

The activity of AdoMet synthetase isozyme in rat liver in hereditary hepatitis was assayed in the presence or absence of Me_2SO after birth. With time, the activity in the LEC rat liver decreased, although the stimulation ratio by Me_2SO of this activity in rat liver was not changed (Table 2).

Separation of the α- and β-form Isozymes of AdoMet Synthetase from Livers by Phenyl-Sepharose Chromatography

We tried to separate both isozymes in order to determine which activity of liver isozymes changes the α and β forms. For separating the α- and β-forms of AdoMet synthetase, the soluble fraction from the normal liver and LEC

Table 2. Effect of Me_2SO on AdoMet synthetase activity in LEC rat liver with time.

Age (Weeks)	AdoMet synthetase activity (units/mg protein)		Stimulation ratio (+/−)
	$-Me_2SO$	$+Me_2SO$	
LEA (Control strain)			
30	0.094 ± 0.01	1.05 ± 0.09	11.1
LEC (Hereditary hepatitis)			
29	0.080 ± 0.007	0.93 ± 0.08	11.6
42	0.038 ± 0.004	0.41 ± 0.04	10.5

liver (with hereditary hepatitis) from rats of the same age were loaded onto a column of phenyl-Sepharose. When the column was washed with Buffer A, the first peak (the α-form) of AdoMet synthetase was eluted (Fig. 1), and showed only a 1.5-fold activation by 10% (v/v) Me_2SO. A second peak (the β-form) of the enzyme was eluted from the column with Buffer A/50% Me_2SO. This fraction was markedly activated by the addition of more Me_2SO to the standard reaction mixture (Fig. 1a). The activities of the first and second peaks decreased strikingly in 30-week-old LEC rat liver (Fig. 1b).

The reduction in specific activities of AdoMet synthetase isozymes in the liver of hereditary hepatitis was accompanied by a decrease in the AdoMet concentration in the liver. AdoMet concentrations in livers from normal rats and from those with hereditary hepatitis were 110 ± 13 nmol/g dry liver and 50 ± 7 nmol/g dry liver (the mean of the results obtained from 4 to 5 rats and the standard deviations). The same decreased activity of AdoMet synthetase isozymes in the liver was observed in rats adminis-tered CCl_4 (Fig. 2).

The values of AdoMet in the cells were almost parallel with the change in the activity of the α-form isozyme [19]. On the other hand, the activity of the β-form in mouse liver was increased following intraperitoneal trans-plantation of Ehrlich ascites tumor cells, although the levels of AdoMet did not significantly change in the liver [20]. These results suggested that only the α-form is principally functional in the liver.

In malignant cells, increased activity of tRNA-methyl-transferase and decreased activity of glycine-methyl-transferase found mainly in the liver have been demonstrated [21–24]. However, in these preparations, both activities in rat liver with hereditary hepatitis showed no significant change (Table 3).

Summary

Isozyme patterns of S-adenosylmethionine synthetase have been measured with or without dimethylsulfoxide in livers of the LEC rat with hereditary hepatitis. The activities of the α- and β-forms are decreased with age after

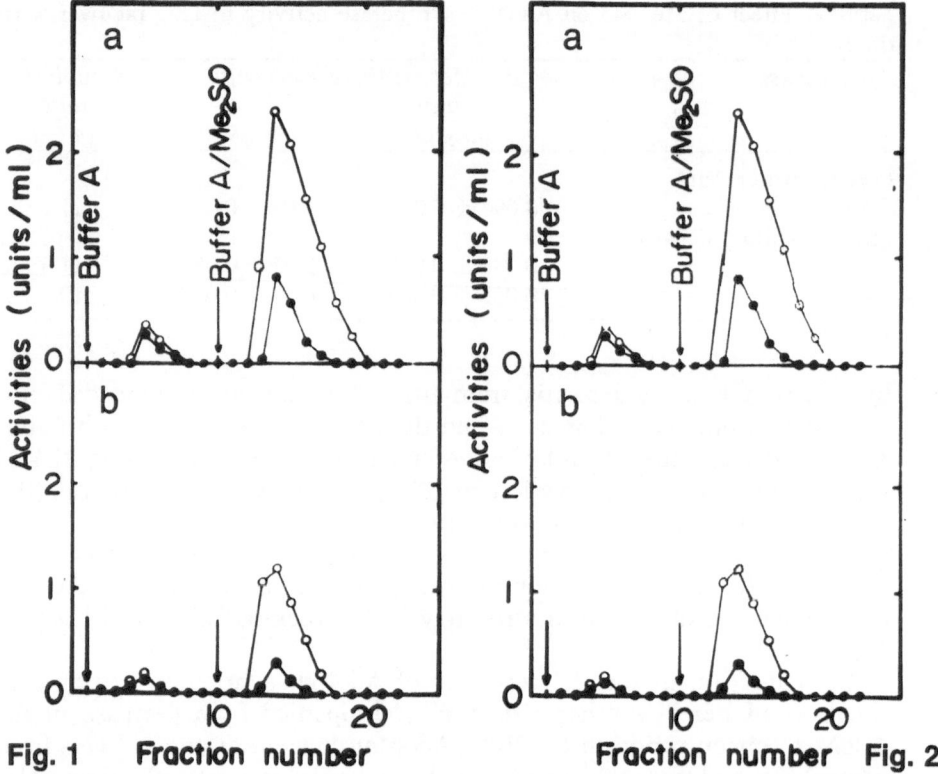

Fig. 1   Fraction number   **Fraction number   Fig. 2**

Fig. 1. Phenyl-Sepharose chromatography of AdoMet synthetase from livers of LEA and LEC rats. The soluble fraction (1 ml) saturated with 20% ammonium sulfate was applied onto a phenylsepharose column (1 × 3 cm) equilibrated with 0.05 M Tris-HCl (pH 7.8), 0.2 mM dithiothreitol, 0.1 mM EDTA, 10 mM MgCl$_2$ (Buffer A) containing 20% saturated (NH$_4$)$_2$SO$_4$. The α-form of AdoMet synthetase was eluted with 10 ml Buffer A, and then the column was eluted with 10 ml Buffer A/50% Me$_2$SO to recover the β-form. Fractions of 0.5 ml were collected. An aliqout (0.01 ml) from each fraction was taken to determine the enzyme activity with (○) or without (●) 10% (v/v) Me$_2$SO. **a** LEA (control strain) liver, **b** LEC (hereditary hepatitis) liver. Both rats were sacrificed at 36 weeks of age

Fig. 2. Phenyl-Sepharose chromatography of AdoMet synthetase from livers of CCl$_4$-treated rats. **b** A normal Wistar rat was injected a CCl$_4$ 50% olive oil solution (0.4 ml/100 g body weight) intraperitoneally 48 h before being sacrificed. **a** Only olive oil was used for a control injection. The liver soluble fractions used for the column chromato-graphy are described in Fig. 1

birth, reaching one-half the normal level on 36 weeks after birth. Concentration of S-adenosylmethionine in the liver is almost one-half the level of control rats. However, the activity of glycine- and tRNA-methyltransferases in the liver shows no significant change.

Table 3. Specific activiy of glycine and tRNA-methyl trans-
ferases in liver of LEC rats with time.

Ages (weeks)	Methyltransferase activity (cpm)	
	Glycine	tRNA
LEA (Control strain)		
30	6120 ± 580	4300 ± 410
LEC (Hereditary hepatitis)		
42	6010 ± 600	4150 ± 420
	6210 ± 690	4100 ± 400

The values of glycine methyl transferase activity are cpm [methyl–^{3}H]
incorporated to glycine per 20 min, and the value of tRNA methyltransferase activity are cpm [methyl–^{3}H] incorporated per 20 μg E. coli
tRNA (MRE 600, Böhringer Mannheim) per 40 min. Each value is the
means ±S.D. of 3 or 4 determinations

References

1. Cantoni GL (1953) S-adenosylmethionine: A new intermediate formed en-
   zymatically from L-methionine and adenosine-triphosphate. J Biol Chem 204:
   403–415
2. Cantoni GL, Durell J (1957) Activation of methionine for transmethylation; II.
   The methionine activating enzyme: Studies on the mechanism of the reaction.
   J Biol Chem 225:1033–1048
3. Mudd SH (1963) Activation of methionine for transmethylation; VI. Enzyme-
   bound tripolyphosphate as an intermediate in the reaction catalyzed by the
   methionine activating enzyme of Baker's yeast. J Biol Chem 238:2156–2163
4. Markham GD, Hafner EW, Tabor CW, Tabor H (1980) S-adenosyl-methionine
   synthetase from Escherichia coli. J Biol Chem 255:9082–9092
5. Shimizu K, Maruyama I, Iijima S, Tsukada K (1986) Tripolyphosphatase associated with S-adenosylmethionine synthetase isozymes. Biochim Biophys Acta
   883:293–298
6. Hoffman JL, Kunz GL (1977) Differential activation of rat liver methionine
   adenosyltransferase isozymes by dimethyl-sulfoxide. Biochem Biophys Res
   Commun 77:1231–1236
7. Liau MC, Lin GW, Hurbert RB (1977) Partial purification and characterization
   of tumor and liver S-adenosylmethionine synthetases. Cancer Res 37:427–435
8. Okada G, Sawai Y, Teraoka H, Tsukada K (1979) Differential effects of
   dimethylsulfoxide on S-adenosylmethionine synthetase from rat liver and
   hepatoma. FEBS Lett 106:25–28
9. Liau MC, Chan CF, Belanger L, Grenier A (1979) Correlation of isozyme
   patterns of S-adenosylmethionine synthetase with fetal stages and pathological
   states of the liver. Cancer Res 39:162–169
10. Abe T, Yamano H, Teraoka H, Tsukada K (1980) Changes in the activities of S-
    adenosylmethionine synthetase isozymes from rat liver on ethionine adminis-
    tration. FEBS Lett 121:29–32

11. Okada G, Teraoka H, Tsukada K (1980) Multiple species of mammalian S-adenosylmethionine synthetase: Partial purification and characterization. Biochemistry 20:934–940
12. Sullivan DM, Hoffman JL (1983) Fractionation and kinetic properties of rat liver and kidney merhionine adenosyltransferase isozymes. Biochemistry 22:1636–1641
13. Okada G, Watanabe Y, Tsukada K (1980) Changes in patterns of S-adenosylmethionine synthetases in fetal and postnatal rat liver. Cancer Res 40:2895–2897
14. Abe T, Okada G, Teraoka H, Tsukada K (1982) Immunological distinction of S-adenosylmethionine synthetase isozymes from rat liver and kidney. J Biochem 91:1081–1084
15. Suma Y, Shimizu K, Tsukada K (1986) Isozymes of S-adenosylmethionine synthetase from rat liver: Isolation and characterization. J Biochem 100:67–75
16. Tsukada K, Okada G (1980) S-adenosylmethionine synthetase isozyme patterns from rat hepatoma induced by N-2-fluorenylacetamide. Biochem Biophys Res Commun 94:1078–1082
17. Cabrero C, Duce AM, Ortiz P, Alemany S, Mato JM (1988) Specific lost of the high-Mr form of S-adenosylmethionine synthetase in human liver cirrhosis. Hepatology 8:1530–1534
18. Shimizu K, Abe M, Yokoyama S, Takahashi H, Sawada N, Mori M, Tsukada K (1990) Decreased activities of S-Adenosyl-methionine synthetase isozymes in hereditary hepatitis in Long-Evans rats. Life Sci 46:1837–1842
19. Matsumoto C, Suma Y, Tsukada K (1984) The α-form of S-adenosylmethionine synthetase isozymes from liver is principally functional. J Biochem 95:1223–1226
20. Abe T, Tsukada K (1981) S-adenosylmethionine synthetase isozymes in the liver of tumor-bearing animals. J Biochem 90:571–574
21. Borek E, Kerr SJ (1972) Atypical transfer RNAs and their origin in neoplastic cells. Adv Cancer Res 15:163–190
22. Craddock UM (1972) Increased activity of transfer RNA N^2-guaninedimethylase in tumors of liver and kidney. Biochim Biophys Acta 272:288–296
23. Kuchino Y, Endo H, Nishimura S (1975) Comparison of the specificity and extent in vitro methylation by guanylate residue-specific transfer RNA methylases isolated from ascites hepatoma, 3'-methyl-4-dimethylaminoazobenzene-induced hepatoma, and normal rat liver. Cancer Res 32:1243–1250
24. Kerr SJ (1972) Competing methyltransferase system. J Biol Chem 247:4248–4252

17 — LEC Rats Mimic LEA Rats Fed a Choline-Deficient Diet

Toshihiro Sugiyama, Mikako Matsunaga, Yoshitaka Ikeda, and Naoyuki Taniguchi[1]

Introduction

Previous studies [1,2] have shown that the composition and the activities of enzymes involved in drug metabolism in LEC rats are quite similar to those observed in hyperplastic foci and nodules induced by chemical carcinogens [3,4]. Dietary deficiencies of methionine and choline have been shown to enhance the activities of several hepatocarcinogens, and ethionine is known to be both a hepatocarcinogen and an anti-metabolite of methionine. Therefore, we thought choline deficiency and ethionine treatment might provide useful model systems. In the present study, we used immunochemical and biochemical methods to investigate the hepatic enzyme alterations in LEC rats fed a choline-deficient diet or in LEC rats treated with ethionine.

Effect of Choline Deficiency and Ethionine Treatment on Hepatic Drug Metabolism in LEC Rats

Growth and Hepatitis

The choline-deficient diet led to weight decreases in both LEC and LEA rats. No significant growth was seen in any rats which were fed this diet (Fig. 1). A choline-deficient diet appears to strongly enhance hepatitis development in LEC rats. The short-term (4 weeks) administration of a choline-deficient diet produced a high incidence of hepatitis and severe jaundice was developed in two-thirds of the LEC rats which died. On the other hand, all of the LEA male rats were still alive without any significant clinical symptoms after the 4 experimental weeks.

---

[1] Department of Biochemistry, Osaka University Medical School, Suita, Osaka, 565 Japan

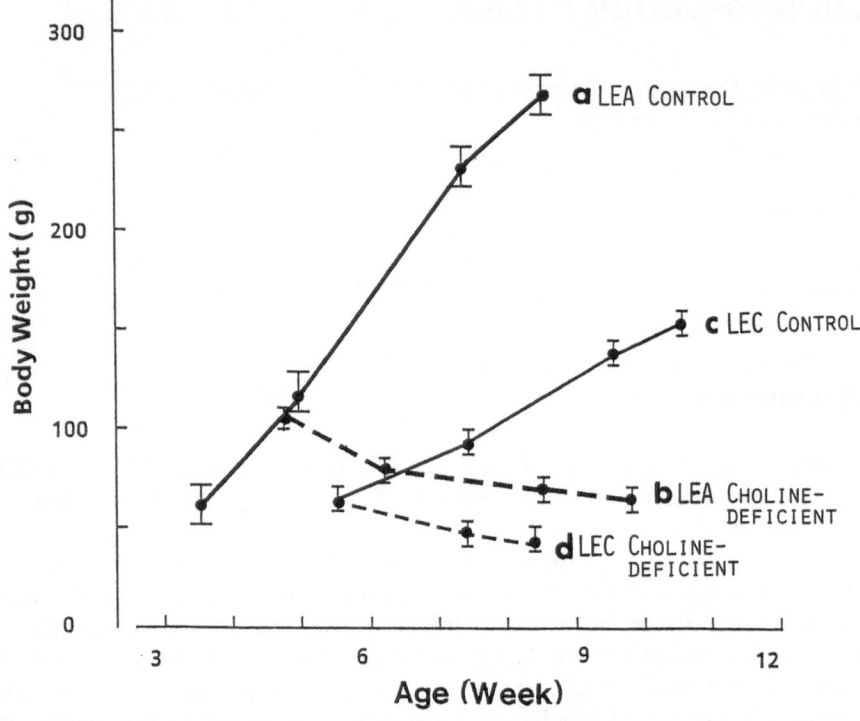

Fig. 1. Effects of a choline-deficient diet on the growth of LEC and LEA male rats. **a** (●—●), LEA control diet; **b** (●--●), LEA choline-deficient diet; **c** (●—●), LEC control diet; **d** (●--●), LEC choline-deficient diet. *Points,* mean of 9–15 values; *bar,* SD

Figure 2 shows the effect of the administration of ethionine on the body weight and serum glutamic-oxaloacetic transaminase (GOT) activity in the LEC rats. The ethionine-treated LEC rats showed a severe weight loss and a marked increase in GOT for 10 days.

Hepatic Drug-Metabolizing Enzymes in LEC and LEA Rats Fed a Choline-Deficient Diet

Figure 3 shows the changes in the hepatic drug-metabolizing enzymes in LEC and LEA rats after being on a choline-deficient diet for 4 weeks. Total microsomal cytochrome P-450 levels were decreased to about 35% of control in LEC male rats. Ethoxyresorufin O-deethylase and pentoxyresorufin O-depentylase activities were markedly decreased to 14% and 13% of the control, respectively. In contrast, γ-glutamyltranspeptidase activity was dramatically increased to 570% of the control level. A small elevation of serum GOT activity was observed in LEC rats fed the choline-deficient diet, suggesting the presence of liver cell injury. The choline-deficient diet decreased the cytosolic glutathione S-transferase activity of LEC rats to about 48% of the control.

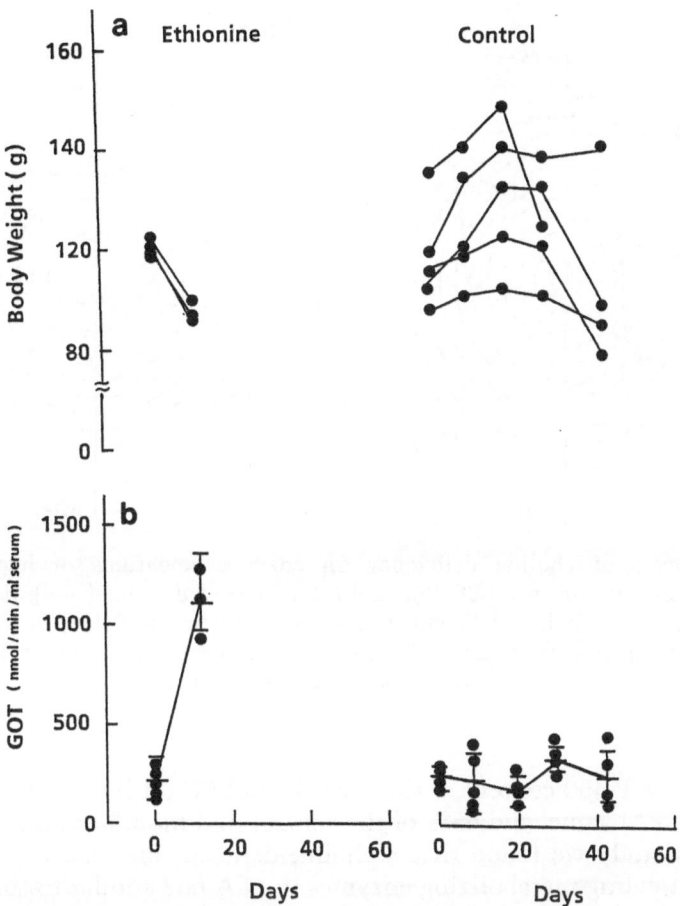

Fig. 2. Effects of ethionine treatment (L-ethionine 200 mg/kg body weight/day, and saline for control, i.p.) on the growth and serum glutamic oxaloacetic transaminase (GOT) activity of LEC rats

In LEA rats, the effects of choline-deficient feeding on these enzymes were quite similar to those observed in LEC except for ethoxyresorufin O-deethylase activity (Fig. 3b). The P-450 content, pentoxyresorufin O-depentylase activity, and glutathione S-transferase activity decreased to 39%, 23%, and 47% of the levels in control LEA rats, respectively, whereas ethoxyresorufin O-deethylase activity remained the same as in LEA control rats. γ-Glutamyltranspeptidase activity increased to almost the same level as that in LEC rats fed the choline-deficient diet.

In this study, we demonstrated that cytochrome P-450 in hepatic microsomes from LEC and LEA rats fed a choline-deficient diet has reduced capacity to catalyze the oxidation of pentoxyresorufin rather than ethoxyresorufin. Similar selective changes in other mixed function oxidase activities may occur in spontaneous hepatic carcinogenesis of LEC rats [4]; the

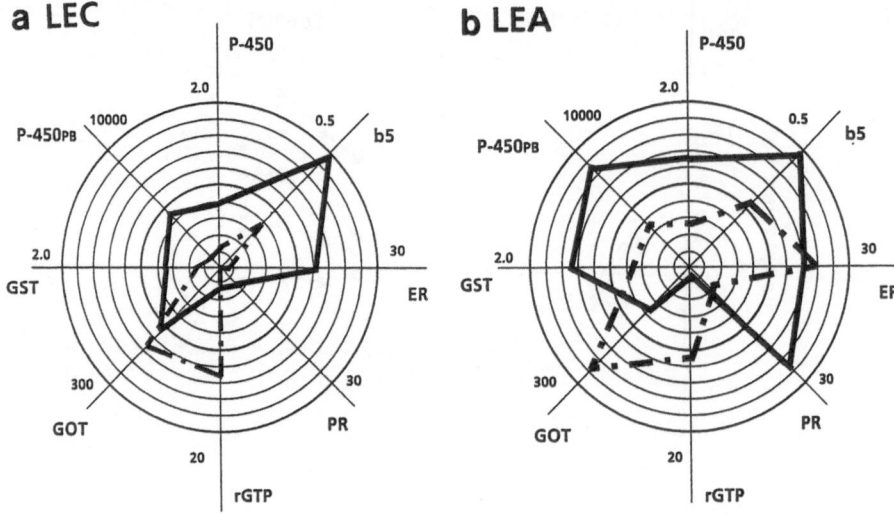

Fig. 3. Effects of choline deficiency on enzyme deviations of hepatic drug-metabolizing system in **a** LEC rats and **b** LEA rats. *Solid line* (——), normal diet; *dashed line* (....), choline-deficient diet. *P-450*, cytochrome P-450; b_5, cytochrome b_5; *ER*, ethoxyresorufin O-deethylase; *PR*, pentoxyresorufin O-depentylase; γ*GTP*, γ-glutamyltranspeptidase; *GST*, glutathione S-transferase

cytochrome P-450 content of the 4-week-old LEC rat liver was 43% of the control (LEA) value, and 65% of the control in 3-month-old rats.

In this study we found that a choline-deficient diet caused changes in the hepatic drug-metabolizing enzymes in LEA rats similar to those occurring spontaneously in LEC rats. The similarity between the patterns of enzyme alterations in the choline-deficient feeding LEA (*dashed line*, Fig. 3b) and the normal diet LEC rats (*solid line*, Fig. 3a) suggests that LEC rats mimic LEA rats fed a choline-deficient diet and that LEC rats have endogenously initiated cells which spontaneously develop hepatitis and hepatoma. This is the first demonstration of a common cellular responses to a methyl-group-devoid diet and endogenous factors acting as inducers of hepatitis.

Western Blot Analysis of the Drug-Metabolizing Enzymes in LEC Rats Fed the Choline-Deficient Diet and Treated with Ethionine

The expression of glutathione S-transferase P (GST-Yp) protein in the LEC rats was investigated after rats were subjected to a choline-deficient diet and ethionine treatment. A typical Western blot is shown in Fig. 4a. Compared to the LEC rats fed the normal diet, the LEC rats fed a choline-deficient diet and treated with ethionine had 33-fold and 26-fold increases in the level of GST-Yp protein, respectively (Fig. 4b).

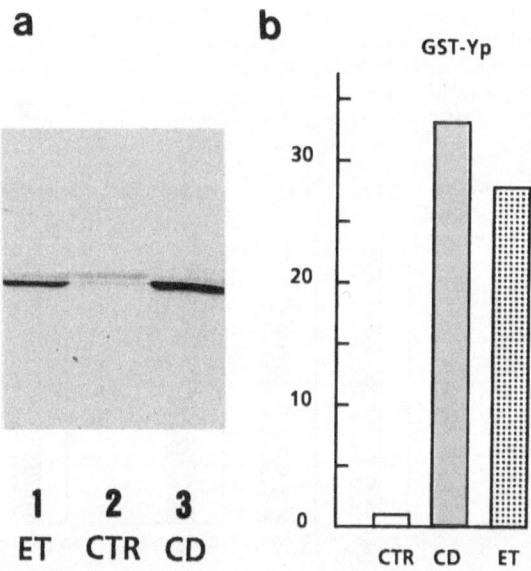

Fig. 4. Expression of glutathione *S*-transferase P (GST-Yp) in the cytosols from the LEC rats fed a choline-deficient diet (*CD*) or treated with ethionine (200 mg/kg body weight, daily i.p.). **a** Western blotting by rat GST-Yp antibody. Immunoblots were carried out using 20 µg protein per lane for each cytosolic fraction. *Lane 1: ET*, ethionine treatment; *Lane 2: CRT*, control diet; *lane 3: CD*, choline-deficient diet. **b** Relative levels of GST-Yp protein in the LEC cytosols

Immunoquantitations of hepatic drug-metabolizing enzymes were carried out (Fig. 5). Levels of the $P\text{-}450_{PB}$ and $P\text{-}450_{MC}$ forms of cytochrome P-450 were markedly decreased in liver microsomes from LEC rats fed the choline-deficient diet. The cytochrome $P\text{-}450_{PB}$ level was only 35% of that in control microsomes, and the $P\text{-}450_{MC}$ level was decreased to 16% of the control. There was a marked difference in the relative composition of glutathione *S*-transferase subunits between LEC rats fed the choline-deficient and the control diets. Following choline-deficient feeding, LEC rats had 26-fold higher levels of GST-Yp protein than LEC rats fed the control diet. In contrast, the levels of GST-Ya, Yb1, and Yb2 decreased to 59%, 77% and 42% of the control, respectively.

Conclusions

Marked alterations of hepatic drug-metabolizing enzymes were observed in hepatitis- and hepatoma-predisposed rats (LEC rats) fed a choline-deficient diet. The diet enhanced the development of hepatitis with severe jaundice.

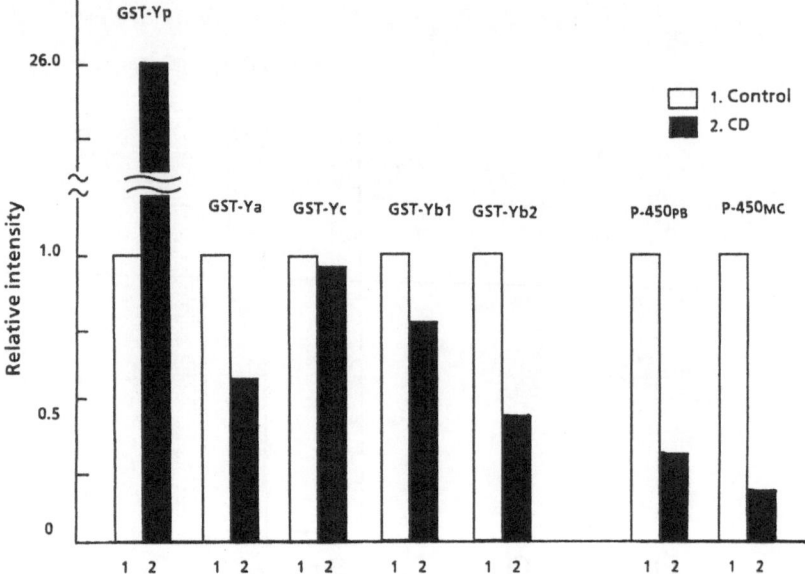

Fig. 5. Relative immunoquantitation of glutathione S-transferase subunits, and cytochromes P-450$_{PB}$ and P-450$_{MC}$ in LEC rat fed a control diet and a choline-deficient diet (*CD*). The *columns* represent the staining intensity relative to the samples from LEC rats fed a normal diet

Cytochrome P-450 in hepatic microsomes from LEC and LEA rats fed a choline-deficient diet has reduced capacity to catalyze the oxidation of pentoxyresorufin rather than ethoxyresorufin. Similar selective changes in other mixed function oxidase activities may occur in the spontaneous hepatic carcinogenesis of LEC rats. The great difference in the cytochrome P-450$_{PB}$ content of liver microsomes between LEC and LEA rats and the maintained constitutive levels of hepatic cytochrome P-450$_{MC}$ in the LEC rats at 4 weeks and 3 months of age had been previously shown. The choline-deficient diet caused marked decreases of the levels of two major classes of cytochrome P-450, P-450$_{PB}$ and P-450$_{MC}$. GST-Yp was dramatically increased, whereas GST-Ya, Yb1, and Yb2 were decreased. LEC rats mimic LEA rats (the control rats to LEC) fed a choline-deficient diet in terms of the above enzyme alterations. The enzyme changes in LEC rats treated with ethionine are also similar to those observed in LEA rats fed a choline-deficient diet. These results suggest that LEC rats have some defects in methyl-group metabolism, including DNA hypomethylation. It is likely that hypomethylation is involved in the pathogenesis of hepatitis and hepatoma in LEC rats. Such hypomethylation may initiate the hepatocytes that spontaneously develop hepatitis and hepatoma.

References

1. Sugiyama T, Takeichi N, Kobayashi H, Yoshida MC, Sasaki M, Taniguchi N (1988) Metabolic predisposition of a novel mutant (LEC rats) to hereditary hepatitis and hepatoma: Alterations of the drug metabolizing enzymes. Carcinogenesis 9:1569–1572
2. Sugiyama T, Suzuki K, Ookawara T, Kurosawa T, Taniguchi N (1989) Selective expression and induction of cytochrome P-450$_{PB}$ and P-450$_{MC}$ during the development of hereditary hepatitis and hepatoma of LEC rats. Carcinogenesis 10:2155–2159
3. Cameron R, Sweeney GD, Jones K, Lee G, Farber E (1976) A relative deficiency of cytochrome P-450 and ary hydrocarbon [benzo (a) pyrene] hydroxylase in hyperplastic nodules induced by 2-acetylaminofluorene in rat liver. Cancer Res 36:3888–3893
4. Åström A, DePierre JW, Eriksson L (1983) Characterization of drug-metabolizing systems in hyperplastic nodules from the livers of rats receiving 2-acetylaminofluorene in their diet. Carcinogenesis 4:577–581

18 — Hypomethylation-Associated Expression of Cytochrome P-450 and γ-Glutamyl Transpeptidase During Hereditary Hepatocarcinogenesis in LEC Rats

SURESH K. JAIN[2], KENJI SUZUKI[3], SADHANA JAIN[2],
TOSHIHIRO SUGIYAMA[1], and NAOYUKI TANIGUCHI[1]

Introduction

Recent evidence suggests that the methylation of specific cytosine residues in DNA is an important factor in regulating gene expression and differentiation in eukaryotes [1,2]. Alterations in the levels and patterns of 5-methyldeoxycytidine have been implicated in many of the basic gene processes of mammalian cells involved in embryogenesis, carcinogenesis, and cell differentiation [3,4]. Hypomethylation of regulatory regions of genes is often associated with enhanced transcriptional activity during carcinogenesis [5,6]. The compiled evidence for this view is based mainly upon the development of tumors elicited by choline-deficient diets which decrease the availability of substrates for DNA methylations in animal models.

A nucleotide analog, 5-azacytidine, is a potent inhibitor of DNA methylation by incorporation into DNA. It can selectively activate eukaryotic gene expression and alter the differentiation stage of cells [7,8]. The possibility that DNA methylation concerns the tissue-specific expression of drug metabolizing enzymes has also been suggested [9,10]. Gooderham and Mannering [11] observed that enzyme activities related to cytochrome P-450 were significantly decreased upon treatment of mice with 5-azacytidine, and we have found that LEC rats are highly sensitive to 5-azacytidine [12].

In previous studies [13,14] we observed that LEC rats have a metabolic predisposition with respect to drug metabolizing enzymes and that the pattern is very similar to that of pre-neoplastic lesions, such as hyperplastic foci or nodules in chemical hepatocarcinogenesis. LEC rats had decreased activities of the phase I enzymes, such as cytochrome P-450, and increased

[1] Department of Biochemistry, Osaka University Medical School, Osaka, 565 Japan
[2] Department of Molecular Pharmacology, Albert Einstein College of Medicine, Bronx, NY 10461, USA
[3] International Research Laboratories, CIBA-GEIGY Japan, Takarazuka, 665 Japan

activities of phase II enzymes, such as γ-glutamyl transpeptidase (γ-GTP) as was observed in chemical hepatocarcinogenesis or in DNA-hypomethylated states. In the present study we elucidated the correlation between DNA methylation and the expression of cytochrome P-450 and γ-GTP in LEC rats.

High Sensitivity of LEC Rats to 5-Azacytidine in the Hepatic Drug-Metabolizing System

The 5-methylcytosine (5-mCyt) content in hepatic DNA of LEC rats was measured in order to determine the mechanism by which changes in the cytochrome P-450 content and γ-GTP occur (Table 1). In comparing LEC and LEA rats, almost no difference was observed between the two strains at 10 and 16 weeks in terms of basal 5-mCyt levels. In addition, the level of 5-mCyt in the 16-week-old LEC rats did not change irrespective of the presence or absence of hepatitis. A single injection of 5-azacytidine (25 mg/kg) caused a statistically significant reduction in the 5-mCyt content of liver DNA of LEC rats, whereas almost no effect of 5-azacytidine was observed in LEA rats.

In both strains of rats, the cytochrome P-450 content decreased in the liver 24 h after the 5-azacytidine treatment. In the LEC rats, the cytochrome P-450 content was markedly reduced in hepatic microsomes to a level of 38% and 56% of the control at ages 10 and 16 weeks, respectively. On the other hand, γ-GTP activity was increased in the LEC rats, whereas no such change was observed in the LEA rats.

Expression of γ-GTP mRNA During Hepatocarcinogenesis

Previous studies have shown that γ-GTP activity in LEC rats was increased 4.3-fold at 3 months, just before the onset of hepatitis [13]. We measured the levels of its mRNA in LEC and LEA rats at different time intervals. Figure 1 shows that there is an age-dependent, biphasic, and increased transcriptional activation of the γ-GTP gene in LEC rats. The level of this mRNA could be barely detected in the livers of either LEA or 8-week-old LEC rats. It is noteworthy that a marked increase in γ-GTP mRNA levels was observed in the LEC rats at around 16 weeks of age, the time of onset of hepatitis.

Different Expression of Cytochrome P-450 Between LEC and LEA Rat Liver

The content of cytochrome P-450 decreased with age in both strains, but was consistently lower in LEC rats [14]. The levels of cytochrome P-450 content in LEC rats were maximal at 8 weeks and decreased steadily by

Table 1. Effect of 5-azacytidine on 5-methylcytosine content and the enzyme alterations in cytochrome P-450 and γ-GTP in LEC and LEA rats

	% Cytosine methylated	P-450 Content (nmol/mg protein)	γ-GTP (nmol/min/mg protein)
LEC 10W	4.01 ± 0.20 (100%)	0.569 ± 0.121 (100%)	1.17 ± 0.32 (100%)
LEC 10W 5AC	3.75 ± 0.15 (94%)*	0.214 ± 0.039 (38%)**	2.00 ± 1.00 (170%)*
LEC 16W	4.07 ± 0.13 (100%)	0.487 ± 0.078 (100%)	2.44 ± 0.82 (100%)
LEC 16W 5AC	3.69 ± 0.07 (91%)**	0.271 ± 0.030 (56%)**	3.06 ± 0.85 (125%)
LEC 16W Jaundice	3.98 ± 0.18 (98%)	0.248 ± 0.069 (51%)	
LEA 10W	3.92 ± 0.22 (100%)	0.975 ± 0.104 (100%)	0.41 ± 0.07 (100%)
LEA 10W 5AC	3.91 ± 0.07 (100%)	0.893 ± 0.150 (92%)	0.50 ± 0.10 (122%)
LEA 16W	4.06 ± 0.11 (100%)	0.730 ± 0.145 (100%)	0.32 ± 0.09 (100%)
LEA 16W 5AC	3.49 ± 0.20 (97%)	0.571 ± 0.112 (78%)	0.31 ± 0.04 (98%)

Animals were given a single i.p. dose of 5-azacytidine (25 mg/kg) and sacrificed at 24 h after the treatment. Student's t-test indicates a statistically significant difference compared to a corresponding value (*$P < 0.05$, **$P < 0.001$)

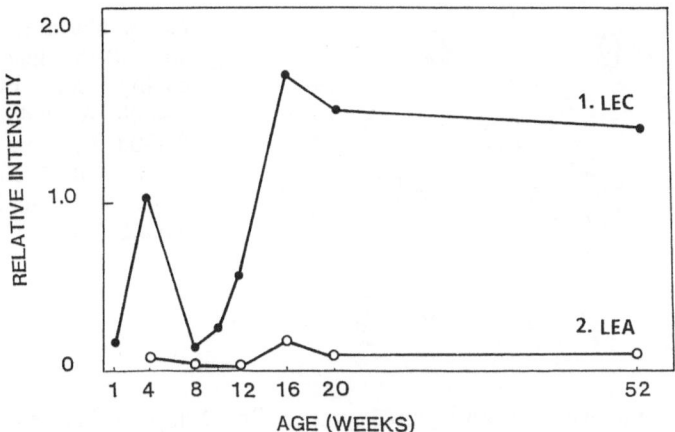

Fig. 1. Age-related levels of hepatic γ-GTP mRNA in LEC (●—●) and LEA (o—o) rats

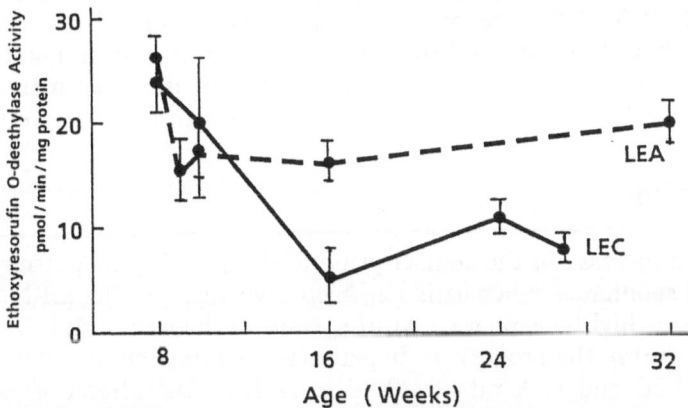

Fig. 2. Age-related changes in microsomal ethoxyresorufin O-deethylase activity in LEC (---) and LEA (●—●) rats

about 50% by 26 weeks of age. The ethoxyresorufin O-deethylase activity in the young (8–10 weeks) LEC rats was greater than that of the young LEA rats, however there was a clear difference in this activity between the LEC and LEA rats after 12 weeks of age (Fig. 2). The decay of the activities of pentoxyresorufin O-depentylase in both strains was similar to the change in ethoxyresorufin O-deethylase activity, except that the pentoxyresorufin O-depentylase activity in the LEC rats was about one-third to that in the LEA rats at all ages studied. The gradual decrease of activities in the LEC rat coincided with the development of spontaneous hepatitis and hepatoma. Apparently the age-related changes in activities for ethoxy-

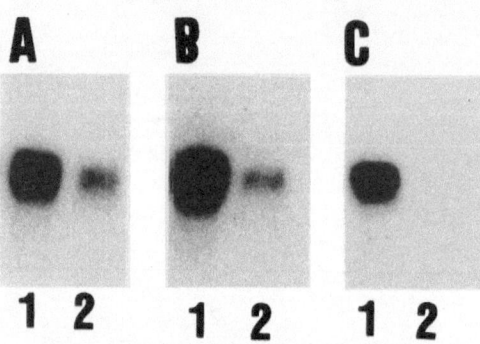

Fig. 3. Northern blotting analysis of hepatic mRNA coding for cytochromes P-450b **A**, P-450c **B**, and P-450d **C**, from LEC rats fed a control diet (*lane 1*) and a choline-deficient diet (*lane 2*)

resorufin *O*-deethylase and pentoxyresorufin *O*-depentylase closely parallel the changes in the cytochrome P-450 isozymes. This suggests that an age-related alteration in decrease in cytochrome P-450 isozymes is responsible for the change in the hepatic microsomal monooxygenase activities.

Following choline-deficient feeding, the levels of two major forms of cytochrome P-450, mainly P-450$_{PB}$ (P450IIB1, P450IIB2) and P-450$_{MC}$ (P450IA1, P450IA2) were markedly decreased in LEC liver microsomes [15]. Northern blots showed that the expression of P-450b, P-450c, and P-450d mRNA in LEC rats fed a choline-deficient diet was markedly suppressed to values of 14%, 1%, and 4% of the control, respectively (Fig. 3).

Discussion

A marked increase in the transcription of the γ-GTP gene during the early stages of spontaneous hepatitis has been investigated. The mRNA level of γ-GTP was highly expressed at the time of hepatitis and was further elevated during the progress of hepatoma. Feeding a choline-deficient diet to both LEC and LEA rats resulted in shifting the alteration of hepatic drug metabolizing enzymes to those characteristic of chemical carcinogen-induced hepatocytes. The levels of two major forms of cytochrome P-450, mainly P-450$_{PB}$ and P-450$_{MC}$, were markedly decreased in the LEC liver. The similar pattern of these enzyme alterations between the LEA rats fed a choline deficiet diet and the LEC rats fed a normal diet suggests that biochemical factors involved in the methyl-group metabolism might comprise a hereditary defect in LEC rats and that such a defect may initiate the altered hepatocytes which are spontaneously developing hepatitis and hepatoma.

DNA hypomethylation has been proposed as a likely regulatory mechanism for the co-ordinate change in pathogenesis. Our observations with dietary methyl-group deficiency tend to support this proposal. In fact, NAD(P)H quinone oxido-reductase [9] and cytochrome P-450 [10] have recently shown hypomethylation to be active during the development of preneoplastic nodules and aging.

The relation of the extent of DNA methylation to eukaryotic gene expression has not been elucidated. Numerous lines of evidence suggest that most genes are undermethylated in tissues where they are expressed and heavily methylated in non-expressing tissues as well as in germ cells [16]. In LEC rats, 5-azacytidine caused a significant decrease in cytochrome P-450 content and an increase in γ-GTP activity. Furthermore, the extent of genomic DNA methylation was decreased only with 5-azacytidine treatment, suggesting that LEC rats which display spontaneous hepatitis and hepatoma are highly sensitive to 5-azacytidine. There are also reports regarding the decreased content of 5-methylcytosine in chemically induced or spontaneous primary hepatocellular carcinoma of genetic origin in mice [17]. Our data on the 5-methylcytosine content of DNA during the progression of hepatocarcinogenesis in LEC rats are in agreement with these reports. Therefore, we suggest that the increased transcription of γ-GTP gene during hepatocarcinogenesis is a consequence of hypomethylation of its gene resulting from the decreased availability of methyl donors.

References

1. Doerflar W (1983) DNA methylation and gene activity. Ann Rev Biochem 52:93–124
2. Jones PA (1986) DNA methylation and cancer. Cancer Res 46:461–466
3. Wilson VL, Smith RA, Ma S, Cutler RG (1987) Genomic 5-methyldeoxycytidine decreases with age. J Biol Chem 262:9948–9951
4. Korba BE, Wilson VL, Yoakum GH (1985) Induction of hepatitis B virus core gene in human cells by cytosine demethylation in the promoter. Science 228: 1103–1106
5. Bhave, MR, Wilson MJ, and Poirier LA (1988) c-H-ras and c-K-ras gene hypomethylation in the livers and hepatomas of rats fed methyl-deficient, amino acid-defined diets. Carcinogenesis 9:343–348
6. Wainfan E, Dizik M, Stender M, Christman JK (1989) Rapid appearance of hypomethylation DNA in livers of rats fed cancer-promoting, methyl-deficient diet. Cancer Res 49:4094–4097
7. Harris M (1983) Induction of thymidine kinase in enzme-deficient Chinese hamster cells. Cell 29:483–492
8. Jones PA, Taylor SM (1980) Cellular differentiation, cytosine analogs and DNA methylation. Cell 20:85–93
9. Wanger G, Pott U, Bruckschen M, Sies H (1988) Effect of 5-azacytidine and methyl-group deficiency on NAD(P)H: quinone oxidoreductase and glutathione S-transferase in liver. Biochem J 251:825–829
10. Umeno M, Song BJ, Kozak C, Gelboin HV, Gonzalez FJ (1988) The rat P450IIE1 gene: Complete intron and exon sequence, chromosome mapping, and correlation of developmental expression with specific 5'cytosine demethylation. J Biol Chem 263:4956–4962
11. Gooderham NJ, Mannering GJ (1985) Depression of the hepatic cytochrome P-450 monooxygenase system by treatment of mice with the antineoplastic agent 5-azacytidine. Cancer Res 45:1569–1572

12. Suzuki K, Sugiyama T, Ookawara T, Kurosawa T, Taniguchi N (1991) High sensitivity to 5-azacytidine in LEC rats, a strain with a metabolic predisposition to hepatitis and hepatoma: Possible involvement of DNA methylation in the expression of cytochrome P-450 and γ-glutamyl transpeptidase. Biochem Int 23:9–14

13. Sugiyama T, Takeichi N, Kobayashi H, Yoshida MC, Sasaki M, Taniguchi N (1988) Metabolic predisposition of a novel mutant (LEC rats) to hereditary hepatitis and hepatoma: Alterations of the drug metabolizing enzymes. Carcinogenesis 9:1569–1572

14. Sugiyama T, Suzuki K, Ookawara T, Kurosawa T, Taniguchi N (1989) Selective expression and induction of cytochrome $P-450_{PB}$ and $P-450_{MC}$ during the development of hereditary hepatitis and hepatoma of LEC rats. Carcinogenesis 10:2155–2159

15. Sugiyama T, Matsunaga M, Jain SK, Jain S, Ikeda Y, Taniguchi N (1991) Enhancing effect of a choline-deficient diet on alterations of hepatic drug-metabolizing enzymes in hepatitis- and hepatoma-predisposed rats (LEC rats). Jpn J Cancer Res 82:390–396

16. Keshet I, Yisraeli J, Cedar H (1985) Effect of regional DNA methylation on gene expression. Proc Natl Acad Sci USA 82:2560–2564

17. Lapeyre JN, Walker MS, Becker FF (1981) DNA methylation and methylase levels in normal and malignant mouse hepatic tissues. Carcinogenesis 2: 873–878

19 — Abnormal Lipid Metabolism in LEC Rats

MASAKO TANIGUCHI[1], TOSHIHIRO SUGIYAMA, and NAOYUKI TANIGUCHI[2]

Introduction

Our previous studies indicated that LEC rats are characterized by a high sensitivity to azacytidine [1], which is a well-known inhibitor of DNA-methyltransferase. In addition, control rats fed choline- and methionine-deficient diets mimic LEC rats, suggesting that the LEC rat has some direct defect in DNA methylation or that the defect is accompanied by a hypomethylated state [2]. Choline deficiency has been reported to induce accumulation of fats in the liver and reduction in circulating phospholipids, triglycerides, and cholesterol in plasma [3–5]. The development of fatty liver in choline-deficient rats could be a result of increased lipid biosynthesis, inhibition of lipid degradation, fatty acid oxidation, or a failure to transfer the newly synthesized triglyceride into the plasma with a resultant increase in liver triglyceride content [5].

No reports have been published, however, on the lipid metabolism of the LEC rats. We expected that the lipid compositions of liver and serum in the LEC rats would be similar to those in rats fed a choline-deficient diet. The present study was undertaken to investigate changes in the serum and liver cholesterol, cholesterol ester, and triglyceride levels during the aging of LEC rats. In addition, the present study will open up a new field for the study of lipid metabolism in human hepatitis and primary hepatoma by providing the first suitable experimental model.

[1] Pre-education Department, Teikoku Women's Junior College, Moriguchi, 570 Japan
[2] Department of Biochemistry, Osaka University Medical School, Suita, Osaka, 565 Japan

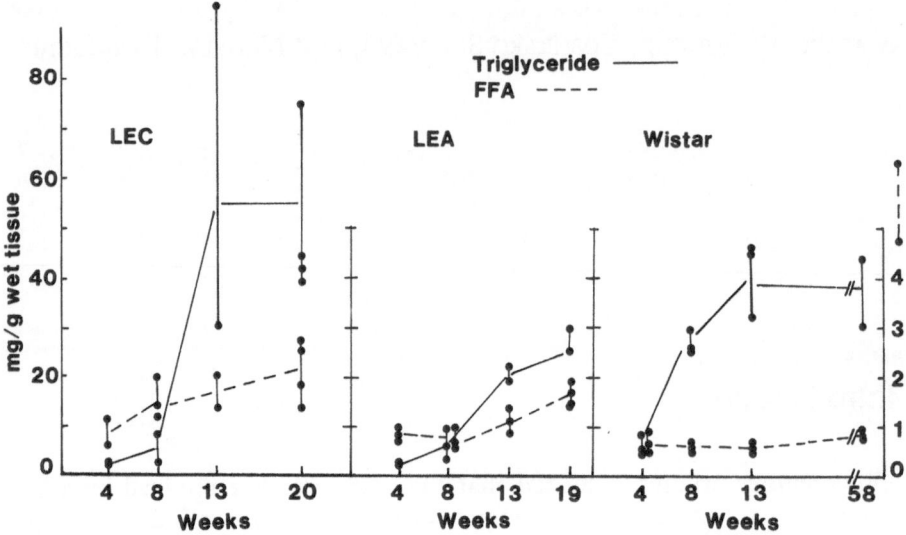

Fig. 1. Triglyceride and free fatty acid levels of LEC, LEA, and Wistar rat livers. The mean and variation of 2–5 rats is shown for each point on the graph

Serum and Liver Lipid Compositions of LEC, LEA, and Wistar Rats

Free Fatty Acid Levels in the Liver

Free fatty acid levels in the LEA and LEC rat livers were higher than those in Wistar rats (Fig. 1), as well as in Sprague Dowley rats (data not shown). The free fatty acid levels were especially high in the LEC rats aged 8–20 weeks. This suggests that free fatty acid is released from triglycerides by triglyceride lipase or that free fatty acid degradation is inhibited in the LEC rat liver.

Triglyceride Levels in the Liver

The liver triglyceride levels in LEC rats at 4 and 8 weeks were significantly low (Fig. 1). At 8 weeks, the value was found to be from one-fifth to one-tenth that of normal Wistar rats. LEA rat livers also had low triglyceride levels at this age.

Increased triglyceride levels in LEC rat liver at 13 and 20 weeks of age could be explained by the following. Serum lipids in the normal control animals are supplied as lipoprotein from the liver and then maintained in the plasma. In the LEC rats, however, the following situations may exist and bring about fatty liver: (1) impairment of the synthesis of protein and lipids due to the inflammation of hepatocytes, (2) abnormal synthesis of

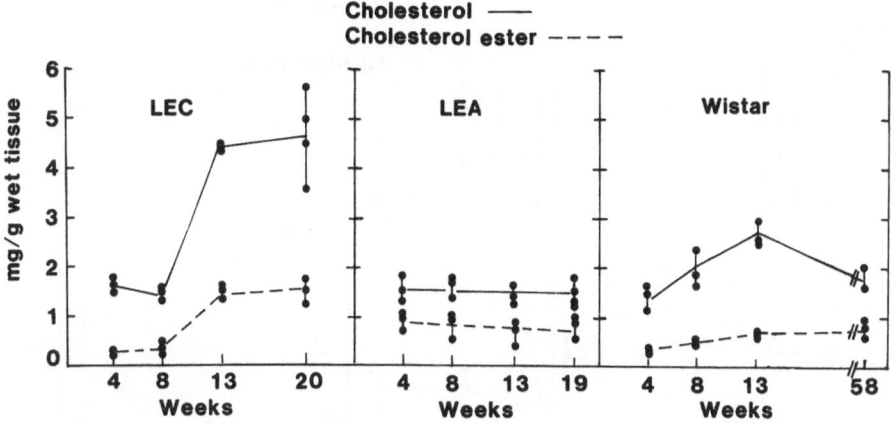

Fig. 2. Cholesterol and cholesterol ester levels of LEC, LEA, and Wistar rat livers. The mean and variation of 2–5 rats in shown

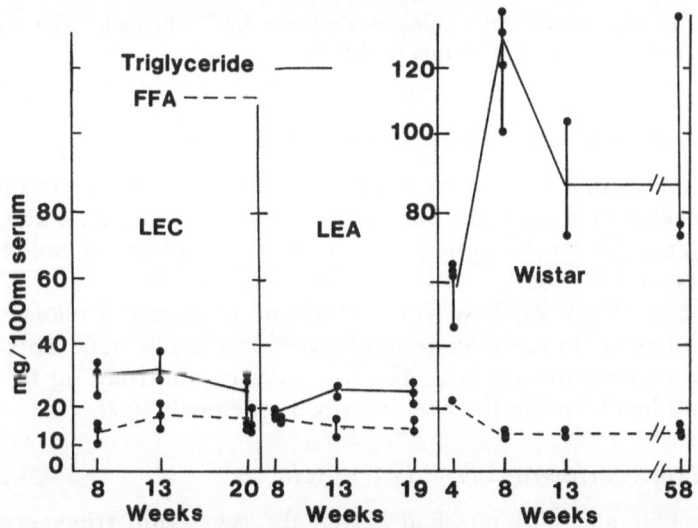

Fig. 3. Serum triglyceride and free fatty acid levels of LEC, LEA, and Wistar rats. The mean and variation of 2–5 rats is shown

lipids affected by bile acids accompanied by cholestasis due to inflammation, and (3) abnormal synthesis of phospholipids and lipoprotein due to hypomethylation or choline deficiency. These situations may affect the lipid metabolism in the liver and result in the release of biliary lipids into plasma.

The wide distribution in triglyceride levels in the LEC rats (Fig. 1) seemed to correlate with the extent of inflammation.

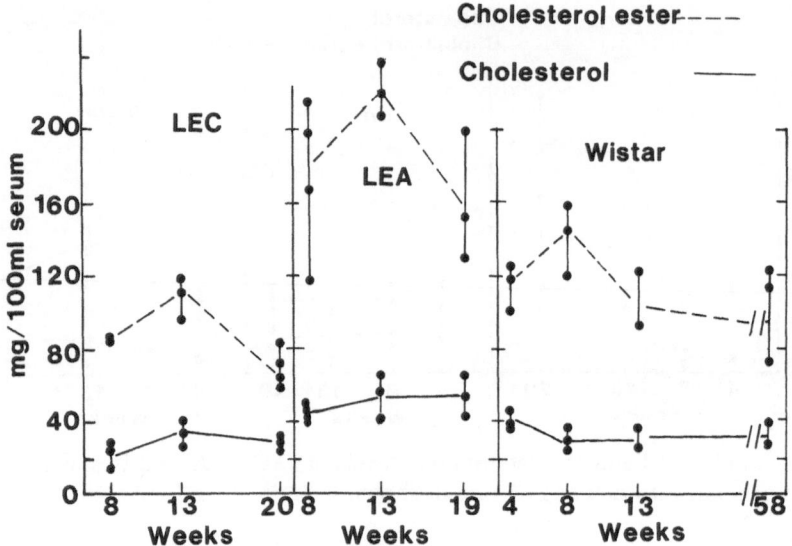

Fig. 4. Serum cholesterol and cholesterol ester of LEC, LEA, and Wistar rat livers. The mean and variation of 2–5 rats is shown.

Liver Cholesterol and Cholesterol Ester Levels

Cholesterol normally exists as a component of the hepatocyte membrane and its level is kept constant during the aging processes. At 4 and 8 weeks of age, no significant difference was observed in cholesterol and choesterol ester levels in LEC, LEA, and Wistar rat livers (Fig. 2)

At 13 and 20 weeks, however, significant increases of cholesterol and cholesterol esters in the liver were observed in the LEC rats. This suggests that high cholesterol levels in the bile may be contributing to the high cholesterol levels in the liver as described previously [6,7].

Serum Triglyceride and Free Fatty Acid

Both the LEC and LEA rats had extremely low serum triglyceride levels compared to the Wistar rat (Fig. 3). This observation is quite interesting, but detailed and definite conclusions require additional study.

No significant difference was found in the serum level of free fatty acid among the three strains.

Serum Cholesterol and Cholesterol Ester Levels

The LEC rats has lower values for both serum cholesterol and cholesterol esters than the LEA rats (Fig. 4). The levels of these lipids in the LEC rat liver were higher than those of the LEA rats at 13 and 20 weeks. These findings are in good agreement with the previous data shown by Sugiyama et al. [3] Mookerjea et al. [4], and Aarsaether et al. [5], who found lower levels of plasma lipids and higher levels of liver lipids in rats fed choline-deficient diets. It is clear that the release of lipoproteins into blood was impaired in the LEC rat livers due to abnormal lipoprotein synthesis.

Discussion

The lipid compositions of the well-perfused liver and serum from LEC rats aged 4, 8, 13, and 20 weeks were compared with those of LEA and Wistar rats. In livers of 13- and 20-week-old LEC rats, in which fulminant hepatitis had been observed, all examined lipid components were found to have higher values than in the LEA rats. In contrast, both cholesterol and cholesterol ester levels in serum in the LEC rats were lower than those in LEA rats, but no difference was seen in the levels of triglyceride and free fatty acid between these rats. These results suggest that the changes in lipid composition in the LEC rats are similar to those in choline-deficient rats. These data supported our previous findings that the LEC rats have hypomethylated states similar to those associated with choline deficiency [1,2].

A low level of triglyceride in plasma and a high level of free fatty acid in liver were found to be characteristics of the lipid metabolism of Long-Evans rats from which the LEA and LEC rats were derived.

Conclusions

Abnormalities of lipid metabolism have been observed in the LEC rats. The lipid patterns of the LEC rats are similar to those of choline-deficient rats, in which the liver may fail to transfer the newly formed triglycerides and cholesterol into the plasma with a resultant increase in liver triglyceride content and a decrease in serum lipid levels.

The LEC rats appear to be a useful animal model for the study of lipid metabolism in hepatocellular diseases including hepatitis and hepatoma.

Acknowledgements. This work was in part supported by Grants-in-Aid for Cancer Research from the Ministry of Education, Science, and Culture, Japan and by a fund from Otsuka Pharmaceutical Co. Ltd. The author (M.T.) thanks Ms. Y. Ohba, Ms. H. Okumura, and Ms. I. Nakama for their skillful technical assistance.

References

1. Suzuki K, Sugiyama T, Ookawara T, Kurosawa T, Taniguchi N (to be published) High sensitivity to 5-azacytidine in LEC rats, a strain with a metabolic predis-

position to hepatitis and hepatoma: Possible involvement of DNA methylation in the expression of cytochrome P-450 and γ-glutamyl transpeptidase. Biochem Int

2. Sugiyama T, Matsunaga M, Jain SK, Jain S, Ikeda Y, Taniguchi N (to be published) Enhancing effect of a choline-deficient diet on alterations of hepatic drug-metabolizing enzymes in hepatitis- and hepatoma-predisposed rats (LEC rats) Jap J Cancer Res

3. Sugiyama K, Mochizuki C, Muramatsu, K (1987) Comparative effects of choline chloride and phosphatidylcholine on plasma and liver lipid levels in rats fed a choline-deficient high cholesterol diet. J Nutr Sci Vitaminol (Tokyo) 33: 369–376

4. Mookerjea S, Park CE, Kuksis A (1975) Lipid profiles of plasma lipoproteins of fasted and fed normal and choline-deficient rats. Lipids 10:374–382

5. Aarsaether N, Berge RK, Aarsland A, Svardal A, Ueland PM (1988) Effect of methotrexate on long-chain fatty acid metabolism in liver of rats fed a standard or defined, choline-deficient diet. Biochim Biophys Acta 958:70–80

6. Taniguchi M, Ishikawa H, Sakagami, T (1986) Phospholipid metabolism in bile duct-ligated rat plasma and erythrocytes. Biochim Biophys Acta 876:631–638

7. Taniguchi M, Tanabe F, Ishikawa H, Sakagami, T (1983) Experimental biliary obstruction of rat. Initial changes in the structure and lipid content of erythrocytes. Biochim Biophys Acta 753:22–31

20 — Identifications of Carbonic Anhydrase III and Triosephosphate Isomerase in the Liver Proteins in LEC Rats on Two-Dimensional Gel Electrophoresis

Toshihiko Nagase[1,2], Toshihiro Sugiyama[1], Shigeki Higashiyama[1], Daitoku Sakamuro[1], Sumio Kawata[2], Seiichiro Tarui[2], and Naoyuki Taniguchi[1]

Introduction

The two-dimensional gel (2-DG) electrophoresis analysis of total cellular proteins as described by O'Farrell [1] is suitable for investigating certain protein changes which precede hepatitis and/or hepatocellular carcinomas (HCCs).

In the present study, we found that although 2-DG electrophoretic patterns of LEA and LEC rat livers were very similar, one new component appeared in LEC rat livers, another was less, and 2 others were greater than in LEA rat livers. One of the latter two, which were much greater in the LEC rats, was identified as a mixture of triosephosphate isomerase (TPI) and carbonic anhydrase III (CA III). Western blotting analysis indicated that only the CA III changed following the episode of hepatitis and the subsequent development of hepatoma, whereas the level of TPI did not change significantly.

Patterns of 2-DG Electrophoresis of 4-Week-Old LEC and LEA Rat Livers

Total cellular polypetides of 4-week-old LEA and LEC rat livers were compared. Figure 1 illustrates the 2-DG electrophoresis separation of Coomassie blue-stained polypeptides from the LEA (Fig. 1A) and LEC (Fig. 1B) rat livers. The electrophoretic patterns of total cellular polypetides from livers of both strains were very similar, but several differences were consistently observed. These differences were explored in detail, with particular attention being directed to one of the components because it changed most dramatically. In LEC rat livers, two components, p29/6.8

---

[1] Department of Biochemistry, and [2] Second Department of Internal Medicine, Osaka University Medical School, Suita, Osaka, 565 Japan

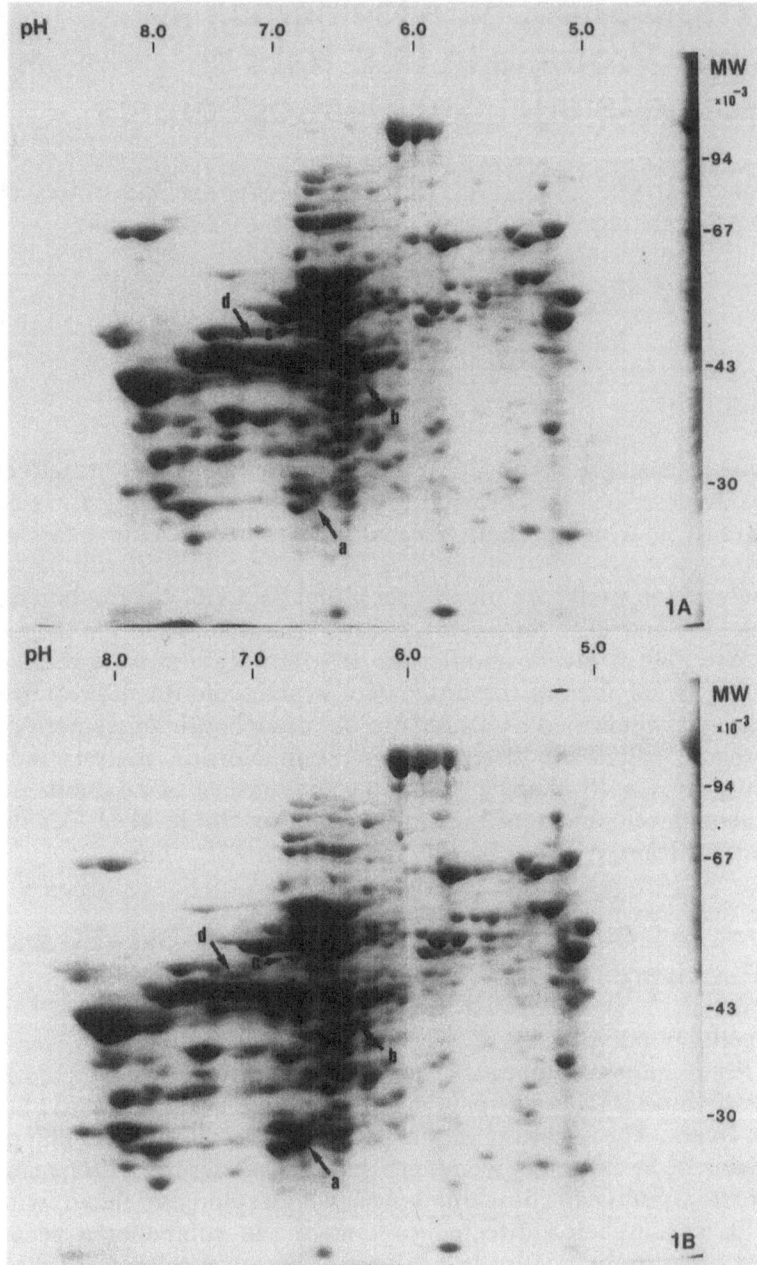

Fig. 1. Two-DG electrophoresis of total cellular proteins from livers of **A** 4-week-old LEA rats and **B** 4-week-old LEC rats. *Arrows:* *a* and *b*, polypeptides which were greater; *c*, polypeptide which was less; *d*, polypeptide which appeared to be new, in 4-week-old LEC rats compared with 4-week-old LEA rats. *Abscissa*, pH range; *ordinate*, molecular weight × 10^{-3}

and p43/6.4 (Fig. 1, *a* and *b*, respectively) were greater and the p51/6.8 (Fig. 1, *c*) component was less compared with those in LEA rat livers, while another, p50/7.2 (Fig. 1, *d*) appeared only in LEC rat livers. These changes were always present when the 5 LEA rats and 6 LEC rats livers were compared. The p29/6.8 component was most strikingly greater in 3 out of 6 LEC rats livers, but the rest were only slightly greater than in the 5 LEA rats livers.

Analysis of Component p29/6.8

The p29/6.8 component increased in livers of both LEA and LEC rats at 16 weeks of age in comparison with those which were 4 weeks old. At 52 weeks of age the polypeptide p29/6.8 tended to decrease in samples from LEC rats, but showed no changes in LEA rats compared with those at age 16 weeks. In 16- and 52-week-old LEC rat livers, the p29/6.8 protein was significantly less than the analogous LEA rat livers (Fig. 2).

A comparison of the amount of this component in the tumorous and non-tumorous tissue from one liver (52 weeks old) showed a marked decrease in the tumorous tissue (Fig. 3). In another pair of samples, no additional difference was observed than that seen in Fig. 3 (data not shown).

The following sequencing procedures of proteins isolated by gel electrophoresis were performed, essentially as described by Cleveland et al. [2] and Matsudaira [3].

Approximately 35 µg of this protein was isolated from 70 Coomassie blue-stained preparative gels using a 4-week-old LEC rat liver as a sample. This was subjected to automated gas-phase peptide sequencing (Applied Biosystems 477A Protein Sequencer), and 14 N-terminal amine acid residues were determined. A search of the National Biomedical Research Foundation (NBRF) Protein Identification Resource revealed that it was homologous to that of TPI [4] (Table 1). A pool of the peptide, p29/6.8, was also digested with V8 protease. The digest was subjected to gel electrophoresis to give the result shown in Fig. 4. The major peptide shown was sequenced for 14 residues. A homology search indicated that this peptide was almost identical to residues 19–33 of rat CA III [5], with the exception of residue 29, serine (Table 1). In order to confirm that both CA III and TPI were present in the component p29/6.8, Western blotting analyses were made on the 2-DG using specific antibodies against these enzymes (Fig. 5). The Western blotting which used the antibody to TPI indicated that the amount of p29/6.8 for the enzyme did not change significantly during aging in LEA rats and during aging and hepatocarcinogenesis in LEC rats compared with the amount indicated in Fig. 5Bc. This correlated with uniform enzyme activities in each liver homogenate at the times examined (data not shown). However, the Western blotting experiments using the antibody to CA III indicated that the amount of the immunoreactive protein changed markedly both within strains and between strains during

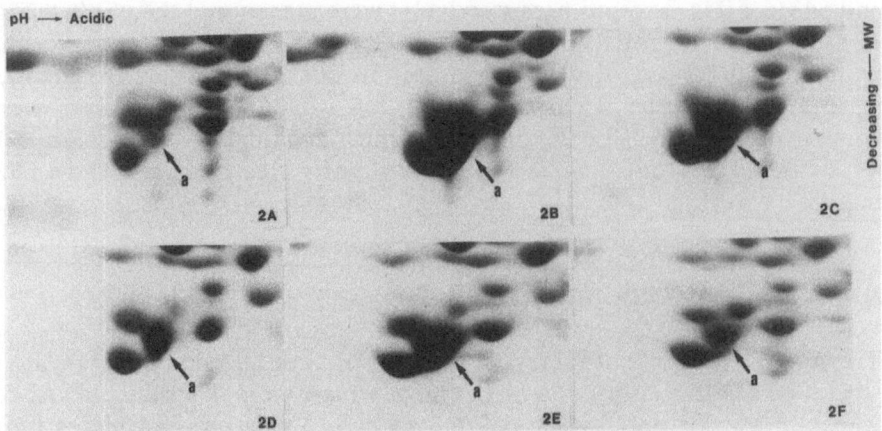

Fig. 2. Enlarged areas containing the spot indicated by the *arrow a*. **A-C** Results for 4-, 16-, and 52-week-old LEA rat livers, respectively. **D-F** Results for 4-, 16-, and 52-week-old LEC rat livers, respectively. The photographs for the 16-week-old rats are for individuals in which the level of GPT is within normal levels in both LEA and LEC rats

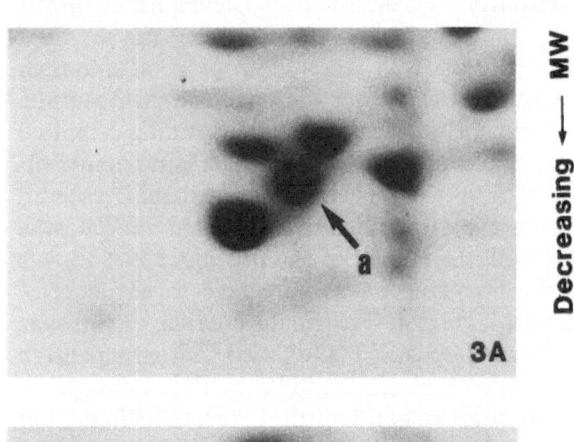

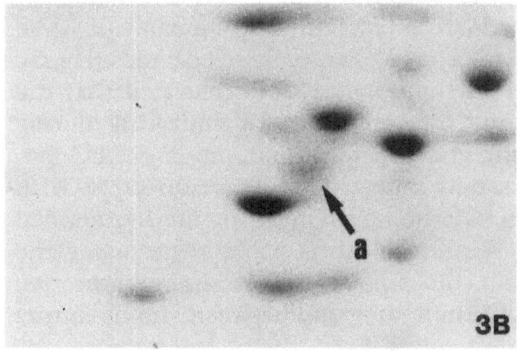

Fig. 3. Enlarged areas containing the component p29/6.8 indicated by the *arrow a* from the liver of a 52-week-old LEC rat. **A** Non-hepatoma and **B** hepatoma tissue

Table 1. N-terminal and internal amino acid sequences of p29/6.8 aligned with carbonic anhydrase III and triosephosphate isomerase.

Source	Enzymes	Sequence, residue number[a]	Reference
p29/6.8 (Internal)			
LEC Rat liver	CA III	Leu-Tyr-Pro-Ile-Ala-Lys-Gly-Asp-Asn-Gln-Xxx-[Pro-Ile-Glu-Leu][b]	
Rat muscle	CA III	Glu-[Leu-Tyr-Pro-Ile-Ala-Lys-Gly-Asp-Asn-Gln]-Ser-[Pro-Ile-Glu-Leu]	[4]
p29/6.8 (N-Terminal)			
LEC Rat liver	TPI	Ala-Pro-Ser-[Xxx-Lys-Phe-Phe-Val-Gly-Gly-Asn]-Xxx-[Lys-Met-Asn-Gly]	
Human placenta	TPI	Ala-Pro-Ser-[Arg-Lys-Phe-Phe-Val-Gly-Gly-Asn]-Trp-[Lys-Met-Asn-Gly]	[5]

Residue numbers above the sequences: 5, 10, 15, 20, 25, 30

[a] Sequencing numbering based on CA III (rat muscle) and TPI (human placenta)
[b] Significant homology is seen between p29/6.8 (internal) and rat muscle CA III and between p29/6.8 (N-terminal) and human placental TPI, as indicated by boxed regions

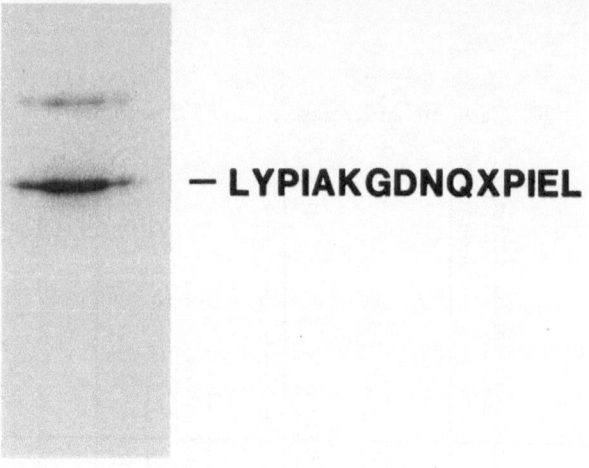

Fig. 4. Coomassie blue staining pattern of p29/6.8 fragments following digestion with V8 protease. Amino acid sequencing of the major polypeptide gave the result shown to the *right*

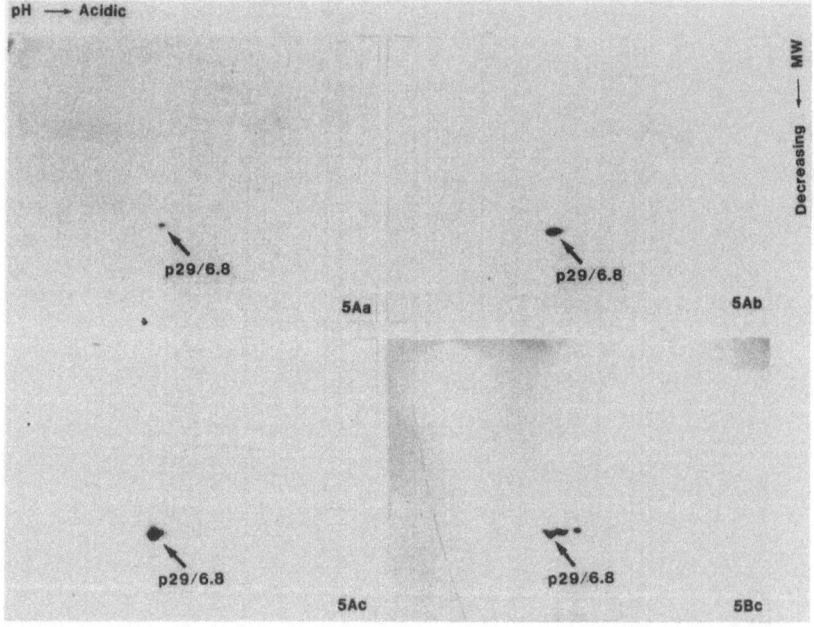

Fig. 5. Immunoblotting analysis of the 2-DG with **A** anti-CA III antibody and **B** anti-TPI antibody. **a**, **b**, and **c** show results for 4-week-old LEA, LEC, and 16-week-old LEC rats livers, respectively. Each spot coincides precisely with the position of p29/6.8. Furthermore, the reactivity with the CA III antibody increased dramatically in the 4- and 16-week-old LEC rat livers compared with 4-week-old LEA rat livers. In the analyses with CA III antibody, the 2-DG electrophoresis utilized 4 μg of total cellular proteins since the application of 400 μg of the proteins resulted in overloading

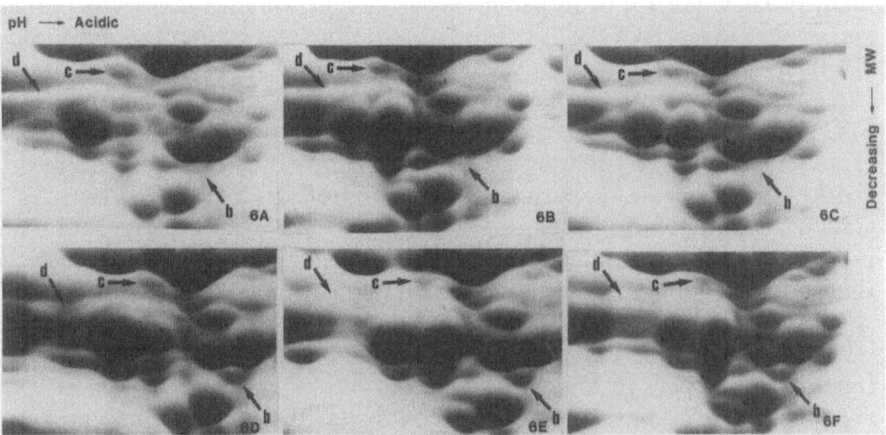

Fig. 6. Enlarged areas containing the spots indicated by the *arrows b,c,d*. **A–C** Results for 4-, 16-, and 52-week-old LEA rat livers, respectively. **D–F** Results for 4-, 16-, and 52-week-old LEC rat livers, respectively

aging in LEA and LEC rats and hepatocarcinogenesis in LEC rats (Fig. 5Aa,b,c). In one (the sample in Fig. 3B) of two HCCs, we could not detect the immunoreactive CA III (data not shown). These results indicated that the apparent changes in intensity of p29/6.8 staining as shown in Figs. 1–3 were attributed to changes in the levels of CA III.

Two-DG Patterns of Polypeptides (p43/6.4, p50/7.2, and p51/6.8) of LEC and LEA Rats at 16 and 52 Weeks of Age

The polypeptides, designated p43/6.4, p50/7.2, and p51/6.8, of five 16- and 52-week-old LEA and LEC rats showed almost the same pattern as the livers of the 4-week-old animals (Fig. 6).

Discussion

CA III levels vary significantly during development and aging of male rats. Prepubescent CA III levels are low and then increase with the onset of puberty before declining in senescent males to levels below those observed in females [6]. Therefore, it is possible that the speed of aging is faster in LEC rats than in LEA rats.

The CA III concentration in the liver is known to be affected by the addition of testosterone or estradiol [7], the levels of androgen receptors in the liver [8–10], or the release pattern of growth hormone [11]. Therefore, an endocrinological disturbance including the receptors might exist in LEC rats.

No data appear to exist on the relationship of HCCs and CA III. However, considering the implications of estrogens or androgens in the development of HCC [12,13] or in the presence of receptors for estrogens [14] and androgens [15] in HCC, it is interesting to note the changes in amounts of CA III in LEC rats.

A single autosomal recessive mutation has evidently occurred in the LEC strain [16,17]. Autosomal recessive hereditary defects of enzymes and proteins such as glucocerebrosidase, sphingomyelinase, and ceruloplasmin are known to cause hepatic dysfunction, reflected by such entities as Gaucher's, Niemann-Pick, and Wilson's diseases, respectively. Autolyzed preparations of ceruroplasmin usually consist mainly of three fragments that have the approximate molecular weights of 67,000, 50,000, and 19,000 [18]. Although such preparations have not been detected in fresh serum [19], it is of interest that p51/6.8 nearly coincides with the 50,000-dalton fragment in respect to molecular weight.

Sugiyama et al. have previously shown that the components and activities of enzymes involved in drug metabolism of the 4-week-old LEC rats were quite similar to those observed in the hyperplastic foci and nodules induced by chemical carcinogens [20]. Up to 52 weeks of age, when LEC rats develop HCCs, three polypeptides, p51/6.8, p43/6.4, and p50/7.2, maintained the same pattern as is seen when they are 4 weeks old. This indicates that there may be proteins which change in HCCs. Wirth et al. [21] have shown that one cytosolic polypeptide, p57/6.8, and three membrane-associated polypeptides, p41/6.25, p24/6.75, and p21/6.05, were expressed in both preneoplastic and neoplastic nodules but not, or at least in very small amounts, in normal tissue. In connection with these data, it is of interest that our polypeptide p43/6.4 apparently coincides with Wirth's polypeptide p41/6.25 and is clearly demonstrable in both neoplastic and extraneoplastic tissues in LEC rat livers in contrast to its being almost absent in LEA rat livers. Furthermore, Wirth et al. [22] reported that two cytosolic polypetides and one cytosolic polypeptide were detected at all ages only in LEA rats and only in LEC rats, respectively, by the two-dimentsional gel electrophoresis in combination with silver staining. Their polypeptides are similar to the p29/6.8 component in terms of molecular weight and isoelectric point. We could not, however, find such polypetides. The reason may be because our staining method, Coomassie brilliant blue, is less sensitive than silver staining. In any event, the three polypeptides were thought to be different from CA III because they did not vary at all during aging.

References

1. O'Farrell PH (1975) High resolution two-dimensional electrophoresis of proteins. J Biol Chem 250:4007–4021
2. Cleveland DW, Fischer SG, Kirschner MW, Laemmli UK (1977) Peptide mapping by limited proteolysis in sodium dodecyl sulfate and analysis by gel electrophoresis. J Biol Chem 252:1102–1106

3. Matsudaira P (1987) Sequence from picomole quantities of proteins electroblotted onto polyvinylidene difluoride membranes. J Biol Chem 262:10035–10038

4. Lu HS, Yuan PM, Gracy RW (1984) Primary structure of human triosephosphate isomerase. J Biol Chem 259:11958–11968

5. Kelly CD, Carter ND, Jeffery S, Edwards YH (1988) Characterisation of cDNA clones for rat muscle carbonic anhydrase III. Biosci Rep 8:401–406

6. Carter ND, Shiels A, Jeffery S, Heath R, Wilson CA, Phillips IR, Shephard EA (1984) Hormonal control of carbonic anhydrase III. Ann NY Acad Sci 429: 287–301

7. Shiels A, Jeffery S, Phillips IR, Shephard EA, Wilson CA, Carter ND (1983) Sexual differentiation of rat liver carbonic anhydrase III. Biochim Biophys Acta 760:335–342

8. Ramaley JA (1982) The neuroendocrinology of puberty. In: Vernadakis A, Timiras P (eds) Hormones in development and aging. Spectrum, New York pp 305–329

9. Adams CE (1972) Aging and reproduction. In: Austin CR, Short RV (eds) Reproduction in mammals: Reproductive patterns, vol. 4. Cambridge University Press, New York, pp 128–156

10. Simpkins JW, Mueller GP, Huang HH, Meites J (1977) Evidence for depressed catecholamine and enhanced serotonin metabolism in aging male rats: Possible relation to gonadotropin secretion. Endocrinology 100:1672–1678

11. Jeffery S, Carter ND, Clark RG, Robinson ICAF (1990) The episodic secretory pattern of growth hormone regulates liver carbonic anhydrase III. Studies in normal and mutant growth-hormone-deficient dwarf rats. Biochem J 266: 69–74

12. Farrell GC, Yoshua DE, Uren RF, Baird PJ, Perkins KW, Kronenberg H (1975) Androgen-induced hepatoma. Lancet I:430–432

13. O'Sullivan JP, Rosswick RP (1976) Oral contraceptives and malignant hepatic tumors. Lancet I: 1124–1125

14. Nagasue N, Ito A, Yukaya H, Ogawa Y (1985) Androgen receptors in hepatocellular carcinoma and surrounding parenchyma. Gastroenterology 89:643–647

15. Nagasue N, Ito A, Yukaya H, Ogawa Y (1986) Estrogen receptors in hepatocellular carcinoma. Cancer 57:87–91

16. Yoshida MC, Masuda R, Sasaki M, Takeichi N, Kobayashi H, Dempo K, Mori M (1987) New mutation causing hereditary hepatitis in the laboratory rat. J Hered 78:361–365

17. Masuda R, Yoshida MC, Sasaki M, Dempo K, Mori M (1988) Hereditary hepatitis of LEC rats is controlled by a single autosomal recessive gene. Lab Anim 22:166–169

18. Takahashi N, Bauman RA, Ortel TL, Dwulet FE, Wang CC, Putman FW (1983) Internal triplication in the structure of human ceruloplasmin. Proc Natl Acad Sci USA 80:115–119

19. Sato M, Schilsky ML, Stockenrt RJ, Morell AG, Sternlieb I (1990) Detection of multiple forms of human ceruloplasmin. A novel Mr 200,000 form. J Biol Chem 265:2533–2537

20. Sugiyama T, Takeichi N, Kobayashi H, Yoshida MC, Sasaki M, Taniguchi N (1988) Metabolic predisposition of a novel mutant (LEC rats) to hereditary hepatitis and hepatoma: Alterations of the drug metabolizing enzymes. Carcinogenesis 9:1569–1572

21. Wirth PJ, Benjamin T, Schwartz DM, Thorgeirsson SS (1986) Sequential analysis of chemically induced hepatoma development in rats by two-dimensional electrophoresis. Cancer Res 46:400–413
22. Wirth PJ, Fujimoto Y, Takahashi H, Mori M, Yoshida MC, Sugimura T, Nagao M (1990) Two-dimensional electrophoretic analysis of hepatitis-associated polypeptides in liver of LEC rats developing spontaneous hepatitis. Jpn J Cancer Res 81:477–482

21 — Two-Dimensional Electrophoretic Analysis of Cellular Polypeptides from Livers of LEC Rats

PETER J. WIRTH[1,3], YOSHINORI FUJIMOTO[1,3], MICHIO MORI[2],
MINAKO NAGAO[1], and TAKASHI SUGIMURA[1]

Introduction

Cancer development in the liver, and most probably in all other organs and tissues as well, is a multistep process occurring over extended periods of time, and which ultimately leads to the frank development of hepatocellular carcinoma. This process has operationally been divided into the stages of initiation, promotion, and progression although the molecular mechanisms responsible for these stages of carcinogenesis are far from being adequately defined [1,2]. In man, it is generally accepted that multiple stages, such as chronic hepatitis, cirrhosis, and hepatocellular carcinoma, also exist during the development of liver cancer, especially due to HB virus infection [3]. Although numerous rodent models have been developed for studies on multistage hepatocarcinogenesis induced by chemical carcinogens, attempts to define stages during spontaneous tumor formation in the livers of rats have been few, due to the extremely low natural occurrence of liver tumors in most rat strains [4,5]. The LEC rat, however, offers a very valuable animal model for such studies, in particular, for defining the relationship between the pathogenesis of hepatitis and hepatocellular carcinogenesis [6–8].

The identification of specific cellular markers prior to the development of hepatitis and the relationship of these markers to specific biologic changes exhibited would be of great importance in understanding the etiology of hepatitis and subsequent cancer development in the LEC rats with possible implications to human cancer development as well. As has been discussed by Yoshida in chapter 1, the molecular mechanism(s) for

[1] Carcinogenesis Division, National Cancer Center Research Institute, Chuo-ku, Tokyo, 104 Japan
[2] Department of Pathology, Sapporo Medical College, Sapporo, 060 Japan
[3] National Cancer Institute, National Institutes of Health, Bethesda, MD 20892, USA

the development of hepatitis and carcinogenesis in the LEC rat is not known at present although genetic analysis has demonstrated that a single autosomal recessive gene, tentatively designated as *hts* (hepatitis), is responsible for the hepatitis [9]. Recently, Li et al. [10] have observed that liver copper levels are markedly increased in LEC rats, and we have confirmed that copper accumulation is associated with hepatitis development in F_1 backcross animals ([LEA × LEC] × LEC) (Sone H, Maeda H, Yoshida M, Takeichi N, Mori M, Sugimura T, Nagao M, unpublished work). These preliminary results suggest that proteins involved in copper binding and metabolism, such as ceruloplasmin and metallothionein, may play a role in hepatitis susceptibility in the LEC rat.

An extremely sensitive and quantitative approach to identify alterations in gene expression which may be integrally involved during the spontaneous development of hepatitis and hepatocarcinogenesis in the LEC rat is the analysis of cellular polypeptides of the liver using high resolution two-dimensional polyacrylamide gel electrophoresis (2D-PAGE). This approach has successfully been used to identify several polypeptides associated both with cellular proliferation and differentiation as well as to identify stage-specific protein alterations during chemical induced hepatocarcinogenesis [11–14].

Two-Dimensional Polyacrylamide Gel Electrophoresis

The technique of 2D-PAGE combines two relatively simple electrophoretic procedures, isoelectric focussing (IEF) and sodium dodecylsulfate (SDS)-polyacrylamide gel electrophoresis, into a single technique. Proteins, actually polypeptides, are separated on the basis of their isoelectric point (pI) in the first dimension and then on the basis of their molecular weight (M_r). Since each separation technique is based on independent physiochemical parameters (e.g., pI and M_r) and since each parameter has an overall resolving power of 100–150 proteins, in theory the overall resolution is 10,000–20,000 proteins [15]. In practice, depending upon the polypeptide spot detection method used (Coomassie blue staining, silver shadowing, or metabolically labeling with radioactive amino acids), one can easily analyze between 1,000–1,500 distinct polypeptide spots on a single 2D-PAGE gel. Utilizing 2D-PAGE, we have analyzed silver-stained cytosolic and particulate polypeptides from LEC and LEA rat livers at ages before and immediately after the development of hepatitis [16]. As might be expected, a typical 2D-PAGE polypeptide spot pattern is quite complex; as a result, our laboratory has developed a computer system to aid in the analysis of such 2D-PAGE patterns. A detailed description of this system is beyond the scope of this monograph. Suffice to say our computer system is capable of resolving all spots visible on a 2D-PAGE gel and is also capable of an accurate quantitation of each individual spot [17].

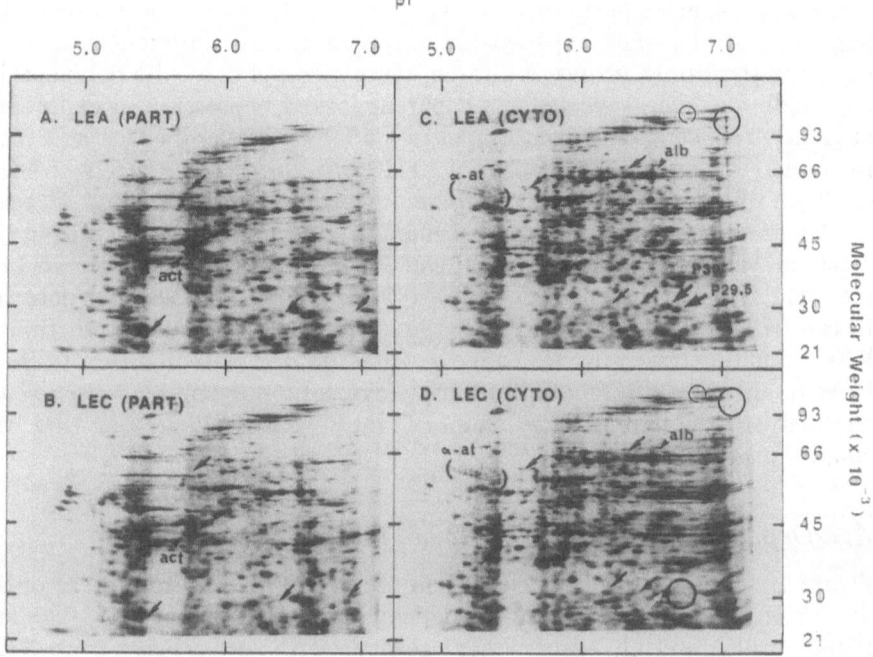

Fig. 1. 2D-PAGE separation of particulate and cytosolic polypeptides from **A, C** 15-week-old LEA and **B, D** 16-week-old LEC rat liver. Polypeptides were separated in the first dimension by equilibrium isoelectric focusing between the pH range of 5 (*left*) to 7 (*right*). *Abscissa*, pH range; *ordinate*, molecular weight (M_r) $\times$ 10^{-3}. *Large arrows* indicate the positions of P29.5 and P30 in the LEA rat liver while *open circles* have been positioned at the expected pI and M_r values for P29.5 and P30 in the LEC rat liver. The *white arrow* illustrates the position of P30-C in the LEC rat liver while the *small arrows* indicate significant quantitative differences. (From [16] with permission)

IEF-Separation of Particulate and Cytosolic Polypeptides from LEA and LEC Rat Liver

Figure 1 illustrates the IEF 2D-PAGE separation of particulate polypeptides (Fig. 1a,b) and cytosolic polypeptides (Fig. 1c,d) from livers of 15-week-old LEA and 16-week-old LEC rats suffering from hepatitis [16]. Approximately 800–1,000 individual polypeptides over the pH range of 4.5–7.0 and M_r 24–100 kd were readily visible on each electrophoretogram. The 2D-PAGE patterns of both particulate and cytosolic polypeptides were quite similar between the hepatitis LEC rat livers and the normal LEA rats with respect to both the total number of polypeptides detected and the overall spot patterns of the individual polypeptides. Although the sensitivity of the silver stain utilized is on the nanogram level (1–5 ng/mm^2) some of the less abundantly expressed polypeptides, e.g., those expressed at less than 10 ng/mm^2, might not be visible on the composite photographs.

A comparison of particulate polypeptides in livers of the normal LEA (Fig. 1a) and LEC (Fig. 1b) revealed only quantitative differences as illustrated by the *small arrows*. A similar comparison of cytosolic polypeptides (Fig 1c,d), however, revealed the apparent loss of expression or expression at greatly reduced concentrations of two polypeptides in hepatitis LEC rat liver (Fig. 1d). These polypeptides, P30 (30 kd/pI 6.70) and P29.5 (29.5 kd/pI 6.73) are illustrated with the *numbered arrows* in Fig. 1c. On Fig. 1d, *open circles* have been placed at the expected M_r and pI values illustrating the apparent lack of expression of P30 and P29.5 in the LEC rat liver. In LEC rats, one cytosolic polypeptide P30-C (30 kd/6.68), which was not detected in the LEA, was expressed in close proximity to the expected position of P30 and is illustrated in Fig. 1d with the *white arrow*. In addition to these three qualitative differences, numerous cytosolic polypeptides were quantitatively modulated in LEA and LEC rat livers as illustrated with the *smaller arrows*.

Age-Dependent Expression of P29.5, P30, and P30-C

Figure 2 is a composite representation of mosaic images from areas of IEF 2D-PAGE gels illustrating the age-dependent expression of P29.5, P30, and P30-C in LEA and LEC rat livers in animals with ages ranging from 1 day to 24 weeks after birth. Both P29.5 and P30 were expressed as early as 1 day after birth in the LEA rat liver (Fig. 2a). Neither P29.5 nor P30 was detected in the LEC rat liver at any age (Fig. 2d–f, j–l). P30-C was detected in the LEC rat at all ages but not in the LEA rat at any age. P29.5 and P30 were also detected in kidney cytosolic preparations from the LEA rat but not from the LEC rat (gels not shown).

NEpHGEL Analysis of Particulate and Cytosolic Polypeptides

In order to analyze for basic polypeptides (pI > 7.0), nonequilibrium pH gradient conditions were utilized in the first dimension and under these conditions two relatively basic polypeptides were detected in the LEC rat liver but not in the LEA rat. P18ne was detected immediately prior to 12 weeks (Fig. 3b) while P27ne was detected immediately after the onset of hepatitis in the LEC rat liver (Fig. 3d). Neither polypeptide was detected in the LEA rat at any age.

Genetic Linkage Analysis of P29.5, P30, and P30-C

In order to determine whether either P29.5, P30, or P30-C was genetically linked to hepatitis susceptibility in the LEC rat, analysis was performed in F_1 backcross ([LEA × LEC] × LEC) rats. In 23-week-old backcross animals 50% (3/6) of the animals showed various degrees of hepatitis as determined from histological evaluation. Severe hepatitis was observed in one animal while the remaining two exhibited much milder signs of hepatitis. No

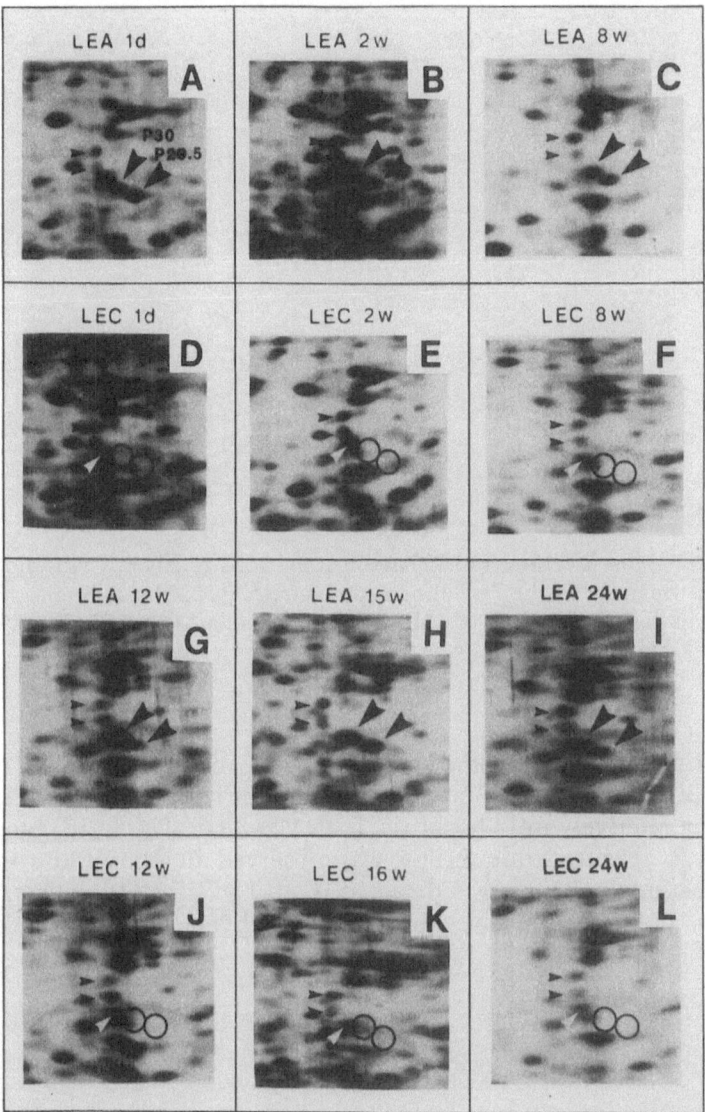

Fig. 2. Age-dependent expression of P29.5, P30, and P30-C. **A–C, G–I** Mosaic enlargements of areas of 2D-PAGE gels from the cytosolic fraction of the LEA and **D-F, J-L** LEC, illustrating the expression of P29.5, P30 and P30-C at **A, D** 1 day (*d*), **B, E** 2 weeks(w), **C, F** 8 weeks, **G, J** 12 weeks, **H, K** 16 weeks, and **I, L** 24 weeks. P29.5 and P30 are indicated with the *large black arrowheads* and P30-C with the *white arrowhead*. To aid in orientation and spot comparison, two constitutively expressed polypeptides found in both LEA and LEC rat livers are illustrated with the *small arrowheads*. (From [16] with permission)

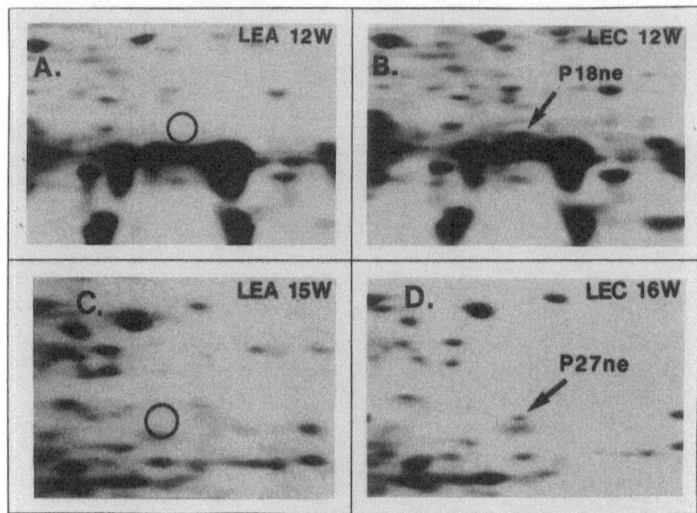

Fig. 3. Expression of P18ne and P27ne LEA and LEC rat liver. Cytosolic polypeptides were separated in the first dimension using NEpHGEL conditions. (From [16] with permission) **A**, 12-week-old LEA; **B**, 12-week-old LEC; **C**, 15-week-old LEA; **D**, 16-week-old LEC

genetic link, however, could be found between the expression of either P29.5, P30, P30-C, or P18ne and hepatitis development. In one animal exhibiting relatively mild hepatitis, both P29.5 and P30 were detected and P30-C was absent, while P18ne was observed in one of the hepatitis-negative animals. P27ne was detected in all backcross animals exhibiting hepatitis, but not in 14-week-old LEC rat livers prior to the onset of hepatitis.

Summary and Conclusions

The LEC rat is a mutant rat strain which exhibits hereditary hepatitis with a very high susceptibility to develop spontaneous hepatocarcinogenesis [6–8]. Genetic analysis has demonstrated that a single autosomal recessive gene, *hts*, is responsible for the hepatitis [9]. Since 2D-PAGE has been successfully used to identify several polypeptides whose expression are highly associated with specific stages of chemically induced hepatocarcinogenesis [11,12], we have used this technique to identify two constitutively expressed LEA rat liver cytosolic polypeptides, P29.5 and P30, which were not detected in the LEC rat. Both polypeptides were expressed as early as 1 day after birth in the LEA rat but not in the LEC rat at any age [16]. In close proximity to P30, however, P30-C was constitutively expressed in LEC rats but not in LEA rats. It is not known whether or not

P30-C is related to P30. The possibility exists that P30-C may represent charge shift modifications of P30 rather than a new polypeptide because the shift in position (toward the acidic end) and the distance in shift in relation to their position to surrounding non-changing polypeptides is near that expected for a single charge difference between polypeptides [15].

In addition, P18ne, a relatively basic polypeptide, was detected in 12-week-old animals immediately prior to the onset of hepatitis but not in age-matched LEA animals. Experiments in F_1 backcross ([LEA × LEC] × LEC) animals, however, failed to demonstrate any genetic link between either the expression or lack of expression of P29.5, P30, P30-C, or P18ne and hepatitis development. An additional polypeptide, P27ne, was detected in all hepatitis-suffering backcross animals but was never observed in rats prior to the onset of hepatitis. Furthermore, during both acute and chronic phases, P27ne was expressed at similar concentrations, suggesting that this polypeptide was a consequence rather than a cause of hepatitis.

Recently, Nagase et al. have utilized 2D-PAGE to identify two polypeptides whose expressions are significantly increased in the LEC rat liver compared to the LEA rat [18]. One of these (p29/6.8) was identified as a mixture of triosephosphate isomerase (TPI) and carbonic anhydrase III (CA III). Subsequent Western immunoblotting analysis demonstrated that only CA III was significantly increased following hepatitis and subsequent hepatoma development [18]. Whether P30-C corresponds to either CA III or TPI awaits future antibody studies.

Sugiyama, et al. have shown that the metabolic activities of numerous Phase I and II enzymes are either increased or decreased in the LEC rat liver, suggesting that these alterations in drug metabolizing enzymes may predispose the LEC rat to hereditary hepatitis and hepatoma development [19]. More specifically, certain biochemical alterations may occur in the liver of LEC rats beginning at birth or shortly after birth and, after the progressive accumulation of a toxic threshold of these alterations, hepatitis may occur [20]. Recently, LEC rats have also been shown to exhibit marked hypogammaglobulinemia [21] as well as markedly increased serum copper concentrations. However, no genetic linkage between the *hts* gene and hypogammaglobulinemia could be demonstrated in the F_1 backcross animals (A. Hattori, personnal communication 1989). Increased liver copper concentrations were, however, observed in F_1 backcross animals, demonstrating a genetic link of this alteration with the *hst* gene mutation.

Examination of cytosolic polypeptides from LEC and LEA rats at the molecular weight regions expected (115–137 kd) for ceruloplasmin, the main copper binding protein in humans and rodents, revealed at least three polypeptides whose expressions were decreased in the LEC rat liver (*circled areas*, Fig. 1c,d). Whether any of these correspond to ceruloplasmin await future antibody studies.

Although the present study failed to detect the expression of any new or the loss of expression of any constitutively expressed polypeptides in the hepatitis-susceptible LEC rat, numerous quantitative changes were noted in both the particulate and cytosolic peptides between the LEC and LEA rat liver. Our initial studies, which were limited to the analysis of approximately 800–1,000 of the most abundantly expressed polypeptides, indicate that gene expression at the protein level is not significantly altered in the LEC rat liver compared to the normal LEA animal. The possibility exists, however, that the maintenance of the normal phenotype in the LEA rat is under the control of polypeptide(s) which are expressed in very minor concentrations or by polypeptides whose molecular weight and pI lie outside the "window" of analysis. Alternatively, the possibility exists that the *hts* mutation in the LEC rat may involved a single neutral amino acid substitution (e.g., alanaine for glycine) which may not result in the change of the apparent pI/M_r of the mutated gene product, yet completely destroys the enzymic or gene regulatory of the protein. Since many of the polypeptides with DNA-binding capacities and gene-regulatory activity are expressed in very low concentrations, the existence of these polypeptides may be obscured by the more abundantly expressed polypeptides and hence go undetected. Future work will require a more precise subcellular fractionation and analysis of specific protein groups in order to detect those polypeptide(s) critically involved in hepatitis development in the LEC rat.

Conclusions

High resolution two-dimensional polyacrylamide gel electrophoresis in combination with ultrasensitive silver staining was used to analyze cellular polypeptides alterations in livers from the LEA and the LEC rat. Analysis of 800–1,000 polypeptides revealed only three qualitative polypeptide differences. Two constitutively expressed cytosolic polypeptides, P29.5 (M_r 29.5 kd/pI 6.73) and P30 (30 kd/6.70) were not detected in livers of the LEC rat while in the LEC rat P30-C (30 kd/6.68) was constitutively expressed in close proximity to P30 but not detected in the LEA rat. In addition, two relatively basic polypeptides, P18ne and P27ne, were detected immediately prior to and immediately after the clinical manifestations of hepatitis, respectively. Genetic analysis, however, failed to demonstrate any genetic linkage between either the expression or lack of expression of P29.5, P30, P30-C, or P18ne and hepatitis development. Although we were unable to identify any unique loss of expression of polypeptides genetically linked to hepatitis development in the LEC rat, numerous polypeptides were observed to undergo significant quantitative modulation.

References

1. Farber E (1980) The sequential analysis of cancer induction. Biochim Biophys Acta 605:149–166
2. Farber E (1984) The multistep nature of cancer development. Cancer Res 44:4217–4223

3. Obata H, Hayashi N, Motoike Y, Hisamitsu T, Okuda H, Kobayashi S, Nishioka K (1980) A prospective study on the development of hepatocellular carcinoma from liver cirrhosis with persistent hepatitis B infection. Int J Cancer 25:741–747

4. Maekawa A, Kurokawa Y, Takahashi M, Kobubo T, Ogiu T, Onodera H, Tanigawa H, Ohno Y, Furukawa F, Hayashi Y (1983) Spontaneous tumors in F344/DuCrj rats. OK 74:365–372

5. Solleveld HA, Haseman JK, McConnell EE (1984) Natural history of body weight gain, survival, and neoplasia in the F344 rat. J Natl Cancer Inst 72: 929–940

6. Sasaki M, Yoshida MC, Kagami K, Takeichi N, Kobayashi H, Dempo K, Mori M (1985) Spontaneous hepatitis in an inbred strain of Long-Evans rats. Rat News Lett 14:4–6

7. Yoshida MC, Masuda R, Sasaki M, Takeichi N, Kobayashi H, Dempo K, Mori M (1987) New mutation causing hereditary hepatitis in the laboratory rat. J Hered 78:361–365

8. Masuda R, Yoshida MC, Sasaki M, Dempo K, Mori M (1988) A transplantable cell line derived from spontaneous hepatocellular carcinoma of the hereditary hepatitis LEC rat. Jpn J Cancer Res 79:250–254

9. Masuda R, Yoshida MC, Sasaki M, Dempo K, Mori M (1988) Hereditary hepatitis of LEC rats is controlled by a single autosomal recessive gene. Lab Anim 22:166–169

10. Li Y, Togashi Y, Sato S, Emoto T, Kang J, Takeichi N, Kobayashi H, Kojima Y, Une Y, Uchino J (to be published) Spontaneous hepatic copper accumulation in LEC rats with hereditary hepatitis: A model of Wilson's disease. J Clin Invest

11. Goldstein D, Djeu J, Latter G, Burkeck S, Levitt J (1985) Abundant synthesis of the transformation-induced protein of neoplastic human fibroblasts, plastin, in normal lymphocytes. Cancer Res 45:5643–5647

12. Celis JE, Madsen P, Nielson S, Celis S (1986) Nuclear patterns of cyclin (PCNA) antigen distribution subdivide S-phase in cultured cells — some applications of PCNA antibodies. Leuk Res 10:237–249

13. Wirth PJ, Benjamin T, Schwartz DM, Thorgeirsson SS (1986) Sequential analysis of chemically induced hepatoma development by two-dimensional electrophoresis. Cancer Res 46:400–413

14. Wirth PJ, Rao MS, Evarts RP (1987) Coordinate polypeptide expression during hepatocarcinogenesis: Comparison of the Solt-Farber and Reddy models. Cancer Res 47:2839–2851

15. O'Farrell P (1975) High resolution two-dimensional electrophoresis of proteins. J Biol Chem 250:4007–4021

16. Wirth, PJ, Fujimoto Y, Takahashi H, Mori M, Yoshida MC, Sugimura T, Nagao M (1990) Two-dimensional electrophoretic analysis of hepatitis-associated polypeptides in liver of LEC rats developing spontaneous hepatitis. Jpn J Cancer Res 81:477–482

17. Vo KP, Miller MJ, Geiduschek EP, Nielson C, Olson AD, Xuong NH (1981) Computer analysis of two-dimensional gels. Anal Biochem 112:258–271

18. Nagase T, Sugiyama T, Kawata S, Taui S, Deutsch HF, Taniguchi N (to be published) Analyses of polypeptides in the liver of a novel mutant (LEC rats) to hereditary hepatitis and hepatoma by two-dimensional gel electrophoresis: Identification of p29/6.8 as carbonic anhydrase III and triosephosphate isomerase. Comp Biochem Physiol

19. Sugiyama T, Takeichi N, Kobayashi H, Yoshida M, Sasaki M, Taniguchi M (1988) Metabolic predisposition of a novel mutant (LEC rats) to hereditary hepatitis and hepatoma: Alterations of the drug metabolizing enzymes. Carcinogenesis 9:1569–1572
20. Majno G, LaGattuta M, Thompson TE (1960) Cellular death and necrosis: Chemical, physical and morphologic changes in rat liver. Virchows Pathol [A] 333:421–465
21. Namieno T, Takeichi N, Dempo K, Mori M, Uchino J, Kobayashi H (1989) Combined immunodeficiency in LEC (Long-Evans Cinnamon) rats with spontaneous hepatitis. Nippon Geka Gakkai Zasshi 6:886–893

3. Immunology

22 — Combined Immunodeficiency in LEC Rats with Spontaneous Hepatitis

Tsutomu Namieno[1,2], Noritoshi Takeichi[2], Motomichi Sasaki[3], Kimimaro Dempo[4], Michio Mori[4], Jun-ichi Uchino[2], and Hiroshi Kobayashi[1]

Introduction

One of the abnormalities in the LEC rat is immunoglobulin G (IgG) formation, and a definite correlation has been found between suppressed IgG formation and the incidence of hepatitis [1,2]. Therefore, we investigated both cellular and humoral immunological competence in relation to the incidence of hepatitis.

Previous reports have indicated the possibility that various immunological abnormalities are involved in the pathogenesis and in the course of human hepatitis [3–5], but many questions remain unanswered. The experimental results performed on LEC rats with regard to their cellular and humoral immunological competence were compared with those performed on a non-hepatitis strain of LEA rats. In the present paper, abnormalities of the immune system in the pathogenesis of the disease will be presented, and will be followed by a discussion on the immunological aspects.

Materials and Methods

Rats

The animals used in this study were 6- and 12-week-old LEC and LEA rats between the 28th and 33rd generation, selected according to their coat colors from the closed-colony inbreeding of the outbred Long-Evans strain at the Center for Experimental Plants and Animals, Hokkaido University.

[1] Laboratory of Pathology, Cancer Institute, [2] First Department of Surgery, School of Medicine, Hokkaido University, Sapporo, 060 Japan [3] Sasaki Cancer Institute, Chiyoda-ku, Tokyo, 101 Japan, [4] Department of Pathology, Sapporo Medical College, Sapporo, 060 Japan

Comparison of the Wet Weights of Organs

Prior to the immunopathological tests, the wet weights of various organs were measured in a comparative study of the LEC and LEA rats. After the body weights of 6-week-old pre-hepatitis LEC and LEA rats were measured, dissection was performed; the livers, spleens and thymuses were removed and their wet weights were measured immediately.

The wet weights of these organs were also measured at the onset of acute hepatitis in the LEC rats, and compared with those of the age-matched LEA rats.

Measurement of Serum IgG and IgM

Peripheral blood was collected from the jugular vein of LEC and LEA rats aged 15 days and 1, 3, 4 and 12 months, and was separated by centrifugation. Blood was again collected from the LEC rats in the same manner at the onset of acute hepatitis. The serum IgG and IgM levels were measured by the single radial immunodiffusion assay in accordance with Mancini's method. In the preliminary studies with the use of an anti-rat IgG (Cosmo-Bio KK), the agarose-gel antibody concentration was determined to be 6%; holes of 3 mm in diameter were made in the 6% agarose plate. Five microliters each of a standard solution and test samples were injected into the holes, and the plates were set stable for 3 h at 37°C in a humidified environment. A calibration curve was drawn based upon the precipitation rings of the standard solution; the diameter of the precipitation ring of the test serum was measured to determine the IgG concentration. Measurements of IgM were done in the same manner, by using anti-rat IgM (Cosmo-Bio KK, Tokyo) in accordance with Mancini's method. Since no standard solution of IgM was available, the diameter of the precipitation ring for the test serum was measured after 3 h incubation, and this value was squared for comparison.

Measurement of IgG- and IgM-Antibody Forming Cells
(Plaque-Forming Cell: PFC)

A plaque test was performed in accordance with Cunningham and Szenberg's Plaque Method. A 50% suspension of sheep red blood cells (SRBC) (Nippon Biotest Laboratories Co., Ltd., Tokyo) was prepared, and 1 ml of the suspension was administrated via the caudal vein of the LEC and LEA rats aged 6 weeks and 12 weeks. On the 4th day after immunization with SRBC, the rats were sacrificed and spleen cells were obtained from them. After the cells were adjusted to 1×10^6 cells/ml in modified Eagle's medium (Nissui Pharmaceutical Co., Ltd., Tokyo), 400 µl was put in a small test tube; 50 µl of the 50% SRBC suspension and 50 µl of complement from marmot blood (Nakarai Chemicals, Ltd., Kyoto, Japan) were added and mixed slowly and thoroughly. Three chambers of equal volume were created using a clean glass slide (75 × 25 mm), coverslips (22 × 22 mm) and 6-mm-wide double-sided sticky tape. A 100 μl sample of the above-mentioned mixture was pipetted into each of the three chambers, which were incubated for about 60 min in a 37°C, 5% CO_2 incubator. Immediately after incubation, plaques formed by hemolysed SRBCs were assessed by microscopic observation. The IgM-producing PFCs were counted (direct method). To detect IgG-producing PFCs, anti-rat IgG was added before the complement, and the assessment of IgG-producing PFCs was performed in the same manner as the IgM-PFCs assessment through microscopic examination (indirect method).

Measurement of Blastogenic Responses

LEC and LEA rats, 6- and 12-week-olds, were sacrificed, and their spleens were removed under sterile conditions. Each spleen was dissected and the spleen cells were separated, washed, and centrifuged 3 times (1,200 rpm, 5 min) in RPMI1640 including 5% newborn calf serum (FCS) (GIBCO, Rhode Island, USA) and adjusted to 5×10^6/ml. For the final cell adjustment, a complete medium, RPMI1640 supplemented with 10% FCS, IM HEPES (0.01 ml/ml), 100-fold-diluted sodium pyruvate (0.01 ml/ml), 100-fold-diluted non-essential amino acid (0.01 ml/ml) and 2-mercaptoethanol (5×10^{-4} ml/ml), was used. Samples (100 μl each) of the spleen cell suspension, and either prepared 200 μg/ml phytohemaglutinin (PHA) (Difco, Detroit) or 20 μg/ml concavalin A (Con A) (Difco, Detroit) were added to the wells of a 96-well flat bottom microtiter plate (Corning, New York) and were incubated for 3 days at 37°C in a 5% CO_2 incubator. As a control, 100 μl of a complete medium was added to 100 μl of the spleen cell suspension (in triplicate). Eighteen hours prior to the end of the incubation period, 0.5 μCi (20 μl)/well of [methyl³H]-thymidine (³H-TdR) (Amersham International plc, Buckinghamshire, UK) was added to each well. A liquid scintillation counter was used for the activity measurements: if ³H-TdR uptake increased more than twofold of the control's, the increase was considered significant.

Measurement of NK Activity

A suspension of the spleen cells prepared in the manner described previously was produced using RPMI1640 with 10% FCS, and adjusted to 2×10^7 cells/ml. Additionally, two more concentrations, 1×10^7 cells/ml and 5×10^6 cells/ml, were produced by serial dilution, which gave a total of 3 different concentrations of the effector cells. K562 cells were used as the target cells. Suspended K562 cells were adjusted to 5×10^6/ml, of which 0.85 ml was pipetted into a 35 mm flask (Corning, New York). Next, 0.15 ml CR-51 sodium chromate (^{51}Cr) (Amersham International plc, Buckinghamshire, UK) was added to the flask, and the mixture was incubated for 1 h in a 37°C, 5% CO_2 incubator and mixed repeatedly every 15 min.

One hour later, the mixture was removed from the incubator, washed 3 times in sterilized phosphate-buffered saline (PBS⁻) (0.2 g KCL, 0.2 g H_2PO_4, 8 g NaCl, and 2.16 g $NaHPO_4 \cdot 7H_2O$ per liter) and centrifuged (1,200 rpm, 5 min). K562 cells were then adjusted to 1×10^5 cells/ml. After these procedures, each 100 µl of the 3 effector cell suspensions and 100 µl of the target cell suspension were placed in the well of a 96-well round bottom microtiter plate (Corning, New York) (in triplicate). The E/T ratios of the 3 different suspension concentrations were 200:1, 100:1, and 50:1, respectively. A spontaneous release was produced by adding 100 µl of the same medium to 100 µl of the target cell suspension, and a maximum release was produced by adding 100 µl 1N hydrochloric acid to 100 µl of the target cell suspension. After the plates were incubated for 4 h in a 37°C, 5% CO_2 incubator, they were centrifuged (2,000 rpm, 10 min); 100 µl of the supernatant was collected and the ^{51}Cr activity was measured. The percentage of cytolysis was calculated according to the following formula:

$$\% \text{ Cytolysis} = \frac{\text{Experimental release} - \text{spontaneous release}}{\text{Maximum release} - \text{spontaneous release}} \times 100$$

Measurement of Cytostatic Activity of Intraperitoneal Macrophages

After the abdomen of the LEC and LEA rats was opened and the abdominal cavity was washed with cold PBS⁻, intraperitoneal macrophages were collected. The collected macrophages, i.e., the effector cells, were washed 3 times in PBS⁻ and adjusted to 2×10^6, 1×10^6, and 5×10^5 cells/ml in RPMI1640. The target cells were mouse fibrosarcoma cells (BMT-11) which were adjusted to 1×10^5 cells/ml in RPMI1640. The E/T ratios were 20:1, 10:1, and 5:1 in each concentration, respectively. Each 100 µl of the 3 concentrations of effector cells and of the target cells was put into the wells of a 96-well flat bottom microtiter plate (Corning, New York). Control groups were also made for effector or target cells (in triplicate). The plates were incubated for 24 h in a 37°C, 5% CO_2 incubator. Six hours before the end of the incubation period, 20 µl ^3H-TdR (0.4 µCi) was added into each well. A liquid scintillation counter was used for the activity measurements, and the percentage of cytostasis was calculated according to the following formula:

$$\% \text{ Cytostasis} = \left(1 - \frac{\text{cpm Target cells with M\O} - \text{cpm M\O alone}}{\text{cpm Target cells alone}}\right) \times 100$$

Statistical Analysis

The results were expressed as mean values ± standard deviation, and Student's t-test was used in evaluating significant differences between the groups.

Table 1. Autopsy findings of 6-week-old male LEC ($n = 5$) and LEA ($n = 5$) rats.

Weight (g)	LEA	LEC	P value*
Body	156 ± 16.1	149 ± 8.2	N.S.
Liver	6.9 ± 0.8	5.5 ± 0.98	<0.05
Spleen	0.90 ± 0.12	0.33 ± 0.02	<0.001
Thymus	0.41 ± 0.06	0.12 ± 0.02	<0.001

* by Student's t-test; wt, weight; N.S., not significant

Results

Comparison of the Wet Weights of Various Organs

No significant difference was found between the body weights of 6-week-old LEC ($n = 5$) and LEA ($n = 5$) rats; however, the wet weights of the livers showed a significant difference ($P < 0.05$). The mean wet weights of the spleens and the thymuses, which play a role in the immune system, indicated a significant difference ($P < 0.001$) between the two strains (Table 1). The ratios between the wet weight of the liver and the body weight were also calculated ($\times 10^2$) as was done for the LEC rats with hepatitis and the age-matched LEA rats: it was 3.29 ± 0.49 ($n = 21$) in the LEC rats, whereas in the LEA rats it was 4.37 ± 0.57 ($n = 9$), showing a significant difference ($P < 0.001$) (Fig. 1).

From these results, it was clear that the wet weights of the spleens, thymuses, and livers of LEC rats were significantly reduced in comparison to those of LEA rats.

Comparative Study of IgG Levels

The IgG level (mg/ml) was 4.9 ± 0.7 ($n = 4$) in the LEC rats, and 4.5 ± 1.1 ($n = 6$) in the LEA rats 0.5 month after birth. The IgG level decreased in 1-month-old LEA rats and rose in the following months. However, in the LEC rats, the IgG level remained elevated starting at the age of 1 month until it decreased at the ages of 3 and 4 months. Thus, in the LEC rats, a reduced utilization of IgG seemed to accompany a marked suppression of its autogenesis, and this tendency was observed in the long-term survivors (aged 12 months) as well. This phenomenon presents a prominent contrast in the changes of IgG levels between the LEC and LEA rats (Fig. 2).

Comparative Study of IgM Levels

In a monthly comparison of the IgM levels in the LEC and LEA rats, it was found that the IgM levels of LEC rats were relatively higher than those of

Fig. 1. Comparison of liver/body weight ratios between LEC rats with hepatitis and age-matched LEA rats

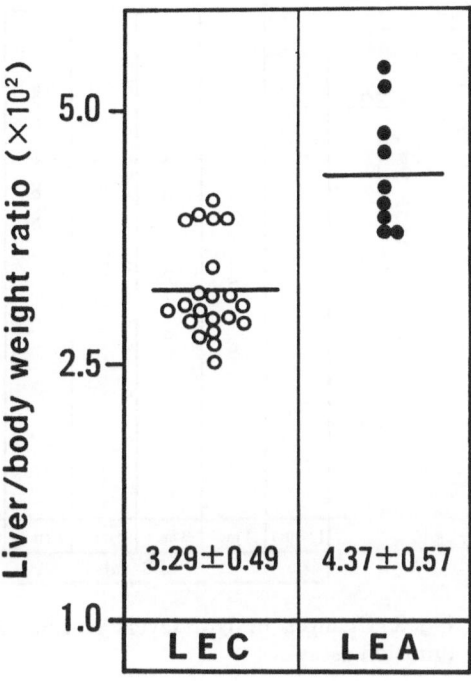

Fig. 2. Changes in IgG levels of LEC and LEA rats by single radial immuno-diffusion assay

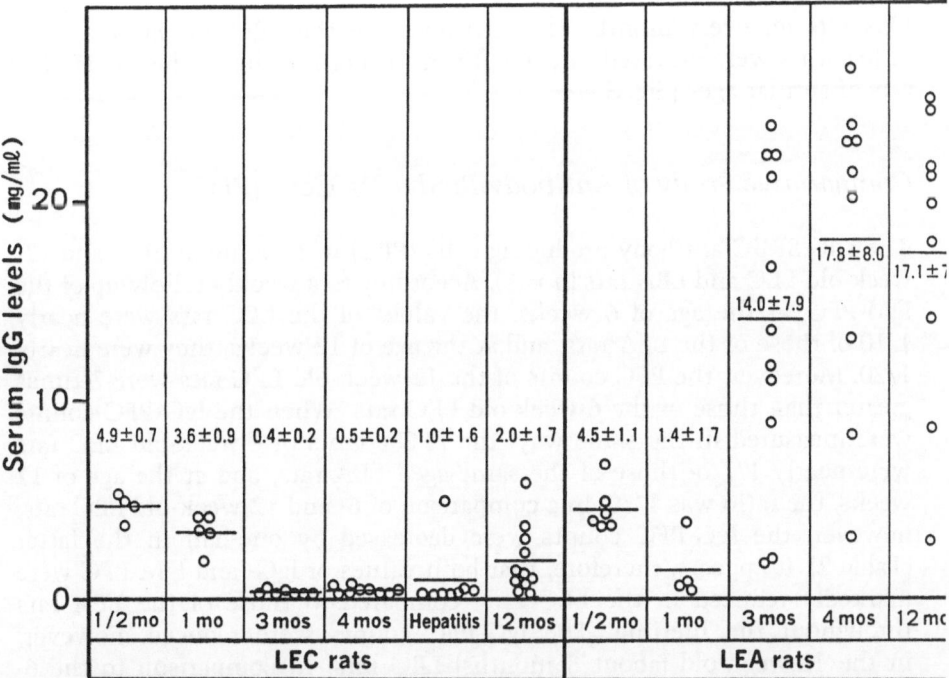

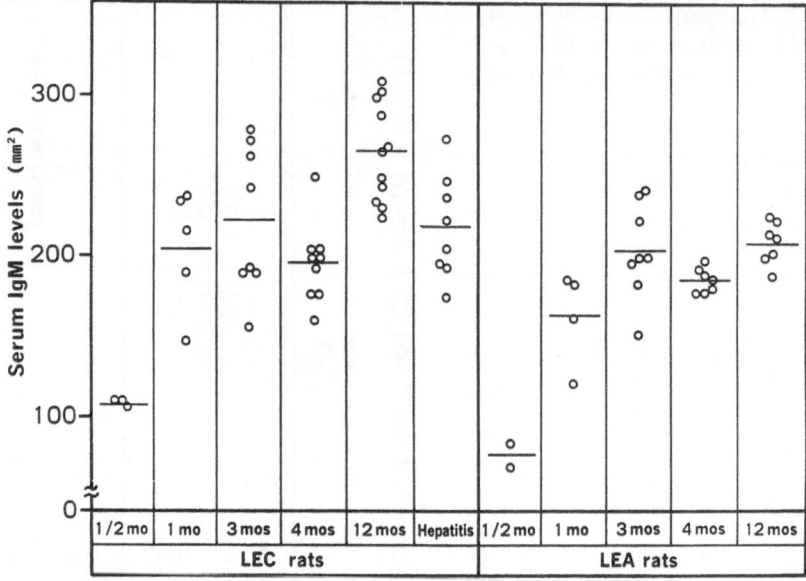

Fig. 3. Changes in IgM levels of LEC and LEA rats by single radial immuno-diffusion assay

LEA rats for every month. The IgM levels in the LEC rats at the onset of hepatitis were elevated in comparison to those of the pre-hepatitis LEC rats of similar ages (Fig. 3).

Comparative Study of Antibody-Producing Cells (PFC)

The anti-SRBC antibody producing cells (PFC) were counted in 6- and 12-week-old LEC and LEA rats ($n = 5$). According to a weekly follow-up of the IgM-PFC, at the age of 6 weeks, the values of the LEC rats were nearly 1/10 of those of the LEA rats, and at the age of 12 weeks, they were nearly 1/20. Moreover, the PFC counts of the 12-week-old LEC rats were 7 times greater than those of the 6-week-old LEC rats. When the IgG-PFC counts were measured in the same way, the PFC counts of 6-week-old LEC rats were nearly 1/7 of those of the same-aged LEA rats, and at the age of 12 weeks, the ratio was 1/70. In a comparison of 6- and 12-week-old LEC rats, however, the IgG-PFC counts were decreased by one-half in the latter (Table 2). It appears, therefore, that both values of IgG- and IgM-PFC were markedly reduced in the LEC rats, compared to those of the LEA rats throughout the lifetime. The IgG-PFC counts were reduced, however, in the 12-week-old (about 3 months) LEC rats, in comparison to the 6-week-old LEC rats, which seems to indicate a correlation between the above-described serum IgG levels and the IgG production abnormalities.

Table 2. Comparison of plaque-forming (anti-SRBC antibody) cells (PFC) using spleen cells in LEC and LEA rats.

Strain[a]	Age (weeks)	Mean PFC ± S.D./10⁶ IgM	Spleen cells IgG
LEC	6	10 ± 18	26 ± 18
LEA	6	961 ± 176	176 ± 98
LEC	12	71 ± 28	11 ± 3
LEA	12	1380 ± 150	762 ± 107

[a] Five rats were used in each group

Table 3. Comparison of blastogenic responses in spleen cells between LEC and LEA rats.

Strain of rats[a]	Age (weeks)	³H-thymidine uptake (Mean cpm ± S.D.) PHA	ConA	Control
LEC	6	3593 ± 1510[b]	5891 ± 3046[c]	1482 ± 426
LEA	6	7518 ± 2111	74148 ± 5456	1908 ± 85
LEC	12	11075 ± 7182[b]	21993 ± 8235[c]	2715 ± 679
LEA	12	48137 ± 25167	119877 ± 21346	2430 ± 853

[a] Five rats were used in each group
[b] $P < 0.05$ (by Student's t-test)
[c] $P < 0.001$ (by Studnet's t-test)

Comparative Study of Blastogenic Responses

We tested T-cell function by the blastogenic reaction by using PHA and Con A. In a comparison of 6-week-old LEC with LEA rats ($n = 5$), the blastogenic reaction to PHA in the spleen cells of LEC rats was reduced to nearly 1/2, and to nearly 1/13 to Con A. At the age of 12 weeks ($n = 5$), the blasto-genic reaction to PHA was reduced to nearly one-fourth, and nearly one-fifth to Con A in the LEC rats. In comparison to the control, the blasto-genic reactions of the LEC rats were also reduced in all of the mitogens throughout the whole period (Table 3). The above results showed the reduced lymphatic cell reaction to PHA and Con A in the LEC rats at the ages of 6 and 12 weeks.

Comparative Study of NK Activity

The natural killer (NK) activity of the spleen cells in the 6- and 12-week-old LEC and LEA rats ($n = 5$) was measured. The E/T ratios were 200:1, 100:1, and 50:1. At the age of 6 weeks, a significant elevation of NK activity was found in the LEC rats at a 200:1 E/T ratio and in the LEA rats at 50:1 E/T ratio, but no significant differences were otherwise detected.

Table 4. Comparison of NK activity in spleen cells between LEC and LEA rats.

Strain[a]	Age (weeks)	% Cytotoxicity at E/T Ratio[b]		
		200:1	100:1	50:1
LEC	6	19.7 ± 4.2	8.5 ± 2.6	0.6 ± 0.5
LEA	6	10.2 ± 1.5	7.3 ± 0.9	4.2 ± 1.0
LEC	12	15.3 ± 1.1	10.8 ± 1.2	4.0 ± 1.0
LEA	12	15.2 ± 2.5	11.6 ± 1.4	4.0 ± 1.0

[a] Five rats were used in each group
[b] K562 cells were used as target cells for 4-h ^{51}Cr-release assay

Table 5. Comparison of cytostatic activity of peritoneal macrophages between LEC and LEA rats.

Strain[a]	Age (weeks)	% Inhibition of ^{3}H-thymidine uptake at E/T ratio[b]		
		20:1	10:1	5:1
LEC	6	54.9	42.0	13.9
LEA	6	18.7	18.7	20.6
LEC	12	53.1	48.5	24.7
LEA	12	25.6	20.7	18.9

[a] Five rats per group
[b] Mouse fibrosarcoma cells were used as target cells for assay

By overall analysis of these results, it seems that no significant differences in the NK activity existed between LEC and LEA rats (Table 4).

Comparative Study of Intraperitoneal Macrophage Cytostatic Activity

The cytostatic activities of the intraperitoneal macrophages was measured as was done for 6- and 12-week-old LEC and LEA rats ($n = 5$). The E/T ratios were 20:1, 10:1, and 5:1. Except for the reduced suppression ratio, 5:1 E/T, in the 6-week-old LEC rats, the suppression ratios were elevated in the LEC rats compared to those of the LEA rats. However, no significant changes were found in the LEC rats between the 6th and the 12th week after birth. Thus, we can conclude that the cytostatic activity of the intraperitoneal macrophages was markedly increased in the LEC rats compared to that in the LEA rats (Table 5).

Discussion

The possibility of correlation between different immunological reactions and the pathogenesis or course of liver disease has been analyzed by various researchers; however, no definite explanation of how the immunological reactions are related to the mechanism of onset of acute, chronic, and fulminant hepatitis has yet been found. Regarding the mechanisms of the change from virus-induced hepatitis to fulminant disease, Almeida's hypothesis (induction of disseminated liver cell necrosis by immunological complexes which result from excessive antibody production [3]) and Duddley's hypothesis (an excessive reaction of T cells against multiple virus infected liver cells [4]) have been advocated. Since then, it has been generally believed that fulminant hepatitis is associated with an abnormal condition of the immune system, and that the disease is provoked by an immunological surplus. More recently, however, it has been suggested that fulminant hepatitis is associated with acceleration of humoral immunity [5]. It has also been reported that in an acute hepatic failure model, in which the disease was induced by iv. infusion of heat-killed *Propionibacterium acnes*, no blastogenesis of the immunocompetent cells were found among the infiltrative cells in the liver, apart from adhesive cells; instead, there was an immunosuppression of all other immunocompetent cells (intrahepatic adhesive cells, peritoneal exudate macrophages, peripheral monocytic cells, and spleen cells), as well as a suppression of antibody production within the spleen [6]. From these findings we can deduce that the change from hepatitis to a fulminant disease is associated with abnormalities both in the humoral and the cellular immune systems, i.e., a state of excessive reaction of the former, and a state of suppression of the latter. In other words, fulminant hepatitis may be mainly accounted for hepatic cell-impairing mechanisms ascribable to chemical mediators such as cytokines (monokines, lymphokines, etc.), which also include humoral antibodies. These hepatic cell-impairing mechanisms may also be ascribed to macrophages or NK cells dominating non-specific immunity, in contrast to mechanisms involving killer T-cell destruction of cells which plays an important role in acute hepatitis. Prior to investigating the immunological competence, we compared the wet weights of the organs which are considered to play a part in the immune system, i.e., the spleen and thymus [2]. The result, a significant weight reduction of these organs in the LEC rats, is sufficient enough to suggest an abnormality of the immune system. The wet weights of the livers, as well, tended to be reduced in the LEC rats, which is also attributable to insufficient development or atrophy. A correlation between the suppressed IgG levels and the onset of hepatitis has been described in our previous report [2]. In addition, through a follow-up of the IgG levels over a period of a few months, we have found that the shift to acute hepatitis in the LEC rats followed a failure to recover from the state of physiological immunodeficiency, and that even in the individuals which were spared, or those in which the hepatitis was in remission, the suppression of the autogenesis of IgG was apparent. This fact corresponds with the increased suppression of the IgG-PFC found at the age of 12 weeks, in comparison to that at the age of 6 weeks. In the experiments in which a strain from crossbreeding of LEC and LEA rats was used, we were observed that the lower the IgG level was, the higher the incidence of hepatitis was [2]. Any cause-and-effect relationship between the IgG level suppression and the onset of hepatitis has not yet been clarified, but we infer that the suppression of IgG, a part of the immune system, participates in one form or another in the onset and course of hepatitis. On the other hand, in the comparative study of the IgM in the LEC and the LEA rats, an elevation tendency was found only in the former, whereas the IgM-PFC counts were significantly reduced in the LEC rats.

From our present experimental results, we set out the following two points regarding abnormalities of immunoglobulin production in the LEC rats. (1) The discrepancy between the elevated serum IgM level and the reduced IgM-PFC indicates an insufficient maturation of the immature B cells after immunization and elevation of the serum IgM level through production of IgM by the immature B cells. Since maturation of B cells is insufficient, the absolute number of mature B cells with μ chains, which are capable of "class transformation" to the cells which will process γ chains, decrease. There is also a suppression of the IgG-PFC; as a result, the serum IgG level is reduced. (2) The presentation of antigens by antigen-presenting cells (APC) as well as the participation of helper T cells is required for the maturation of B cells. We suggest that, in the LEC rats, the participation of one or both of them is insufficient.

The blastogenic reaction evoked by PHA and Con A is markedly suppressed in the LEC rats in comparison to the LEA rats, which generally delineates a suppressed T-cell function. Therefore, it seems that one factor in the abnormalities in B cell maturation is the suppressed T-cell function. From the measurements of the cytostatic activity of macrophages, it appears that the antitumor activity of the macrophages is significantly elevated in the LEC rats in comparison to that in the LEA rats, and that there are no distinct changes in macrophage function between the two strains. It is not clear, however, whether cell-to-cell contact is required for the initiation of the macrophage cytostatic effect, or whether a secreted factor is required for the effect. Another study has reported that the cytostatic macrophages actually belong to a subpopulation different from the other macrophages [7]. Taking these opinions into consideration, if we assumed that the macrophages in the LEC rats do present sufficient antigen, we would still emphasize that the suppression of the T-cell function would cause the inhibition of B-cell maturation, resulting in the onset of hepatitis in the LEC rats.

Lastly, we will discuss immunity as a defense mechanism of the living body. In the LEC rats, there was a marked suppression of specific antibody (IgG) production, as well as a marked suppression of the T-cell function. On the other hand, a part of the non-specific cellular immunity — the NK activity — was found to be almost identical in both the LEC and LEA rats, while the macrophage antitumor activity was elevated in the LEC rats. It is evident that defense mechanisms against infections, a type of specific immunity, is relatively suppressed in the LEC rats, and that non-specific cellular immunity plays an important role.

The relationships among the onset of hepatitis, the suppressed function of T and B cells, and the elevated function of the cells associated with non-specific immunity have not yet been clarified. We assume that there is a correlation between abnormalities of the immune system and facilitation of liver diseases, which will be important subjects for our future research. Understanding the pathogenesis of acute or fulminant hepatitis in the LEC rats may provide us with insights for the pathology of human hepatitis.

Conclusions

We carried out immunopathological studies of the pathogenesis of LEC rats which spontaneously develop acute hepatitis and fulminant hepatitis, in comparison with non-hepatitis LEA rats as a control group. Our findings are as follows:

1. In comparison between 6-week-old LEC and LEA rats, the wet weights of the spleens, thymuses, and livers of the LEC rats were significantly lighter than those of the LEA rats.
2. Serum IgG levels and IgG antibody formation capacity were suppressed in the LEC rats, and this kept the animals physiologically immuno-deficient. On the other hand, serum IgM levels in the LEC rats were relatively elevated, although IgM antibody formation capacity was suppressed; in addition, the immature B cells did not appear to mature completely.
3. Blastogenic responses of spleen cells to PHA and Con A, as well as the B cell function, were much suppressed in the LEC rats.
4. Cytostatic activity of intraperitoneal macrophages against tumor cells was more evident in the LEC rats, but there was no difference in natural killer (NK) activity between the two rat strains.

These findings suggest that the immunodeficiency involving the function of T and B cells and the elevated macrophage function may directly or indirectly affect development of hepatitis in the LEC rats.

Acknowledgment. This work was supported by grants from the Ministry of Education, Science and Culture of Japan.

References

1. Namieno T, Takeichi N, Sasaki M, Dempo K, Mori M, Uchino J, Kobayashi H (to be published) Clinical and pathological characteristics of Long-Evans Cinnamon (LEC) rats with spontaneous development of hepatitis

2. Namieno T, Takeichi N, Sasaki M, Dempo K, Mori M, Uchino J, Kobayashi H (to be published) Pathogenesis of spontanteous hepatitis in Long-Evans Cinnamon (LEC) rats
3. Almeida JD, Waterson AP (1969) Immune complexes in hepatitis. Lancet II: 983–986
4. Dudley FJ, Fox RA, Sherlock S (1972) Cellular immunity and hepatitis-associated Australia antigen liver disease. Lancet I:723–726
5. Singh NK, Goyal AK, Srivastava PK, Gupta RM, Tripathi KK (1984) Immunological status in acute viral hepatitis and fulminant hepatic failure. J Indian Med Assoc 82:281–283
6. Tsutsui H, Mizoguchi Y, Yamamoto S, Morisawa S (1986) Studies on experimentally-induced acute hepatic failure: Possible involvement of activated liver adherent cells. In: Kirn A, Knook DL, Wisse E (eds) Cells of hepatic sinusoid. The Kupffer Cell Foundation, The Netherlands, pp 307–314
7. Chapes SK, Stezhen H (1983) Role of *Corynebacterium parvum* in the activation of peritoneal macrophages. II. Identification of distinguishable anti-tumor activities by macrophage subpopulation. Cell Immunol 76:49–57

23 — Genetic Analysis of Immunodeficiency and Hereditary Hepatitis in LEC Rats

ATSUO HATTORI, YASUHIRO KONISHI, HIROSHI ISOMURA, KOUKI INAOKA, YUN ZHONG, and MICHIO MORI[1]

Introduction

The new mutant LEC rat suffers from hereditary hepatitis with severe jaundice, anemia, subcutaneous bleeding, weight loss, and oliguria at around 4 months after birth [1,2]. About one-half of the LEC rats die within 1 week after the onset of hepatitis, whereas the remaining LEC rats survive much longer with chronic hepatitis and subsequently develop liver cancer at a high frequency [3,4].

Genetic analysis performed on various crossed breedings of LEC and LEJ rats has revealed that a single autosomal recessive gene designated *hts* (hepatitis) is responsible for the development of hepatitis [5]. However, the causative abnormality transmitted by this gene has not yet been identified. On the other hand, the presence of combined immunodeficiency caused by another autosomal recessive gene has been shown in the LEC rat [6]. In this paper, we performed a genetic analysis of both the hereditary hepatitis and the immunodeficiency, in an attempt to elucidate the relationship between these two disorders possessed genetically by the LEC rat.

Histological and Immunohistological Characteristics of the Immunodeficiency in LEC Rats

The lymphoid tissues of 2- to 14-week-old LEC rats, were examined histologically and immunohistologically before the onset of hepatitis. For controls, the lymphoid tissues of LEA rats of the same ages were used.

The most striking histological finding of the LEC rat was observed in the thymus, in which the medulla was severely hypoplastic (Fig. 1a). Such a change in the thymic medulla was already observed at 4 weeks of age. On

---

[1] Department of Pathology, Sapporo Medical College, Sapporo, 060 Japan

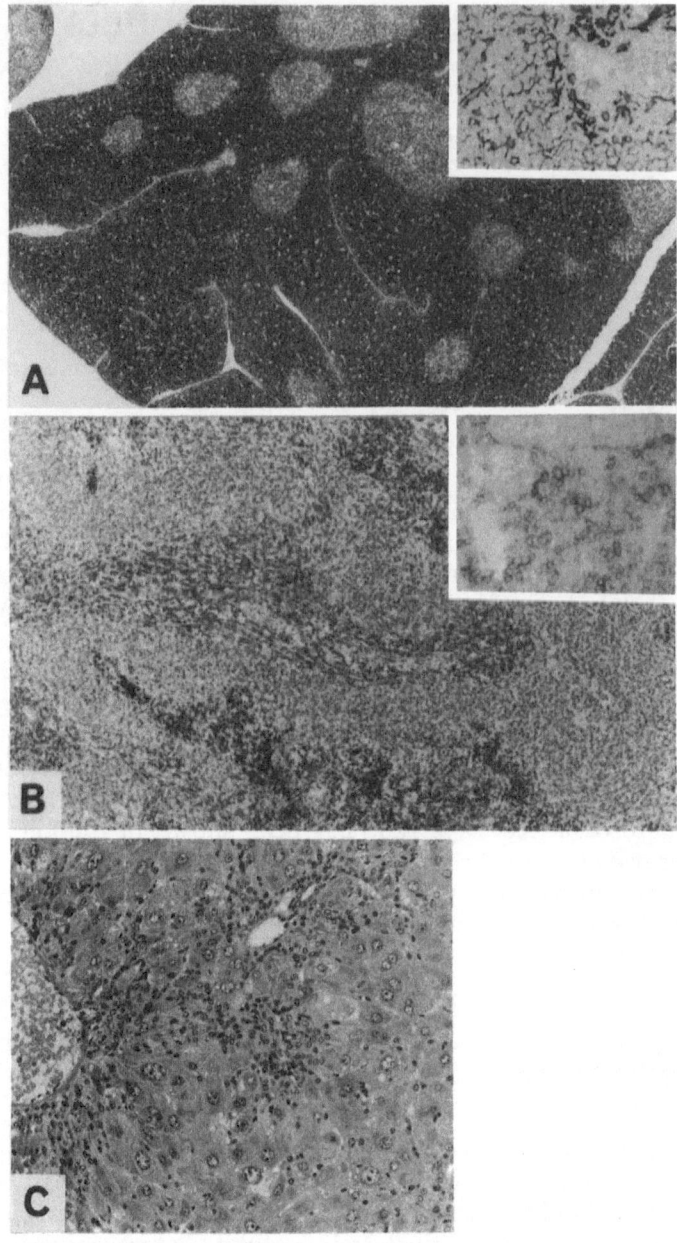

Fig. 1. Marked deletion of the thymic medulla in a 8-week-old LEC rat (H and E stain.). **A** *Insert* shows the deletion of the thymic epithelium (keratin immuno-staining). **B** Marked deletion of T cell area (perivascular area) in the LEC rat spleen. The deletion is mainly due to the deletion of W3/25 positive cells. **C** Hepatitis of LEC rat at the age of 20 weeks: enlarged nuclei and degenerating of hepatocytes are seen

Table 1. The mean ratio percent of lymphocyte subsets (percent ± SEM*)

		Source of lymphocytes								
		Thymus			Lymph nodes			Spleen		
Age of rats in weeks (n = 4)		4	8	12	4	8	12	4	8	12
3B3 (Lyt-1)	LEC	95.3 (±1.9)	97.9 (±0.5)	93.6 (±3.8)	39.2[b] (±2.2)	43.8[c] (±3.3)	38.9[a] (±2.7)	16.2 (±1.5)	14.1 (±1.8)	23.0[c] (±1.2)
	LEA	89.9 (±10.6)	95.0 (±3.0)	93.5 (±3.1)	65.0 (±5.8)	71.8 (±3.2)	58.4 (±4.2)	25.2 (±5.2)	34.7 (±9.1)	38.1 (±1.8)
10B5 (Lyt-2)	LEC	93.4 (±1.6)	97.0 (±0.9)	93.7 (±2.6)	31.5 (±3.3)	32.8[a] (±4.0)	26.5 (±2.7)	22.9 (±2.1)	11.8 (±1.3)	17.8 (±0.6)
	LEA	88.3 (±10.0)	90.6 (±2.8)	88.4 (±3.4)	24.0 (±6.9)	53.7 (±6.9)	22.5 (±6.1)	20.3 (±5.1)	22.1 (±4.9)	19.0 (±1.6)
W3/25	LEC	93.6 (±1.8)	95.2 (±0.9)	89.6 (±4.7)	23.5[a] (±6.6)	23.6[c] (±2.1)	23.0[a] (±3.5)	11.4[a] (±0.9)	8.2[a] (±1.5)	14.0[a] (±0.6)
	LEA	92.5 (±4.9)	91.1 (±4.5)	89.4 (±2.8)	50.1 (±6.5)	55.4 (±5.4)	43.4 (±3.1)	21.3 (±2.7)	22.5 (±5.3)	29.0 (±4.1)
OX-6	LEC	21.0 (±7.1)	25.8 (±6.2)	17.3 (±6.6)	46.0[c] (±2.2)	37.9 (±6.5)	46.4[a] (±1.5)	40.2 (±0.8)	64.1 (±3.9)	60.9 (±2.5)
	LEA	27.5 (±2.3)	26.4 (±2.1)	20.7 (±4.2)	23.2 (±2.2)	24.2 (±3.6)	32.2 (±2.7)	44.4 (±9.4)	37.8 (±0.8)	52.0 (±3.0)

Comparison of the percentage of lymphocytes positive for the monoclonal antibodies (3B3 for Lyt-1, 10B5 for Lyt-2 as described [12] and W3/25 for helper/inducer T cell, OX-6 for I-A antigen of lymphocytes) between LEA and LEC rat
[a] $p < 0.01$, [b] $P < 0.05$, [c] $P < 0.001$, when compared to those matched LEA rats by using Student's t-test
* SEM, Standard error of the mean

the other hand, the thymic cortex showed essentially the same normal development as that in the LEA rat. Anti-keratin antibodies utilized to distinguish the epithelial cells in the thymus clearly revealed that there were few epithelial cells and Hassall's bodies in the thymus of LEC rats (Fig. 1a *insert*). The thymus is a central lymphoid organ which plays a principal role in the generation of diverse T lymphocytes in mammals [7,8]. T lymphocytes are considered to differentiate in the thymus by making contact with reticular networks of thymic epithelial cells under the influence of substances, such as thymosin, thymopoietin, thymic humoral factors, and interleukins [9–11]. On the other hand, in the peripheral lymphoid organs of LEC rats, such as the spleen and lymph nodes, there was a marked depletion of T lymphocytes in the periarterial regions at 8 and 12 weeks of age (Fig. 1b). There was a marked decrease in the number of medium-sized lymphocytes positive for immunohistochemistry with W3/25 antigen (Fig. 1b *insert*), whereas the number of Ig M- and Ig A-positive lymphocytes did not show any significant changes. The results of the fluorescent-activated cell sorter (FACS) analysis supported the above-mentioned histological findings in that the percentages of lymphocytes labeled with anti-Lyt-1, -Lyt-2, -W3/25, and -OX-6, in the thymus, spleen, and lymph nodes of LEC rats changed by the same magnitude [12] (Table 1). In the thymus, 94%–99% of the cells were positive for Lyt-1, Lyt-2, and W3/25 in both the LEC and LEA rats. Contrarily, in the peripheral lymphoid tissues, the number of lymphocytes positive for Lyt-1 and W3/25 in the LEC rat was about one-half of that seen in the LEA rat at every age examined, whereas there were more cells labeled with Lyt-2, OX-6, and immunoglobulins found in the LEC rat than in the LEA rat. These findings strongly suggest that the maturation of T lymphocytes is impaired at the sites between the thymus and the peripheral lymphoid organs.

The results of blastogenesis studies are shown in Table 2. The lymphocytes of LEC rats did not respond well to blastogenic stimulation. Briefly, the response of LEC rat lymphocytes against concanavalin A (Con A) was one-fifth of that found in LEA rat lymphocytes. Also, lymphocytes of the

Table 2. Comparison of blastogenic responses in spleen cells of LEC and LEA rats.

Mitogenic stimulator[a]	^{3}H-Thymidine uptake (cpm ± SEM*)	
	LEA Rats (control)	LEC Rats (control)
Concanavalin A	39,843 ± 4,551 (1,408 ± 275)	6,034 ± 193[b] (1,217 ± 193)
Lipopolysaccharide	5,748 ± 1,042 (1,841 ± 275)	996 ± 165[b] (1,328 ± 226)

[a] Four 8-week-old male rats each of LEA and LEC rats were used. Spleen cells were cultured with 4 µg/ml Con A and with 12.5 µg/ml LPS for 72 h in a 96-well culture plate. The cell concentration was 4×10^5/well. ^{3}H-thymidine (1 µCi/well) was added to each well for 12 h

[b] $P < 0.001$, when compared with those of LEA rats by using Student's t-test.

* *SEM* Standard error of the mean

LEC rat did not respond to lipopolysaccharide (LPS), suggesting that both T and B lymphocytes of LEC rats can not respond well to mitogenic stimuli. The results of the mixed lymphocyte reaction showed that the lymphocytes of LEC rats had virtually no response to the spleen cells from LEA rats. These findings seem to be supported by the evidence that when the hepatocytes of LEA rats were transplanted into the spleen of LEC rats, the hepatocytes survived for more than 18 weeks without rejection. Taken together, it seems reasonable to consider that the immunologic development of both T and B lymphocytes of LEC rats is impaired, probably due to abnormal development of the thymic medulla.

Genetic Analysis of Immunodeficiency and Hepatitis in LEC Rat

The possible interrelation between the hepatitis and immunodeficiency of the LEC rat was investigated by mating LEC rats with LEA rats. The F_1 hybrids from LEC rats and LEA rats were intercrossed to produce F_2 hybrids. In addition, reciprocal backcrosses of (LEC × LEA) F_1 × LEC, and (LEA × LEC) F_1 × LEC were bred. Peripheral blood lymphocytes were collected from each rat at 12–16 weeks of age by the Ficoll-Conray method [13]. The T-cell subsets were analyzed after labeling with monoclonal antibodies with the FACS analyzer. When clinical signs, such as jaundice and oliguria appeared, the rat was sacrificed immediately for histological, biochemical, and laboratory examinations. Asymptomatic rats were sacrificed at the age of 24–28 weeks for the same examinations. The FACS analysis revealed that the ratio of W3/25 to Lyt-2 (helper/inducer T:cytotoxic/suppressor T cell) was higher than 1.00 in the LEA rat (normal type), whereas in the LEC rat it was lower than 1.00 (abnormal type). Eight pairs of F_1s were bred and 30 F_2 hybrids, 15 each for male and female, were obtained. Four pairs of reciprocal backcrosses were bred and 13 backcrosses, 4 males and 9 females, were obtained. The results are shown in Table 3. Among the 15 male F_2 hybrids, 12 were of a normal type, leaving 3 of an abnormal type in the T-cell subset ratio. Among the female F_2 hybrids, 1 was of a normal type, while 2 were of an abnormal type. In the reciprocal backcrosses, male F_2 hybrids were divided into 1 normal and 3 abnormal types, whereas female F_2 hybrids were divided into 5 normal and 4 abnormal types. In the F_2 hybrids, the abnormal/normal ratio was 5:25. In the reciprocal backcross F_2 hybrids, the abnormal/normal ratio was 7:6. These results are essentially in accordance with a previous report which found that the immunodeficiency of the LEC rat is controlled by an autosomal recessive gene [6].

The relation between the occurrence of such an abnormal ratio in T-cell subsets and the development of hepatitis was then investigated. Histological and laboratory findings were used as the indicator of hepatitis (Fig.

Table 3. Inheritance mode of hepatitis and immunological abnormality (T-cell depletion) in F_2 and backcross rats.

		F_2 (30 Rats) Rats showing T-cell depletion (n)					Backcross (13 rats) Rats showing T-cell depletion (n)		
		(+)	(−)	Total			(+)	(−)	Total
Rats showing hepatitis (n)	(+)	2	3	5	Rats showing hepatitis (n)	(+)	3	3	6
	(−)	3	22	25		(−)	4	3	7
	Total	5	25			Total	7	6	

1c). An elevated serum GPT level over 100 iu/ml, the presence of hepatocytes in necrosis, Councilman bodies, and enlarged nuclei of hepatocytes were used as the cirteria for the diagnosis of hepatitis. Among the 30 F_2 hybrids, 5 rats showed evidence of hepatitis. In the reciprocal backcross rats, 6 F_2 hybrids showed evidence of hepatitis. F_1 hybrids showed no evidence of hepatitis, in accordance with the previous report [5]. In the F_2 generation (Table 3) the frequency of rats showing T-cell depletion was 16.6%, equal to the frequency of rats showing hepatitis. These results indicated that the immunodeficiency in the LEC rat is also inherited through an autosomal recessive gene as in hepatitis. However, as is shown in Table 3, there is no obvious relationship between the manifestation of hepatitis and the development of immunodeficiency, at least when T-cell (helper/inducer) depletion is used as an indicator of immunodeficiency. Therefore, our study indicated that the genes responsible for the hepatitis and immunodeficiency in LEC rats are different.

Conclusions

We described the histological features of the immunodeficiency of LEC rats, which are characterized by hypoplasia of the thymic medulla, due mainly to the decrease in the thymic epithelial cells. Depletion of T cells in the thymus-dependent areas in the spleen and lymph nodes was also observed. FACS analysis revealed a marked decrease in the number of T cells, especially of helper/inducer T cells in the spleen and lymph nodes. The spleen cells of LEC rats had virtually no response to blastogenic stimulators. Such histological changes of lymphoid tissues and the abnormalities of T-cell differentiation were similar to the findings experimentally induced by the potent immunosuppressing agent, cyclosporin A (Cs A), in the mouse and rat [14,15], suggesting that the same mechanisms may interfer with T-cell differentiation in the thymus of the LEC rat as in Cs A-treated animals.

We also reported that the immunodeficiency of the LEC rat is characterized by helper/inducer T-cell depletion in the peripheral blood and that this is controlled by a single autosomal recessive gene. There was no relationship between the occurrence of hepatitis and the appearance of T-cell (helper/inducer) deletion in the LEC rat. Our data suggested that the hepatitis of LEC rats is controlled by an autosomal recessive gene different from that responsible for the development of immunodeficiency.

References

1. Sasaki M, Yoshida MC, Kagami K, Takeichi H, Kobayashi H, Dempo K, Mori M (1985) Spontaneous hepatitis in an inbred strain of Long-Evans rats. Rat News Letter 14:4−6
2. Yoshida MC, Masuda R, Sasaki M, Takeichi N, Kobayashi H, Dempo K, Mori M (1987) New mutation causing hereditary hepatitis in the laboratory rat. J Hered 78:361−365
3. Masuda R, Yoshida MC, Sasaki M, Dempo K, Mori M (1988) A transplantable cell line derived from spontaneous hepatocellular carcinoma of hereditary hepatitis LEC rat. Jpn J Cancer Res 79:250−254
4. Masuda R, Yoshida MC, Sasaki M, Dempo K, Mori M (1988) High susceptibility to hepatocellular carcinoma development in LEC rats with hereditary hepatitis. Jpn J Cancer Res 79:828−835
5. Masuda R, Yoshida MC, Sasaki M, Dempo K, Mori M (1988) Hereditary hepatitis of LEC rats is controlled by a single autosomal recessive gene. Lab Anim 22:166−169
6. Yamada T, Natori T, Izumi K, Sakai T, Agui T, Matsumoto K (to be published) Inheritance of T helper immunodeficiency (thid) in LEC mutant rats. Immunogenetics
7. Cantor H, Weissman II. (1976) Development and function of subpopulations of thymocytes and T lymphocytes. Prog Allergy 20:1−64
8. VanEwijk W (1984) Immunohistology of lymphoid and nonlymphoid cells in the thymus in relation to T lymphocyte differentiation. Am J Anat 170:311−330
9. Low TLK, Goldstein AL (1984) Thymosins: Isolation, structural studies and biological activities. In: Goldstein AL (ed) Thymic hormones and lymphokines. Plenum, New York, pp 21−36
10. Goldscheider I, Ahmed A, Bollum FJ, Goldstein AL (1981) Induction of terminal deoxynucleotidyl transferase and Lyt antigen with thymosin: Identification of multiple subsets of prothymocytes in mouse bone marrow and spleen. Pro Natl Acad Sci USA 78:2469−2473
11. Chen SS, Treng JS, Gills S, Good RA, Hadden JW (1983) Changes in surface antigens of immature thymocytes under the influence of T-cell growth factor and thymic factors. Proc Natl Acad Sci USA 80:5980−5984
12. Matsuura A, Ishii Y, Yuasa H, Narita H, Kon S, Takami T, Kikuchi K (1984) Rat T lymphocyte antigens comparable with mouse Lyt-1 and Lyt-2,3 antigenic systems: Characterization by monoclonal antibodies. J Immunol 132:316−322

13. Böyum A (1968) Isolation and removal of leukocytes from bone marrow of rats and guinea-pigs. Scand J Clin and Lab Invest 21 (Suppl 97):91–106
14. Demetris AJ, Nalesnik MA, Kunz HW, Gill TJ III, Shinozuka H (1984) Sequential analyses of the development of lymphoproliferative disorders in rats receiving cyclosporine. Transplantation 38:239–246
15. Hattori A, Kunz HW, Gill TJ III, Shinozuka H (1987) Thymic and lymphoid changes and serum immunoglobulin abnormalities in mice receiving cyclosporine. Am J Pathol 128:111–120

24 — Remarkable Reduction of Serum IgG2a Subclass in LEC Rats

YOSHITAKA IKEDA, TOSHIHIRO SUGIYAMA, and NAOYUKI TANIGUCHI[1]

Introduction

Spontaneous hepatitis and hepatoma in LEC rats have been demonstrated as being associated with severe jaundice and immunodeficiency. The immunodeficiency that occurs in LEC rats is characterized by a low level of serum IgG and T-cell dysfunction. Serum IgG levels of the LEC rats remain markedly low after the age of 2 months, although IgM levels are the same as those of the control LEA rats. The spleen and thymus were found to be atrophic before the onset of jaundice [1]. Although the genetic basis has been shown to be a single autosomal recessive mutation, no apparent linkage was observed between at least two genes coding for hepatitis and immunodeficiency [2].

IgG antibodies can be divided into four subclasses, IgG1, IgG2a, IgG2b, and IgG2c, in rats as well as in mice and humans [3]. Subclass selection is influenced by various stimuli, including lymphokines from helper T cells and unknown factors.

The pattern of IgG subclasses in serum is considered to partly reflect the T-cell function involved in subclass or isotype selection. It is, therefore, valuable to analyze the pattern of IgG subclasses in serum in relation to T-cell dysfunction in LEC rats with hypogammaglobulinemia or low levels of serum IgG. In the present study, we examined the serum levels of three IgG subclasses, IgG2a, IgG2b and IgG2c, in LEC and LEA rats at 52 weeks using the sodium dodecyl sulfate-polyacrylamide gel electrophoresis technique (SDS-PAGE), immunoblotting, and enzyme-linked immunosorbent assay (ELISA).

[1] Department of Biochemistry, Osaka University Medical School, Suita, Osaka, 565 Japan

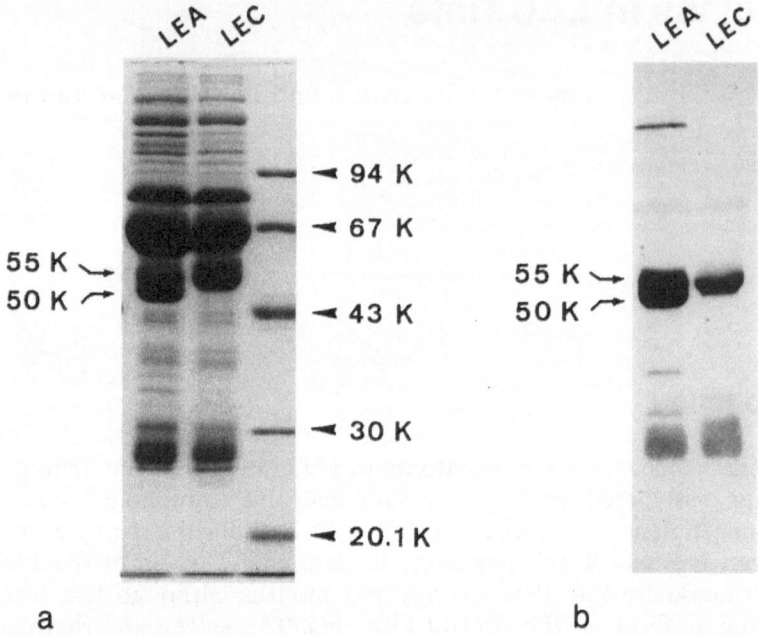

Fig. 1. Analysis of immunoglobulin γ chains on SDS-PAGE and immunoblotting in 52-week-old LEC and LEA rat sera. A polyacrylamide gel of 10% was used. Rat sera were diluted 20-fold with sample buffer containing 5% 2-mercaptoethanol, and boiled. Five μl of the treated samples were loaded in each lane. **a** The gel was stained with Coomassie brilliant blue. **b** The blot of the gel in **a** is shown. Anti-rat Igγ polyclonal antibody was used to probe IgG heavy chains

Identification of the Immunoglobulin γ Chain

Figure 1 shows representative profiles of SDS-PAGE and immunoblotting analysis of LEC and LEA rats sera. SDS-PAGE of rat sera was performed according to Laemmli's method under reduced conditions and the gel was stained with Coomassie brilliant blue (Fig. 1a). In order to identify the γ chains (heavy chains of IgGs), proteins in the gel were transferred onto a nitrocellulose membrane and probed with an anti-rat immunoglobulin γ chains polyclonal antibody (Fig. 1b).

The γ chains of IgG2a and IgG2c exhibited relative molecular masses of 50,000–52,000, and those of IgG1 and IgG2b about 55,000 on SDS-PAGE [4]. As shown in Fig. 1a, LEC rats lacked a band corresponding to 50 kd, whereas LEA rats had bands of both 50 kd and 55 kd, identical to the γ chains in Fig. 1b. The LEC rats did have the 55 kd species of γ chains, which indicates that only certain subclasses of IgG are decreased in these rats.

Fig. 2. Serum levels of IgG subclasses in 52-week-old LEC and LEA rats measured by ELISA. IgG subclass level is expressed as mg per ml of serum. The *columns* and *bars* express the mean values and standard errors, respectively, for five rats in each group. *Asterisks* indicate $P < 0.05$ (by Student's t-test)

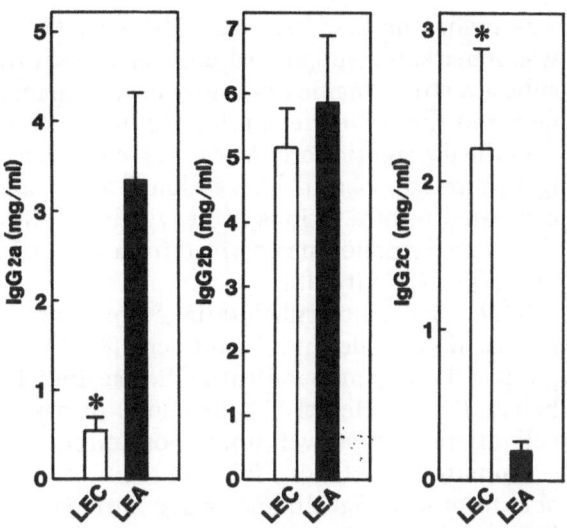

Quantitation of IgG Subclasses

In the ELISA system used, IgG subclass-specific antibodies that react with antigenic determinants particular to the γ chain of each subclass were immobilized on 96-well microtiter plates. The immobilized antibodies captured the heavy chains of serum IgGs. A horseradish peroxidase-conjugated anti-light chain antibody was then used to create a sandwich. o-Phenylenediamine was used as a coloring reagent. Standard samples of IgG subclasses were purified from LEA rat sera with Protein A-Sepharose by pH-stepwise elution, and were further purified with diethylaminoethyl (DEAE) cellulose according to Rousseaux et al. [5].

The level of IgG2a was significantly lower in LEC rats than in LEA rats (Fig. 2). Contrarily, the IgG2c level of LEC rat sera was higher than that of LEA rat sera. No significant difference between LEC and LEA rats was observed in the IgG2b level.

These results indicate that hypogammaglobulinemia in LEC rats is mainly due to a decrease of serum IgG2a, at least at 52 weeks after birth.

Discussion

It has already been reported that immunodeficiency in LEC rats is highly associated with T-cell dysfunction and a low level of serum IgG [1,2,6]. Our results show that not all IgG subclasses are lower in LEC rats than in the control LEA rats. Only one subclass, IgG2a, among three subclasses examined in this study was lower in LEC rats. The IgG2b level in LEC rat sera was almost the same as that in control (LEA) sera, and the IgG2c level was higher in LEC rat sera. Although the IgG2a level in LEC rat sera was remarkably suppressed compared with the level in LEA rat sera, this subclass still remained at a low level. Therefore, the presence of a genetic defect in the coding region for γ2a (heavy chain of IgG2a) seems unlikely.

In the differentiation process of B cells, gene recombination occurs in the IgH (immunoglobulin heavy chain) locus, and μ chains of antibodies are converted to other kinds of heavy chains. Studies in mice have indicated that some lymphokines derived from helper T cells cause a class switch in vivo [7] and in vitro [8].

IgG2a is a major subclass in normal rat serum and is primarily active against thymus-dependent antigens (TDA) such as bovine serum albumin [9]. B cells may produce antibodies against TDA with the participation of helper T cells. Helper T cells could, in part, determine the direction of B cell differentiation even under non-immunized conditions.

Immature B cells of LEC rats seem to be normal because LEC rats are able to produce IgG2b and IgG2c antibodies. Presumably if the B cells of LEC rats were given appropriate stimuli by helper T cells, they would produce sufficient levels of IgG2a antibodies. Consequently, the low level of IgG2a in LEC rats appears to result mainly from T-cell dysfunction.

In mice, interleukin-4 (IL-4) can stimulate IgG1 antibody production [10], and interferon-γ (IFN-γ) can stimulate IgG2a production [11]. IL-4 is produced by a subpopulation of helper T cells, termed Th2, and IFN-γ by TH1 [12]. Thus, the pattern of IgG subclasses might be determined by the balance of subpopulations of helper T cells and the degree of their activation.

In LEC rats, as mentioned above, hypogammaglobulinemia could be a result of T-cell dysfunction leading to reduced levels of serum IgG2a. T-cell dysfunction in the LEC rats could be explained by the inability of a certain subpopulation of helper T cells to cause B-cell activation or differentiation.

Conclusions

In this study, we examined the pattern of three IgG subclasses, IgG2a, IgG2b, and IgG2c, in 52-week-old LEC rats using SDS-PAGE, immuno-blotting, and ELISA. The IgG2a level was remarkably low in LEC rats compared with LEA rats as normal control. On the other hand, the IgG2b level in LEC rats was not significantly different from that in LEA rats, and the IgG2c level in LEC rats was higher than that in LEA rats. These results suggest that some subpopulation of helper T cells is poorly developed in the LEC rats.

Acknowledgements. This work was in part supported by a Grant-in-Aid for Cancer Research from the Ministry of Education, Science and Culture,

Japan. We wish to thank Mrs. S. House for editing and correcting this manuscript.

References

1. Namieno T, Takeichi N, Dempo K, Mori MC, Uchino J, Kobayashi H (1989) Combined immunodeficiency in LEC (Long Evans Cinnamon) rats with spontaneous hepatitis (in Japanese). Nippon Geka Gakkai Zasshi 90:886–893
2. Matsumoto K, Takeichi N, Izumi K, Otsuka H (1989) Quantitative variation in immunoglobulin G (Igsr-1) in LEC rats associated with spontaneous hepatitis and hepatoma. Transplant Proc 21:3259
3. Bazin H, Beckers A, Querinjean P (1974) Three classes and four (sub)classes of rat immunoglobulins: IgM, IgA, IgE and IgG1, IgG2a, IgG2b, IgG2c. Eur J Immunol 4:44–48
4. Bazin H, Rousseaux J (1979) Rat immunoglobulins. Vet Immunol Immunopathol 1:61–78
5. Rousseaux J, Picque MT, Bazin H, Biserte G (1981) Rat IgG subclasses: Differences in affinity to protein A-sepharose. Mol Immunol 18:639–645
6. Matsumoto K, Ono E, Izumi K, Otsuka H, Yoshida MC, Sasaki M, Takeichi N, Kobayashi H (1987) Expression of new esterases and pathologic profile in LEC rats with spontaneous fulminant hepatitis. Transplant Proc 19:3207–3211
7. Finkelman FD, Holmes J, Katona IM, Urban JF Jr, Beckmann MP, Park LS, Schooley KA, Coffman RL, Mosmann TR, Paul WE (1990) Lymphokine control of in vivo immunoglobulin isotype selection. Annu Rev Immunol 8:303–333
8. Esser C, Radbruch A (1990) Immunoglobulin class switching: Molecular and cellular analysis. Annu Rev Immunol 8:717–735
9. McGhee JR, Michalek SM, Ghanta VK (1975) Rat immunoglobulins in serum and secretions: Purification of rat IgM, IgA and IgG and their quantitation in serum, colostrum, milk and saliva. Immunochemistry 12:817–823
10. Vitetta ES, Ohara J, Myers CD, Layton JE, Krammer PH, Paul WE (1985) Serological, biochemical, and functional identity of B cell-stimulatory factor 1 and B cell differentiation factor for IgG1. J Exp Med 162:1726–1731
11. Snapper CM, Paul WE (1987) Interferon-γ and B cell stimulatory factor-1 reciprocally regulate Ig isotype production. Science 236:944–947
12. Mosmann TR, Cherwinski H, Bond MW, Giedlin MA, Coffman RL (1986) Two types of murine helper T cell clone: 1. Definition according to the profiles of lymphokine activities and secreted proteins. J Immunol 136:2348–2357

25 — Genetic Analysis of IgG Deficiency and T-Helper Immunodeficiency in LEC Rats

Kozo Matsumoto and Takahisa Yamada[1]

Introduction

The discovery of nude mice, asplenic mice, and severe combined immuno-deficiency (*scid*) mice has greatly accelerated studies on basic and applied immunology, because nude mice lack functional T cells by agenesis of the thymus, and asplenic mice show depressed immunoglobulin levels [1]. *Scid* mice lack T cells, B cells, and immunoglobulin [2] because of no rearrangement of the configuration of T-cell receptors (TCR), beta-chain genes [3], or immunoglobulin genes [4]. Recently, we have found novel mutations showing large decreases of serum IgG, but not of IgA and IgM, and arrest of maturation from CD4$^+$8$^+$ to CD4$^+$8$^-$ thymocytes accompanied with CD4$^+$ T-cell deficiency in the peripheral organs in the LEC rat [5−7] which spontaneously develops heptatic injury and hepato-cellular carcinoma [8,9]. The genes responsible for the decrease of serum IgG and deficiency of helper T cells were designated as *Igsr-1* and *thid*, respectively [6,7]. We were interested in investigating whether helper T-cell deficiency affects the decrease of serum IgG levels or the occurrence of hepatic injury and/or hepatocellular carcinoma, since it is thought that CD4$^+$ T-cell deficiency and dysfunction of CD4$^+$ T cells reduce the pro-duction of antibodies by B cells and may accelerate tumor growth. We consider that the discovery of these novel mutations in LEC rats should contribute to the studies on basic and applied immunology as well as to those of mutant mice established previously. This chapter describes the genetic nature of the mutant genes occurring in LEC rat.

Serum IgG Deficiency

Levels of serum immunoglobulins were detected by the double immuno-diffusion and enzyme-linked immunosorbent assay (ELISA) system. Since serum immunoglobulin levels are generally influenced by infection from

[1] Institute for Animal Experimentation, University of Tokushima School of Medicine, Tokushima, 770 Japan

Fig. 1. Double immuno-diffusion tests for serum immunoglobulin from LEC and normal rats. Subclass specific anti-rat immunogloblulin anti-serum was put in the center well. Individual serum was put in the outside well. **A** The outside wells of *1–4* contained LEC rat sera at 4 weeks of age while those of *5* and *6* con-tained the age-matched WKAH sera. Tenfold dilution sera were used for anti-IgG2a, IgG2b, and IgG2c. **B** The outside wells of *8*, *11*, and *12* contained LEC rat sera at 6–7 weeks of age, while those of *7*, *9*, and *10* contained the age-matched WKAH rat sera. Four- and two-dilution sera were used for anti-IgG2a and anti-IgG2b, respectively

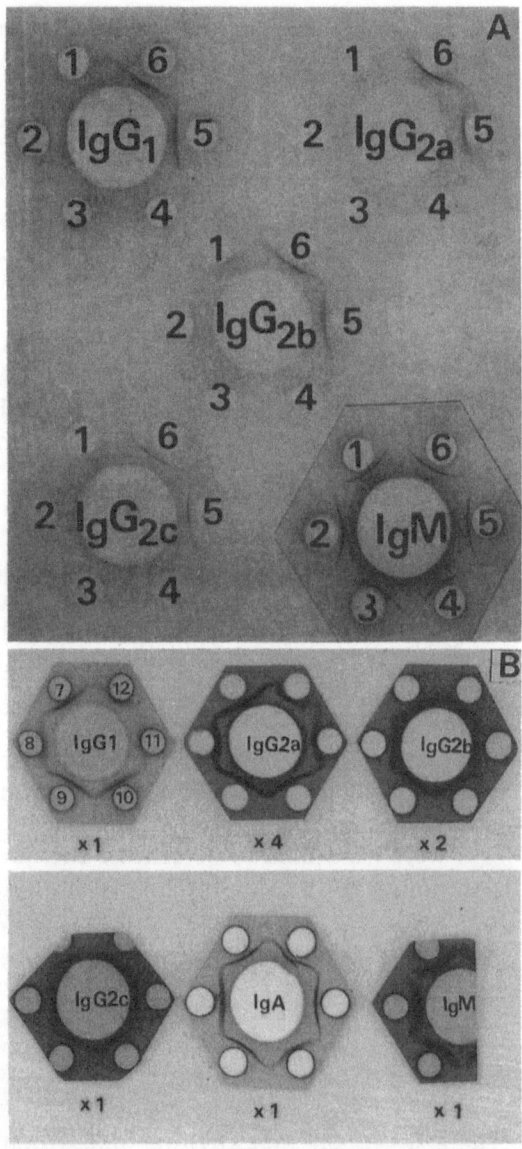

virus and bacteria, it is essential to breed rats under a specific pathogen-free (SPF) condition. Serum immunoglobulin levels between LEC/Tj mutant and WKAH/Slc or LEA/Tj normal rats were compared by the double immunodiffusion test. No IgG subclasses were detectable in LEC rats at the age of 4 weeks, while they were detected in age-matched WKAH rats, with a ten-fold dilution of the sera for IgG2a, IgG2b, and IgG2c. (Fig. 1a). In spite of the marked decrease of serum IgG, levels of serum IgM in LEC rats were similar to those of WKAH rats. However, IgG2a, IgG2b, and

Table 1. Segregation data for Igsr-1B and Igsr-1AB among backcross progeny of (LEC × LEA) F_1 × LEC. (From [6] with permission).

| | Igsr-1 | | | |
| | B | | AB | |
Mating	Female	Male	Female	Male
1. (LEA × LEC) F_1	0	0	3	4
2. (LEC × LEA) F_1 × LEC	6	11	10	7

IgG2c became detectable using a one- to four-fold dilution of sera from 6- to 7-week-old LEC rats (Fig. 1b). IgG1 still showed a faint precipitation line with the same sera. Levels of IgA and IgM of LEC and LEA rats were similar at this age. In order to test additional aging effects on IgG1 content, serum IgG1 levels were determined by the sandwich ELISA system. Serum IgG1 levels in old LEC and WKAH rats (6 months old) were significantly different from the young LEC and WKAH rats. Significantly, LEC rats constantly showed a marked decrease (approximately 1/15) in the IgG1 levels compared to the age-matched WKAH rats at 4 weeks and 6 months of age (data not shown). Since the levels of IgA and IgM were normal in LEC rats, the B cells seemed to be normal. Indeed, B cells responded well to the B-cell-specific antigen, Ficoll [5]. This polymorphism for quantitative difference of IgG levels was tentatively designated as immunoglobulin subclass regulator-1 (Igsr-1). LEC rats carried Igsr-1B (low expression of IgG) while the other strains of rats thus far tested carried Igsr-1A (normal expression of IgG). Backcross progeny of (LEC × LEA) F_1 × LEC were examined to determine the mode of inheritance of quantitative variation of IgG1 using the double immunodiffusion test. Segregation data indicated that Igsr-1 was a single gene (X^2 analysis resulted in $P > 0.5$) (Table 1). The nuclear gene symbol is designated *Igsr-1*, and the two alleles are *Igsr-1a* and *Igsr-1b* for the Igsr-1A and Igsr-1B phenotypes, respectively.

Helper T-Cell Deficiency

The sizes of LEC rat thymus and lymph nodes were approximately one-half of normal thymus and lymph nodes. This suggested some thymic or T-cell defects. In order to test them, thymocytes and peripheral T cells from LEC and WKAH rats at the age of 6 weeks were analyzed by either one- or two-color flow cytometry (FACScan, Becton Dickinson) with FITC-conjugated W3/25 (anti-rat CD4 mAb) and PE-conjugated OX 8 (anti-rat CD8 mAb). As we expected, we found a novel defect in thymocytes and peripheral T cells in LEC rats [5]. Namely, the percentage of CD4$^+$8$^-$ thymocytes was negligibly small (<1%) at the age of 6 weeks, while CD4$^-$8$^+$ thymocytes seemed to be at a normal level (Fig. 2). Accordingly, the percentage of CD4$^+$8$^+$ thymocytes was relatively higher in LEC rats

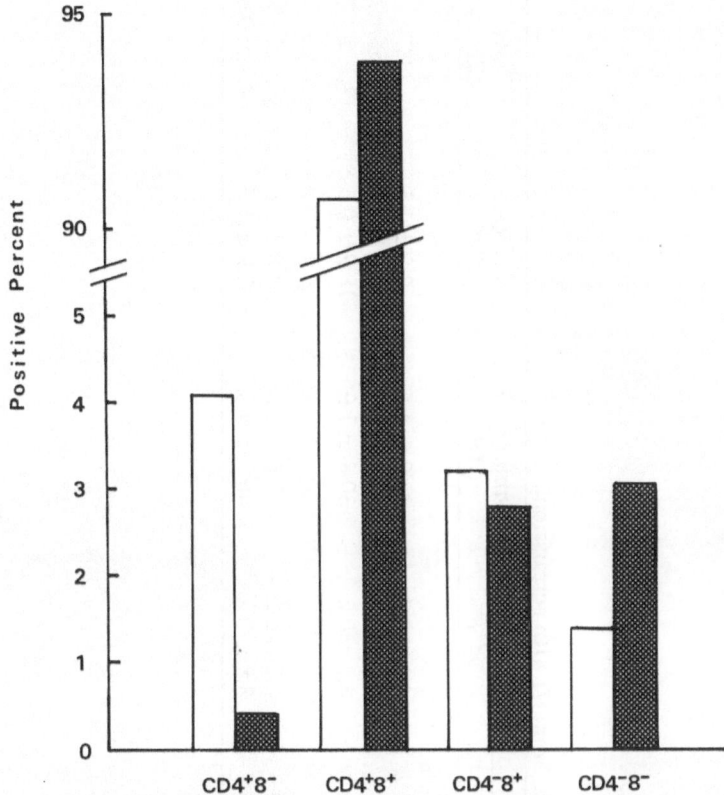

Fig. 2. Ratio of T-cell sub-populations in thymocytes from LEC and WKAH rats at the age of 6 weeks. Thymocytes were prepared and stained with FITC-conjugated anti-CD4 and PE-conjugated anti-CD8 mAbs. These cells were analyzed by FACScan. *Open bars* show results from WKAH rat thymocytes and *shaded bars* show data from LEC rat thymocytes. Data represent the mean of results from 3–4 rats

than that in WKAH rats. This indicated that the arrest of maturation from CD4$^+$8$^+$ to CD4$^+$8$^-$ thymocytes occurred in young LEC rats. In the peripheral organs, such as spleen, CD4$^+$ T cells were also decreased, but the number of CD8$^+$ cells appeared to be normal [5].

Aging effects of the deficiency in CD4$^+$ T cells were investigated in LEC rats at the age of 3–12 months (Table 2). The percentage of CD4$^+$8$^-$ thymocytes in adult LEC rats remained at extremely low levels such as in the young LEC rats (4 weeks old). In contrast, the percentages of CD4$^+$ T cells in the peripheral organs slightly increased with age. The lymph nodes of LEC rats contained an increasing number of CD4$^+$ T cells (20%–34%) with age, but the percentage was still lower than that of normal WKAH rats (47%). The percentage of CD4$^+$ T cells in spleen from adult LEC rats showed two-fold and then three-fold increases at the age of 3–6 months

Table 2. Aging effect on CD4$^+$ T-cell deficiency in LEC rats. (From [7] with permission).

	Thymus				Lymph nodes CD4$^+$	Spleen CD4$^+$	Blood CD4$^+$
	CD4$^+$8$^-$	CD4$^-$8$^+$	CD4$^+$8$^+$	CD4$^-$8$^-$			
LEC							
3 months	0.5 ± 0.5	6.0 ± 0.9	90.2 ± 0.2	4.3 ± 0.7	18.0 ± 4.6	9.8 ± 1.5	N.T.
6 months	1.4 ± 0.9	4.0 ± 0.5	89.2 ± 4.2	6.3 ± 3.0	23.4 ± 3.9	10.9 ± 0.3	11.2 ± 1.7
12 months	0.7 ± 0.2	8.0 ± 0.6	88.2 ± 1.1	3.1 ± 0.2	30.8 ± 1.9	18.9 ± 0.5	12.1 ± 1.0
WKAH							
3 months	7.2 ± 0.6	6.6 ± 0.4	83.0 ± 0.9	4.1 ± 0.2	47.6 ± 3.8	24.8 ± 1.6	39.3 ± 1.2
6 months	9.2 ± 2.6	6.4 ± 0.3	80.1 ± 0.7	3.8 ± 0.2	46.7 ± 4.3	33.2 ± 2.5	44.2 ± 0.6

N.T., not tested

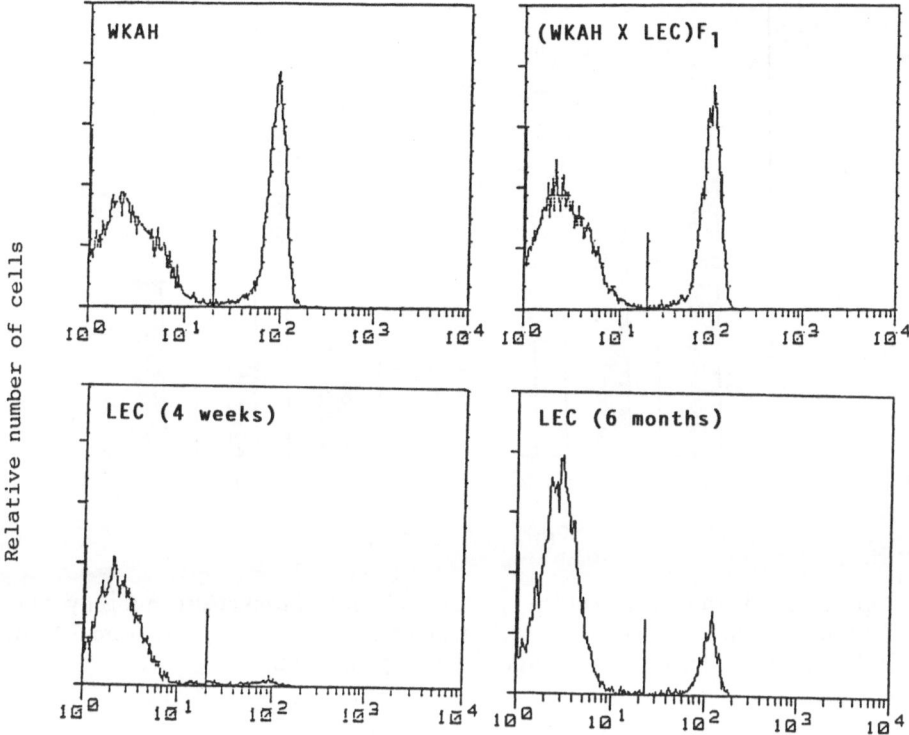

Fig. 3. FACS analysis of CD4 antigen on peripheral blood lymphocytes. Peripheral blood was collected from the tail vein of rats at the age of 6 weeks and 6 months. Cells stained with FITC-conjugated CD4-specific mAb (W3/25) were analyzed with a FACScan (Becton-Dickinson, Mountain View, Calif.). Dead cells were gated out by using two parameters of forward and side light scatters, and then the data for 20,000 cells were collected and analyzed with a Consort 30 software program.

(10%) and 12 months (19%), respectively, when they were compared to that of CD4$^+$ T cells in spleen from young LEC rats (5%). However, these percentages were always lower than that in WKAH rats (24%–35%). The percentage of CD4$^+$ T cells in blood from adult LEC rats (10%) was increased up to two-fold with age. This percentage was much lower than that in blood from adult WKAH rats (39%–44%). From these observations, we chose the percentage of blood CD4$^+$ T cells as a marker to analyze the genetic trait of CD4$^+$ deficiency in LEC rats. Very interestingly, CD4$^+$ T cells in peripheral organs from LEC rats were shown not to have helper T-cell function such as IL-2 and IL-4 productions, and not to be responsive to T-cell-dependent antigens [5]. Details for the nature of CD4$^+$ T-cell deficiency are described in the next chapter.

We examined the mode of inheritance of the T-helper immunodeficiency (*thid*) mutation by studies on the backcross progeny of (WKAH × LEC)F$_1$ ×

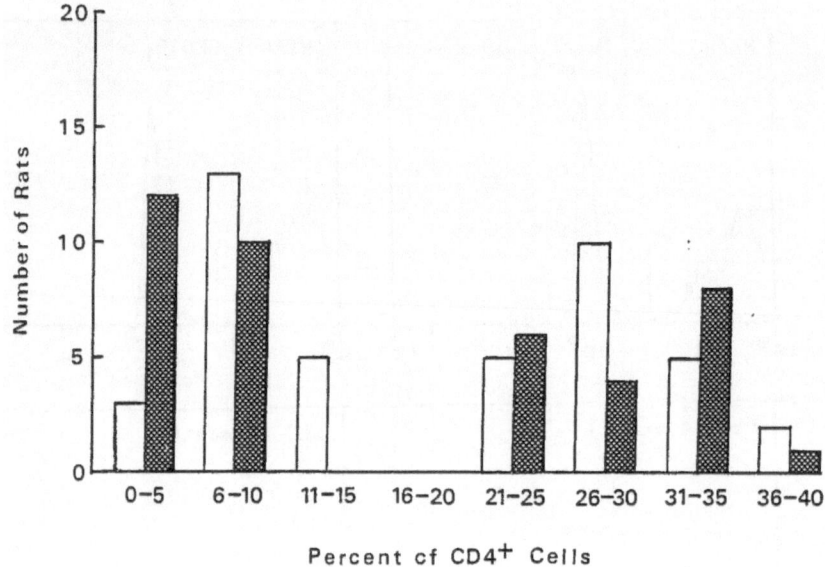

Fig. 4. Distribution of the percentage of CD4$^+$ cells in backcrossed progeny. *Open bars*, data for [(BN × LEC)F$_1$ × LEC] backcrosses; *shaded bars*, data from [(WKAH × LEC)F$_1$ × LEC] backcrosses. (From [7] with permission)

Table 3. Data on segregation of the T helper immunodeficiency (*thid*) gene. (From [7] with permission).

Parental combination	thid/thid	+/thid	Chi square	P
(WKAH × LEC) F$_1$	0	6		
(WKAH × LEC) F$_1$ × LEC	22	19	0.220	NS*
(BN × LEC) F$_1$ × LEC	21	22	0.023	NS

*NS, not significant (P > 0.10)

LEC and (BN × LEC)F$_1$ × LEC. The CD4$^+$ T cells from WKAH/Tj, (WKAH × LEC)F$_1$, young and adult LEC rats were analyzed by flow cytometry using single staining of blood T cells with FITC-conjugated W3/25 (anti-rat CD4). All of the F$_1$ rats had normal levels of CD4$^+$ T cells (Fig. 3). Although CD4$^+$ T cells from aged LEC rats showed somewhat higher levels than immature LEC rats (Fig. 3D), the distribution of the percentages of CD4$^+$ T cells at the age of 4 weeks and 6 months allowed a clear division of the backcross rats into 2 groups (Fig. 4). In both crosses, the segregation ratio was approximately 1:1, indicating that this mutation is caused by a single recessive gene (Table 3). Therefore, we designated this locus as *thid*.

Table 4. Linkages of *thid* with 9 genetic marker loci. (From [7] with permission).

Locus	Linkage group	Recombinant: nonrecombinant	Recombinant frequency ±SE	Chi square
Igsr-1		15:10	0.60 ± 0.10	0.40
RT1	IX	34:34	0.50 ± 0.06	0.11
hts		22:13	0.63 ± 0.08	0.59
Acp-2	X	12:12	0.50 ± 0.10	0.17
Es-6		23:19	0.55 ± 0.08	0.03
h	VI	34:34	0.50 ± 0.06	0.04
Hao-1	IV	24:36	0.40 ± 0.06	1.40
Hbb	I	23:20	0.53 ± 0.08	0.06
p	I	33:35	0.49 ± 0.06	0.04

Genetic Linkage Analyses for IgG Deficiency (*Igsr-1*) and T-Helper Immunodeficiency (*thid*)

Nude mice lack functional T cells, but the IgG and IgM contents seem not to have such low levels [1]. It may suggest that B cells could be helped to produce IgG by a T-cell-independent mechanism. When this is taken into account, the decrease of IgG levels in LEC rats might not be due to only the helper T cell deficiency. However, it is important to investigate whether IgG deficiency (*Igsr-1*) is linked to T-helper immunodeficiency (*thid*) in LEC mutant rats, since helper T cells assist B-cell function in the production of IgG. Unfortunately, we have found no linkages between *Igsr-1* and *thid* genes (Table 4). As suggested above, the origin of IgG deficiency seems to be independent of helper T-cell function. B cells themselves may have some defect in LEC mutant rats.

Linkage study between T-helper immunodeficiency (*thid*) and RT1 haplotype is also important, since several investigations have demonstrated that differentiation of $CD4^+8^+$ thymocytes into either $CD4^+8^-$ (helper precursor) or $CD4^-8^+$ thymocytes requires interactions with major histocompatibility complex (MHC) antigens expressed on thymic stromal cells [10,11]. Especially, class II MHC antigen is essential to develop the double positive to $CD4^+8^-$ thymocytes. From this reason, the abnormality of class II MHC antigen in LEC rat thymus has been suggested as contributing to helper T-cell deficiency. However, the *thid* locus was not linked to the *RT1* locus (Table 4), indicating that the arrest of maturation cannot be attributed to any abnormalities in the class II molecule on thymic stroma cells.

The hereditary hepatic injury in LEC rats is reported as being caused by an autosomal recessive locus designated as *hts* [9,12]. Furthermore, LEC rats develop hepatocellular carcinoma with 100% occurrence at the age of 18 months [13]. This suggests that the occurrence of hepatic injury must be related to the occurrence of the hepatocellular carcinoma. In addition, dysfunction of CD4$^+$ T cells may correlate with the occurrence of hepatocellular carcinoma or tumor growth. Considering this aspect, it is necessary to study the linkage between the immunodeficiency and hereditary hepatic injury. However, we could not detect any linkage between *hts* and *Igsr-1* or *thid* genes (Table 4). This indicates that the development of hepatic injury is independent of genetic immuno-deficiencies, although it may be still possible that the immunodeficiencies may promote development of hepatoma from liver injury.

In conclusion, novel mutant genes causing low levels of IgG and helper T-cell deficiencies were identified in LEC rats, and named *Igsr-1* and *thid* [6,7]. Both genes showed characteristics of single recessive traits, but the loci could not be mapped. In addition, the origins of IgG and CD4$^+$ T-cell deficiencies are still unclear. However, our recent investigation suggests that the arrest of maturation from CD4$^+$8$^+$ to CD4$^+$8$^-$ thymocytes is due to the pre-T-cells mutation derived from bone marrow. Since T-cell development in the thymus is a current topic of interest, study of the mechanism of T-cell development would be enhanced by using LEC or the *thid*-congenic strain of rat. Although immunodeficiency was not linked to the occurrence of hepatic injury, it would be necessary to test any further relationships between the immunodeficiency and tumor growth in LEC rats. Using congenic strains would also be helpful in clarifying this problem. In order to accomplish these studies, we are now developing *thid*-congenic and *hts*-congenic strains of rats.

References

1. Fogh J, Giovanella BC (eds) (1982) The nude mouse in experimental and clinical research, vol 2. Academic, New York
2. Bosma GC, Custer RP, Bosma MJ (1983) A severe combined immunodeficiency mutation in the mouse. Nature 301:527–530
3. Schuler W, Weiler IJ, Schuler A, Phillips RA, Rosenberg N, Mak TW, Kearney JF, Perry RP, Bosma MJ (1986) Rearrangement of antigen receptor genes is defective in mice with severe combined immune deficiency. Cell 46:963–972
4. Fulop GM, Phillips RA (1990) The *scid* mutation in mice causes a general defect in DNA rapair. Nature 347:479–482
5. Agui T, Oka M, Yamada T, Ishida Y, Himeno K, Matsumoto K (1990) Maturational arrest from CD4$^+$8$^+$ to CD4$^+$8$^-$ thymocytes in a mutant strain (LEC) of rat. J Exp Med 172:1615–1624
6. Matsumoto K, Takeichi N, Izumi K, Otsuka H (1989) Quantitative variation in immunoglobulin G (*Igsr-1*) in LEC rats associated with spontaneous hepatitis and hepatoma. Transplant Proc 21:3259
7. Yamada T, Natori, T, Izumi, K, Sakai T, Agui T, Matsumoto K (to be published) Inheritance of T helper immunodeficiency (*thid*) in LEC mutant rats. Immunogenetics

8. Masuda R, Yoshida MC, Sasaki M, Dempo K, Mori M (1988) High susceptibility to hepatocellular carcinoma development in LEC rats with hereditary hepatitis. Jpn J Cancer Res 79:828–835
9. Yoshida MC, Masuda R, Sasaki M, Takeichi N, Kobayashi H, Dempo K, Mori M (1987) A new mutation causing hereditary hepatitis in the laboratory rat. J Hered 78:361–365
10. Kruisbeek AM, Mond JJ, Fowldes BJ, Carmen JA, Bridges S, Longo DL (1985) Absence of the Lyt-2$^-$, L3T4$^+$ lineage of T cells in mice treated neonatally with anti-I-A correlates with absence of intrathymic I-A-bearing antigen-presenting cell function. J Exp Med 161:1029–1047
11. Marusic-Galesic S, Stephany DA, Longo DL, Kruisbeek AM (1988) Development of CD4$^-$CD8$^+$ cytotoxic T cells requires interactions with class I MHC determinants. Nature 333:180–183
12. Masuda R, Yoshida MC, Sasaki M, Dempo K, Mori M (1988) Hereditary hepatitis of LEC rats in controlled by a single autosomal recessive gene. Lab Anim 22:166–169
13. Sawaki M, Enomoto K, Takahashi H, Nakajima Y, Mori M (1990) Phenotype of preneoplastic liver lesions during spontaneous liver carcinogenesis of LEC rats. Carcinogenesis 11:1857–1861

26 — Arrest of Maturation of Helper T Cells in LEC Rats

TAKASHI AGUI and KOZO MATSUMOTO[1]

Introduction

T-cell maturation and its acquisition of the repertory reactive to foreign antigens in the thymus is one of the important topics in recent immunology. T cells are mainly categorized into two subtypes, helper and killer cells. Most of the helper T cells express CD4 antigens on their cellular surface, while killer T cells express CD8 antigens. These two surface antigens play an important role for the adherence to the target cells in helping the T-cell receptor for antigens (TCR) recognize major histocompatibility complex (MHC) antigens. Recently, differentiation of T cells within the thymus has been clarified by using these two surface marker antigens. Bone marrow-derived pre-T cells do not express either CD4 nor CD8 antigen. They express CD8 antigen first, but at this time they still do not express TCR/CD3 antigen complex and are regarded as an immature type. Immature $CD8^+$ cells next express CD4 antigen and the TCR/CD3 antigen complex. This population of the thymocytes ($CD4^+8^+$) are thought to receive both negative and positive selections. $CD4^+8^+$ cells, which escaped from the clonal deletion, differentiate into mature single-positive cells (either $CD4^+8^-$ or $CD4^-8^+$ cells). This sequential maturation of T cells requires the aid of thymic stromal cells.

LEC rats were established as a mutant strain which develops hepatitis and hepatocarcinoma [1]. Besides hepatic diseases, it has been reported that LEC rats have low levels of serum IgG but not IgM [2]. A typical immunodefective mutation is a deficiency in helper T cells and its responsible gene was designated as *thid* (T-helper immunodeficiency) [3]. It has been elucidated that deficiency in peripheral helper T cells is caused by an arrest in T-cell maturation from $CD4^+8^+$ to $CD4^+8^-$ cells in the thymus [4]. This arrest is limited in that it occurs in the formation of

[1] Institute for Animal Experimentation, Tokushima University School of Medicine, Tokushima, 770 Japan

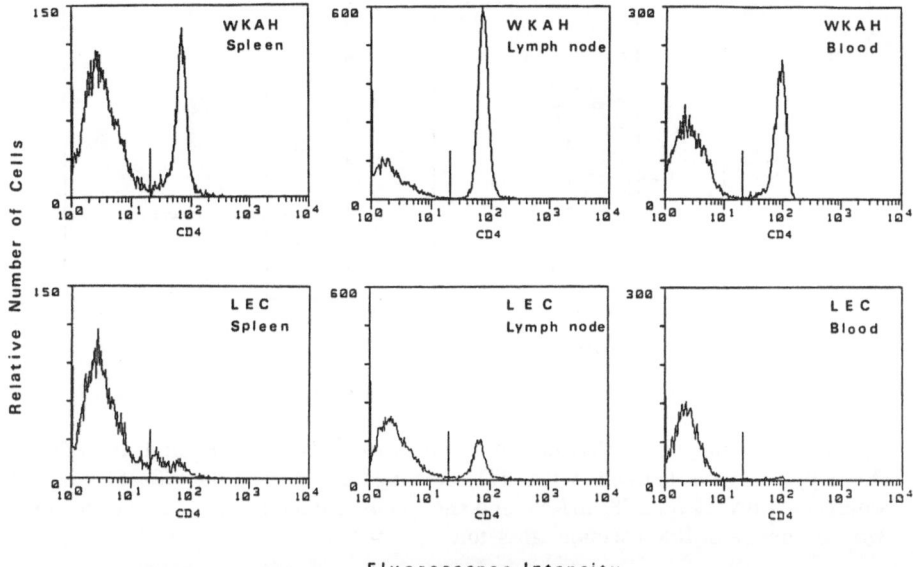

Fig. 1. FACS analysis of the peripheral lymphocytes. Lymphocytes from the peripheral lymphoid organs of normal (WKAH/Slc) and LEC/Tj rats were stained with FITC-conjugated anti-CD4 (W3/25) mAb. Analyses were done with FACScan (Becton-Dickinson and Co., Mountain View, Calif.) after gating out dead cells using forward and side light scatters. (From [4] with permission)

CD4$^+$8$^-$ cells. LEC rats, therefore, seem to be useful as an animal model for elucidating the mechanism of positive selection. In this chapter, the nature of the phenotype of *thid* is described and the cause of this deficiency is discussed.

Aspects of FACS Analysis

Lymphocytes in the peripheral lymphoid organs and blood were analyzed with the fluorescence-activated cell sorter (FACS) (Fig. 1). Normal rats contain CD4$^+$ cells approximated 20% of the spleen lymphocytes, 50% of the lymph node lymphocytes, and 40% of the blood lymphocytes, while CD4$^+$ cells in LEC rats are reduced to ~5%, ~20% and ~4% in the respective lymphoid organs. When thymocytes are stained with fluorescein isothiocynate (FITC)-conjugated anti-CD4 and phycoerythrin (PE)-conjugated anti-CD8 monoclonal antibodies (mAbs), it becomes clear that only the CD4$^+$8$^-$ cell population is deficient in LEC rats (Fig. 2). The percentages of the other populations (CD4$^-$8$^-$, CD4$^-$8$^+$, and CD4$^+$8$^+$ cells) are the same as those of normal rats. This deficiency in CD4$^+$ T cells has been shown to occur from the single recessive mutational gene [3].

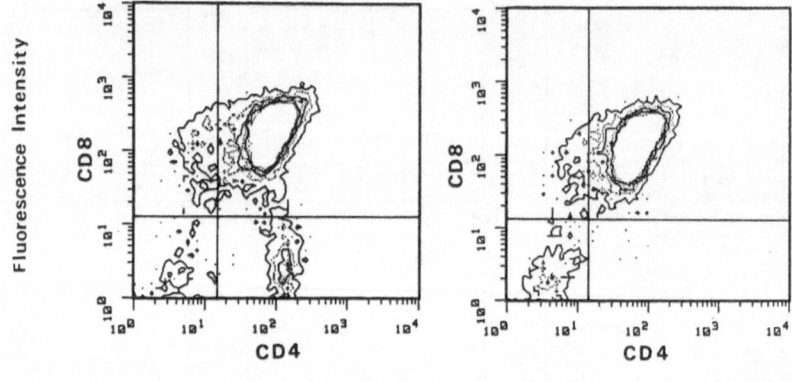

Fig. 2. FACS analysis of thymocytes from normal (WKAH/Slc) and LEC/Tj rats. Thymocytes were stained with FITC-conjugated anti-CD4 (W3/25) and PE-conjugated anti-CD8 (OX8) mAbs, and then analyzed as in Fig. 1, except for using two parameters of fluorescence emission

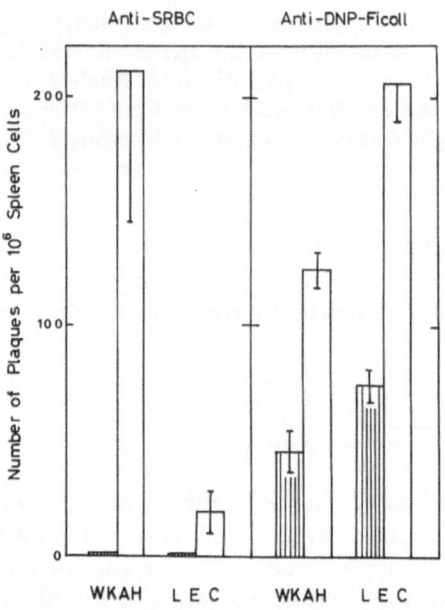

Fig. 3. Plaque-forming cell assay in spleen cells from normal (WKAH/Slc) and LEC/Tj rats. Rats were immunized with either SRBC or dinitrophenyl (DNP)-conjugated Ficoll. After 5 days, spleen cells were prepared from each strain and counted the number of plaque-forming cells responding to either DNP-conjugated SRBC or trinitrophenyl (TNP)-conjugated Ficoll by the method of Jerne and Nordin [8]. The basal levels of plaque formation by spleen cells from nonimmunized rats are shown by vertically striped columns. *Columns* and *bars* represent means ± standard error of the means (SEMs) of values for three rats. (From [4] with permission)

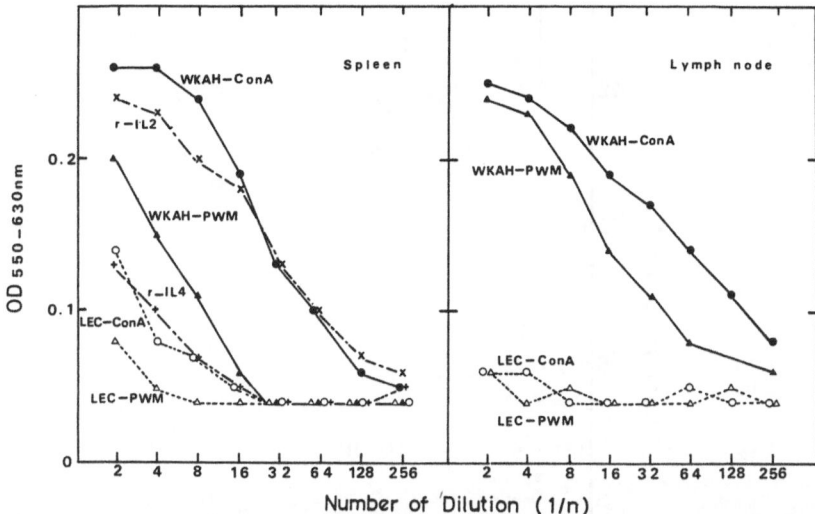

Fig. 4. Cytokine assay in spleen and lymph node cells from normal (WKAH/Slc) and LEC/Tj rats. Spleen or lymph node cells were cultured with either 2.5 μg/ml conconavalin (Con) A or 5 μg/ml pokeweed mitogen (PWM) for 2 days and the supernatants were subjected to the test for the ability supporting growth of CTLL-2 cells by the method of Mosmann [9]. *Filled* and *open* symbols represent data from WKAH and LEC rats, respectively. Murine rIL-2 (×) and rIL-4 (+) were used as positive controls. (From [4] with permission)

Functional Deficiency in Helper T Cells

Most of the CD4$^+$ cells are helper T cells. Therefore, the deficiency in CD4$^+$ cells ought to lead to the dysfunction of the helper T cells. As shown in Fig. 3, when LEC rats had been immunized with T cell-dependent antigen, sheep red blood cells (SRBC), the spleen cells did not produce antibodies specific to SRBC. On the other hand, when immunized with the T-cell-independent antigen, Ficoll, spleen cells could produce antibodies specific to Ficoll as well as the normal rats did. This indicates that helper T cells are dysfunctional, but that B cells themselves can produce antibodies in LEC rats.

Dysfunction of helper T cells in LEC rats was also shown in in vitro experiments. The ability of interleukin-2 (IL-2) production by mitogen stimulation is dramatically reduced in LEC rats when compared to normal rats (Fig. 4). IL-4 production was also shown to be reduced in LEC rats by a Northern blotting experiment [4]. Helper T cells are divided into Th1 and Th2 subtypes by the kinds of cytokines produced [5]; Th1 cells produce IL-2 and interferon-γ, while Th2 cells produce IL-4, IL-5, and IL-6. These results indicate that both subtypes of helper T cells are deficient. Moreover, the deficiency in the productions of IL-2 and IL-4 support the fact that LEC rats have eventually no CD4$^+$ cells, rather than showing alteration of the antigenic epitopes in their CD4 molecules.

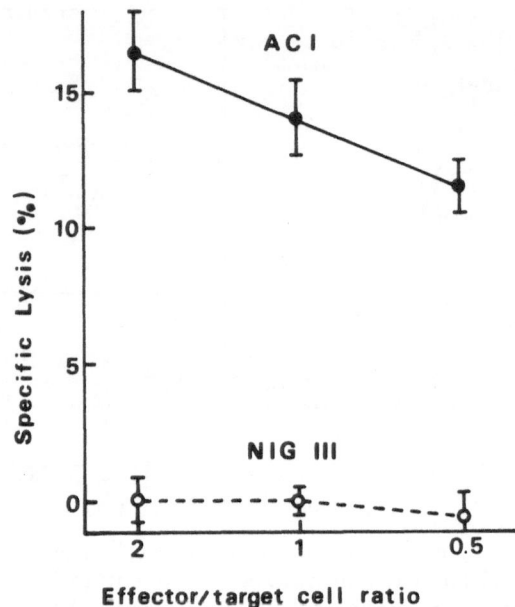

Fig. 5. Allo-reactive killer assay in PEL. LEC/Tj (RT1A^u) rats were immunized with ACI/Tj (TR1A^a) rat spleen cells (40 million) intraperitoneally 4 times with 1-week intervals. At the 5th day after the final immunization, PEL were prepared and subjected to the killer assay. ACI rat spleen Con A blast cells prepared by culturing with 2.5 µg/ml Con A for 2 days and labeled with ^{51}Cr were used as target cells. Killer assay was performed for 6h at 37°C. Data are expressed as specific killing calculated as: $100 \times (a - b)/(t - b)$; where a is the ^{51}Cr release in the presence of effector cells, b is spontaneous release from labeled target cells in the absence of effector cells, and t is the total radioactivity releasable by incubating with 0.1% NP-40. *Closed* and *open* sympbols represent the use of ACI and irrelevant NIG III (RTIA^q) rat spleen cells, respectively, as target cells

Normal Maturation of Killer T Cells

In order to confirm that the arrest of T-cell maturation occurs at the specific stage from CD4$^+$8$^+$ to CD4$^+$8$^-$ cells, peripheral T cells must be shown to have normal killing ability. FACS analysis demonstrated the normal percentages of CD8$^+$ cells in the peripheral lymphoid organs in LEC rats. Furthermore, most of the CD8$^+$ cells were shown to be TCR/CD3$^+$ [4]. Peritoneal exudate lymphocytes (PEL) from LEC rats which had been immunized intraperitoneally with allogeneic splenocytes (RT1A^a) could kill the same target cells but not the irrelevant target cells (RT1A^q) (Fig. 5). The results from mixed lymphocyte culture (MLC) killer assay also support the fact of functional killer ability by CD8$^+$ cells in LEC rats: when lymph node cells of LEC rats were cocultured with allogeneic splenocytes in the presence of exogenous IL-2, allo-specific killer T cells

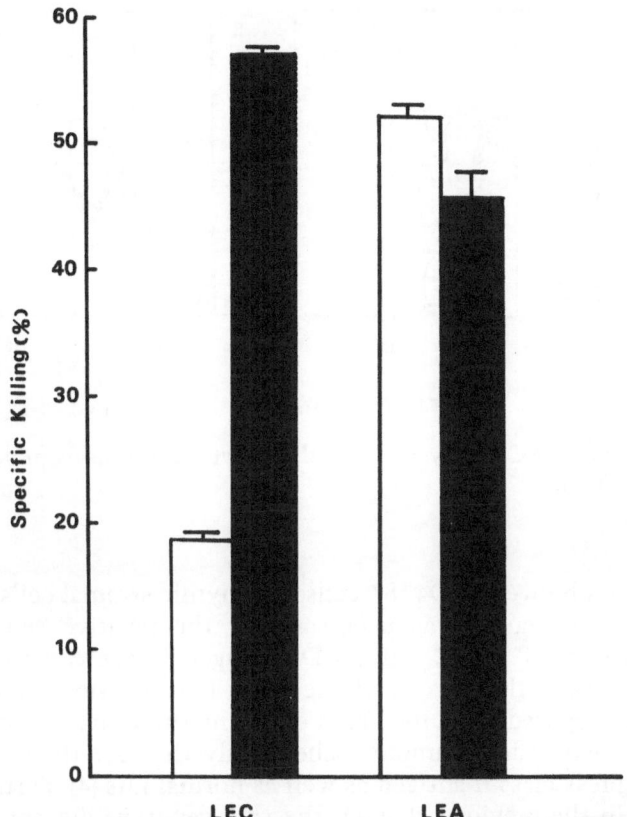

Fig. 6. MLC killer assay in lymph node cells of LEC/Tj (RT1Aᵘ) and LEA/Tj (RT1Aᵘ) rats. Lymph node cells from each strain of rats as responder cells were cocultured with mitomycin C-treated ACI/Tj (RT1Aᵃ) rat spleen cells as stimulator cells for 5 days in the absence (*open columns*) or presence (10%, vol/vol) (*filled columns*) of the supernatant of rat Con A blast spleen cells as an exogenous source of IL-2. Cells were harvested and incubated with ⁵¹Cr-labeled target cells (ACI rat Con A blast spleen cells) for 15 h at 37°C. Data are expressed as specific killing calculated as in Fig. 5. *Columns* and *bars* represent means ± SEMs of triplicated observations. (From [4] with permission)

could be proliferated as well as in normal rats (Fig. 6). These data indicate that the arrest occurs at a specific stage in T-cell maturation in LEC rats.

Class II Expression

Kruisbeek et al. demonstrated that deletion of the CD4⁺8⁻ subset in the two-color FACS analysis by administrating a large quantity of either anti-CD4 or anti-class II mAb to the mouse from birth [6,7]. They proposed that

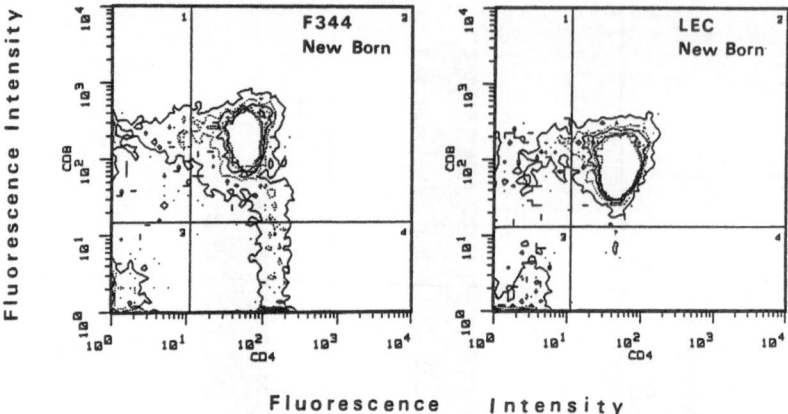

Fig. 7. Two-color FACS analysis of the thymocytes from newborn normal (F344/Tj) and LEC/Tj rats

the interaction between $CD4^+8^+$ cells and thymic stromal cells using CD4 and class II molecules was necessary for the positive selection from $CD4^+8^+$ to $CD4^+8^-$ cells. Since CD4 antigen is expressed on $CD4^+8^+$ cells in LEC rats, the default of the class II expression on the thymic stroma was supposed to be the cause of the maturational arrest. However, it was demonstrated immunohistochemically that the thymic stroma of LEC rats express class II antigen as well as normal rats [4]. Furthermore, as mentioned in the previous chapter, the *thid* genotype did not link to the *MHC* genotype in backcross rats, indicating that any abnormalities in the class II molecule, even if they exist, can not be attributed to the maturational arrest in LEC rats.

Ontogeny of T-Cell Maturation

There is a claim that $CD4^+8^-$ cells may differentiate normally in the prenatal stage and then their deletion begins postnatally. However, $CD4^+8^-$ cells did not appear from day 16 of gestation through the neonatal period. Figure 7 shows the FACS analysis pattern of neonatal thymocytes. Normal rat thymocytes showed the development of both single-positive subsets, while LEC rat thymocytes lacked development of the $CD4^+8^-$ cells. These data indicate that the arrest of T-cell maturation occurs from the early stage of the ontogeny.

Since mature T cells are formed by cooperation between bone marrow-derived pre-T cells and the thymic microenvironment, elucidating which part contributes to the arrest of maturation should be the first step in identifying the origin of the arrest. Preliminary data from the experiment in which LEC rat fetal thymus was transplanted into the kidney subcapsule of the nude rat showed normal maturation of $CD4^+8^-$ cells, suggesting that the LEC rat thymic microenvironment was normal. Further investigations are necessary for complete resolution of what is the cause of this novel mutation.

References

1. Sasaki M, Yoshida MC, Kagami K, Takeichi N, Kobayashi H, Dempo K, Mori M (1985) Spontaneous hepatitis in an inbred strain of Long-Evans rats. Rat News Lett 14:4–6
2. Matsumoto K, Takeichi N, Izumi K, Otsuka H (1989) Quantitative variation in immunoglobulin G (Igsr-1) in LEC rats associated with spontaneous hepatitis and hepatoma. Transplant Proc 21:3259
3. Yamada T, Natori T, Izumi K, Sakai T, Agui T, Matsumoto K (1991) Inheritance of T helper immunodeficiency (thid) in LEC mutant rats. Immunogenetics 33:216–219
4. Agui T, Oka M, Yamada T, Sakai T, Izumi K, Ishida Y, Himeno K, Matsumoto K (1990) Maturational arrest from $CD4^+8^+$ to $CD4^+8^-$ thymocytes in a mutant strain (LEC) of rat. J Exp Med 172:1615–1624
5. Mosmann TR, Coffman RL (1989) TH1 and TH2 cells: Different patterns of lymphokine secretion lead to different functional properties. Annu Rev Immunol 7:145–173
6. Kruisbeek AM, Mond JJ, Fowlkes BJ, Carmen JA, Bridges S, Longo DL (1985) Absence of the Lyt-2$^-$, L3T4$^+$ lineage of T cells in mice treated neonatally with anti-I-A correlates with absence of intrathymic I-A-bearing antigen-presenting cell function. J Exp Med 161:1029–1047
7. Zuniga-Pflucker JC, McCarthy SA, Weston M, Longo DN, Singer A, Kruisbeek AM (1989) Role of CD4 in thymocyte selection and maturation. J Exp Med 169:2085–2096
8. Jerne NK, Nordin AA (1963) Plaque formation in agar by single antibody-producing cells. Science 140:405
9. Mosmann T (1983) Rapid colorimetric assay for cellular growth and survival: Application to proliferation and cytotoxity assays. J Immunol Methods 65:55–63

PART III   Liver Cancer

1. Cytogenetics and Oncogenes

27 — Chromosomal Analysis of Spontaneous Hepatomas, a Derived Cell Line, and Chemically Induced Hepatomas in LEC Rats

Ryuichi Masuda, Takao Ono, Michihiro C. Yoshida[1], and Motomichi Sasaki[2]

Introduction

Recent banding studies of chromosomes in a variety of human and animal tumors have provided a growing body of evidence that certain specific or nonrandom chromosomal changes are causally related to or closely associated with the inhibition, promotion, or progression of malignant neoplasia [1–5]. Despite the vast amount of data now available on nonrandom occurrence of chromosomal abnormalities in human tumors, our knowledge on animal tumors appears to be very limited and the data on hand are rather conflicting.

Even before the advent of banding techniques it had been known that azo-dye-induced rat transplantable ascites hepatomas are usually aneuploid with different modal values and stemline karyotypes [6] or show different patterns of DNA replication of chromosomes greatly deviating from the normal pattern [7]. In contrast, a considerable number of apparently diploid tumors are known to exist in the so-called minimal deviation hepatomas [8] as well as in azo-dye-induced primary hepatomas of the rat [9,10]. At present, however, no reports are available on banded karyotypes of primary liver tumors, either spontaneously developed or induced by chemicals. LEC rats provide very useful material for studying cytogenetic questions on tumorigenesis, because they spontaneously develop not only hepatitis but also hepatocellular carcinomas (hepatomas) at a remarkably high incidence [11].

In this study, the banding pattern analysis of metaphase chromosomes is performed in constitutionally normal somatic cells of LEC and LEA rats as well as in primary hepatomas and in one established hepatoma cell line of LEC rats. Although a sufficient number of analyzable hepatomas to reach any conclusions has not yet been obtained, this report describes that trisomy or partial trisomy of chromosome 10 was observed in a small

[1] Chromosome Research Unit, Faculty of Science, Hokkaido University, Sapporo, 060 Japan
[2] Sasaki Cancer Institute, Chiyoda-ku, Tokyo, 101 Japan

portion of cells from some spontaneous hepatomas of LEC rats. In addition, karyotypes of 4-dimethylamino-3′-methylazobenzen (3′-Me-DAB)-induced hepatomas in LEC rats were examined for comparison with spontaneous hepatomas.

Materials and Methods for Chromosomal Preparations

Chromosomal analysis was performed in bone marrow cells, skin fibroblasts, and regenerating hepatocytes of LEC and LEA rats maintained at the Center for Experimental Plants and Animals of Hokkaido University. In order to obtain bone marrow cells, Colcemid (0.5 μg/g body weight) was injected intraperitoneally into rats. Bone marrow cells were collected 0.5 h after injection from the femur by flushing with hypotonic solution (0.075M KCl). Fibroblasts were obtained from the primary skin culture of a newborn LEC rat. Hepatocytes were obtained with Colcemid treatment for 1 h from regenerating livers of partially hepatectomized LEC rats. Chromosomal preparations from these tissues were made by the conventional air-drying method with hypotonic KCl pretreatment and fixation in 3 : 1 methanol-acetic acid.

Spontaneous primary hepatomas and a transplantable hepatoma cell line LSH206G of LEC rats were obtained as described previously [11,12]. These hepatoma-bearing rats received an intraperitoneal injection of Colcemid (0.5 μg/g body weight) 1 h before operation. Tumorous tissues were carefully dissected from the rats after anesthesia by ether. Each tissue was minced into pieces by scissors and treated at 37°C for 1 h with 0.5% collagenase (CLS 2, 115–163 U/mg, Worthington, USA) dissolved in Eagle's minimum essential medium (Nissui Pharmaceutical Co., Tokyo) containing 10% fetal bovine serum. Treated tissues were pipetted and passed through a 22-gauge 1.5-inch needle. Separated cells were incubated in hypotonic KCl solution at 37°C for 20 min and fixed with 3 : 1 methanol-acetic acid. Chromosomal preparations were made by the conventional air-drying methods. 3′-Me-DAB-induced hepatomas were examined by the same procedure used for spontaneous hepatomas.

Q-banding patterns of chromosomes were demonstrated by the 33258 Hoechst-quinacrine double staining method [13]. G-banding patterns were obtained basically by the method of Seabright [14]. Karyotypes were analyzed in accordance with the standard nomenclature [15] and the proposed numbering system [16].

Karyotypes of Normal Somatic Cells and Spontaneous Hepatomas of LEC Rats

In order to examine the existence of cytogenetic abnormality in somatic cells of LEC rats, karyotypes with G- and Q-banding techniques were performed on bone marrow cells of rats before and after the onset of

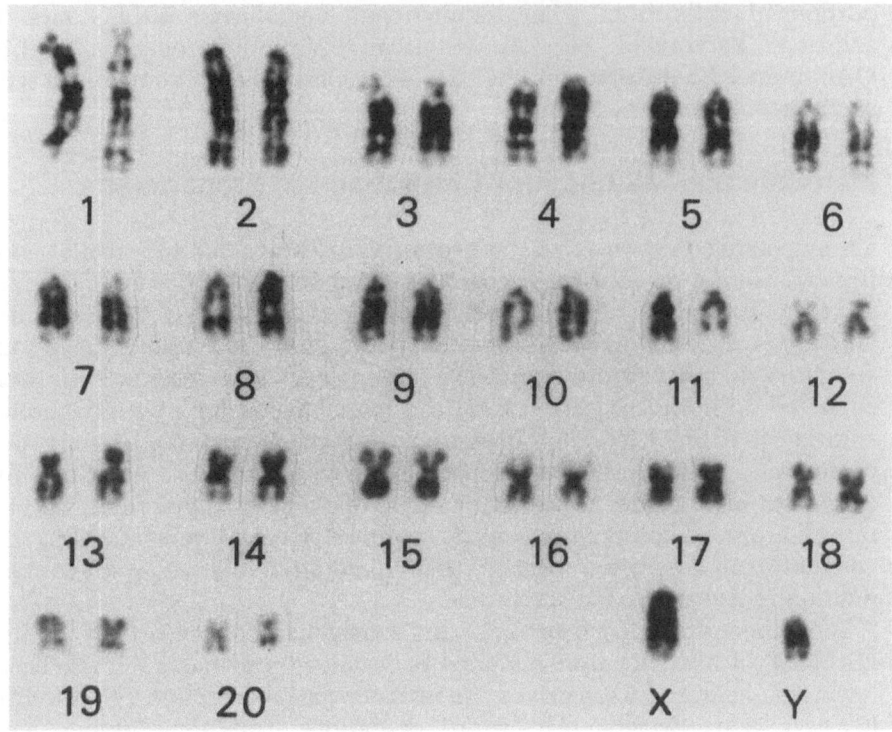

Fig. 1. G-banded chromosomes of a bone marrow cell from a male LEC rat aged 2 months (before the onset of hepatitis), showing a normal karyotype

hepatitis (Figs. 1, 2). No abnormal karyotype was observed. Regenerating hepatocytes (Fig. 3) and skin fibroblasts also showed the normal karyotype.

Chromosomal analysis was successful in seven primary hepatomas, named T1–T7, of LEC rats (Table 1). Of these hepatomas, T3 and T4 contained two and four analyzable hepatoma-nodules, respectively. Most of the cells of these hepatomas were in the diploid range and showed the chromosomal numbers of 40–44. In six of the seven hepatomas, two–four cells were in the tetraploid range, although these cells were not analyzable due to poor spreading of the chromosomes.

Table 2 shows the number of copies in each chromosome pair of the seven hepatomas. Most pairs of chromosomes in these tumors appeared to be disomic, while the monosomic or trisomic condition was observed in chromosomes 4, 9, 10, 11, 12, 18, 19, and 20 in a total of five cases. In addition, certain marker chromosomes were observed in these cases. All abnormal karyotypes which have thus far been observed are shown in Table 3. Of nine cells in T1, three cells had a trisomy for chromosome 10 (Fig. 4). The additional chromosome 10 common in three cells was a derivative chromosome translocated by an unknown segment at the

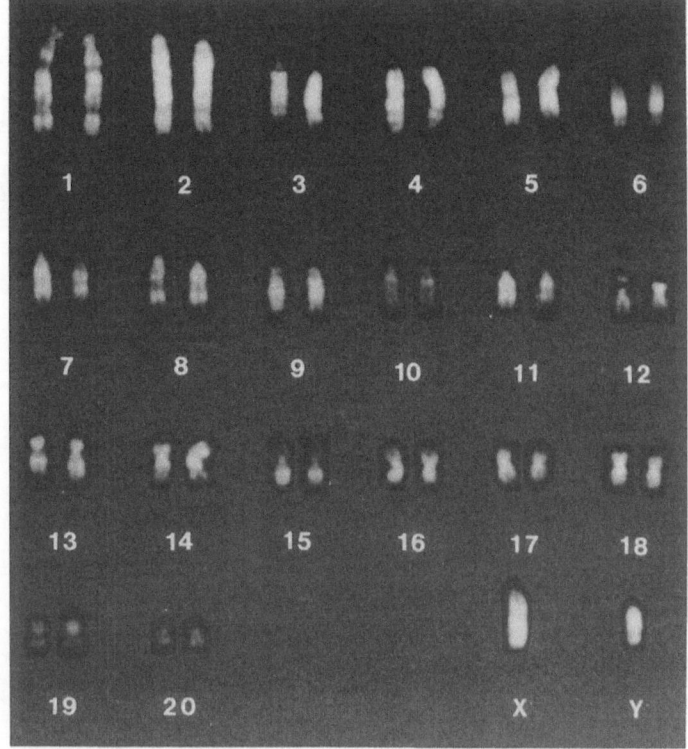

Fig. 2. Q-banded chromosomes of a bone marrow cell from a male LEC rat with fulminant hepatitis at the age of 4 months, showing a normal karyotype

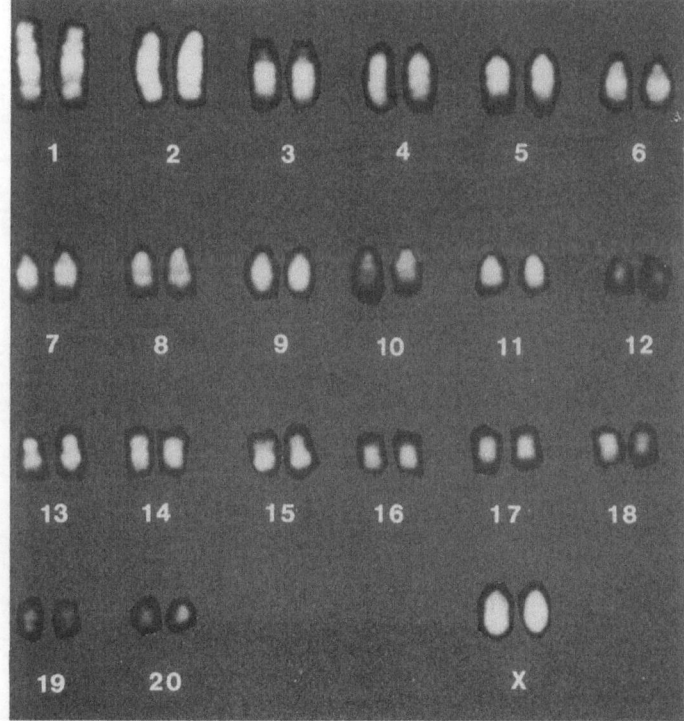

Fig. 3. Q-banded chromosomes of a hepatocyte from a hepatectomized female LEC rat aged 2 months, showing a normal karyotype

Table 1. Chromosomal analysis of spontaneous hepatomas in seven LEC rats.

			No. of cells in the range of 2n					*No. of cells in the range of 4n*
		Total	*Cells with each chromosome no.*					
Tumor	*Sex*[c]	*no.*	*40*	*41*	*42*	*43*	*44*	
T1	M	14	0	1	6	2	0	0[c]
T2	M	42	0	0	8	1	0	2
T3-A[a]	M	44	0	1	5	1	1	2
T3-B	M	38	0	0	2	3	0	2
T4-A[b]	M	34	0	0	5	3	0	2
T4-B	M	35	0	0	10	0	0	2
T4-C	M	30	0	3	9	0	0	0[c]
T4-D	M	36	0	0	3	0	0	0[c]
T5	M	38	0	0	14	1	0	3
T6	M	55	0	0	10	0	0	4
T7	F	31	1	0	8	0	0	2

[a] T3-A and T3-B indicate different nodules from the same liver
[b] T4-A to T4-D indicate different nodules from the same liver
[c] No analyzable cell was observed

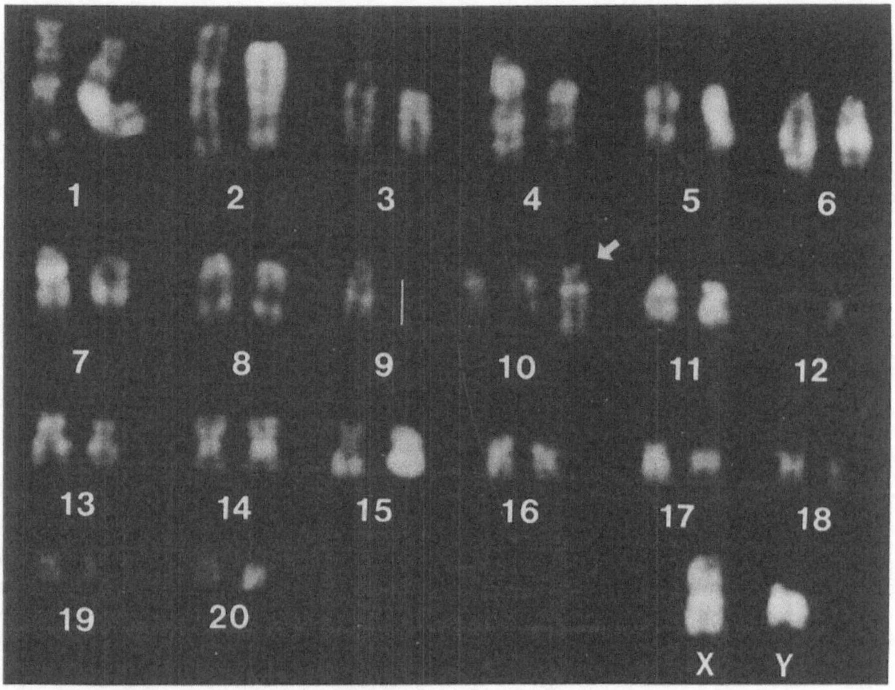

Fig. 4. Q-banded chromosomes of a cell from spontaneous hepatoma, T1, in a male LEC rat, showing a karyotype of 42, XY, −9, +der(10)t(10;?)(q32;?). The *arrow* indicates an abnormal chromosome

Table 2. Number of chromosomal copies in each homologous pair and marker chromosomes of spontaneous primary hepatomas in seven LEC rats.

Tumor	Sex	No. of Cells	Chromosome no.[a]																				X	Y	Markers
			1	2	3	4	5	6	7	8	9	10	11	12	13	14	15	16	17	18	19	20			
T1	M	9	2	2	2	2	2	2	2	2	1,2	2,3	2	2	2	2	2	2	2	2	2	1,2	2	2	1
T2	M	9	2	2	2	2	2	2	2	2	2	2,3	2	1,2	2	2	2	2	2	2	2	2	2	2	0
T3-A	M	8	2	2	2	2	2	2	2	2	2	2,3	2	2	2	2	2	2	2	1,2	2	2	2	2	1
T3-B	M	5	2	2	2	2	2	2	2	2	2	2	2	2	2	2	2	2	2	2	2	2	2	2	1
T4-A	M	8	2	2	2	2	2	2	2	2	2	2	2	2	2	2	2	2	2	2	2	2	2	2	1
T4-B	M	10	2	2	2	2	2	2	2	2	2	2	1,2	2	2	2	2	2	2	2	2	2	2	2	0
T4-C	M	11	2	2	2	2	2	2	2	2	2	2	2	2	2	2	2	2	2	2	1,2	2	2	2	0
T4-D	M	3	2	2	2	2,3	2	2	2	2	2	2	2	2	2	2	2	2	2	2	2	2	2	2	0
T5	M	15	2	2	2	2	2	2	2	2	2	2	2	2	2	2	2	2	2	2	2	2	2	2	0
T6	M	10	2	2	2	2	2	2	2	2	2	2	2	2	2	2	2	2	2	2	2	2	2	2	0
T7	F	8	2	2	2	2	2	2	2	2	2	2	2	2	2	2	2	2	2	2	2	2	2	2	0

[a] Underlines show monosomy (1) or trisomy with or without structural abnormalities (3)

Table 3. Chromosomal analysis of spontaneous hepatomas in LEC rats.

Tumor	Abnormal karyotypes	No. of Cells analyzed[a]
T1	41, XY, −9, −20, +der(10)t(10;?)(q32;?)	1/9
	42, XY, −9, +der(10)t(10;?)(q32;?)	1/9
	43, XY, +der(10)t(10;?)(q32;?)	1/9
	43, XY, +mar	1/9
T2	42, XY, −12, +del(10)(q23)	1/9
	43, XY, +del(10)(q26)	1/9
T3-A	43, XY, +del(10)(q22q26)	1/8
	44, XY, +del(10)(q22q26), +mar	1/8
	41, XY, −18	1/8
T3-B	43, XY, +mar	3/5
T4-A	43, XY, +mar	3/8
T4-C	41, XY, −11	1/11
	41, XY, −19	1/11
T5	43, XY, +4	1/15

[a] 1/9 indicates 1 abnormal karyotype among 9 cells karyotyped

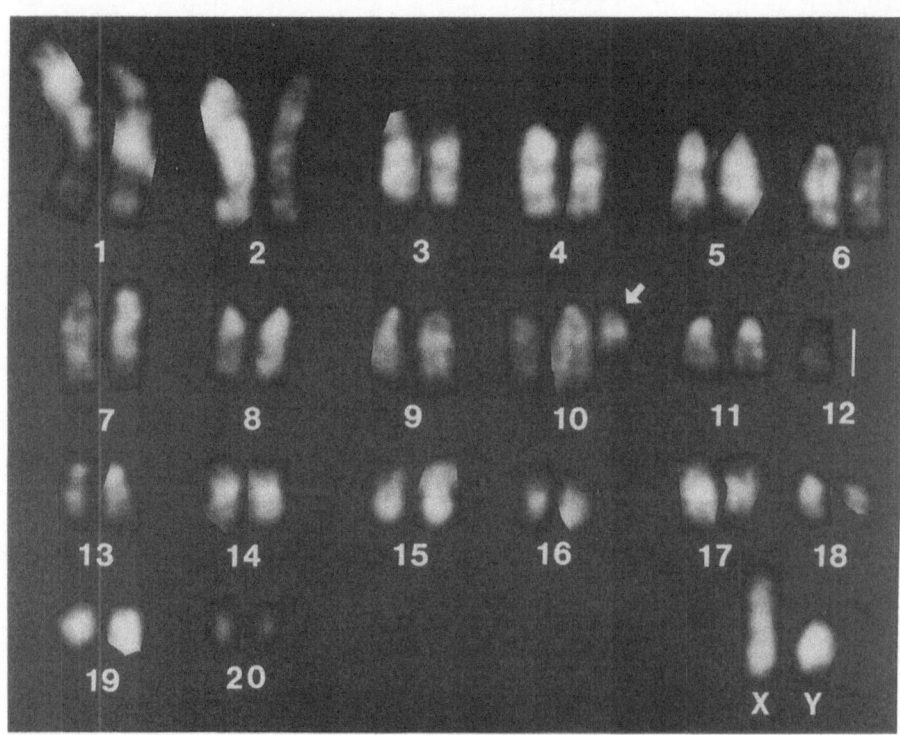

Fig. 5. Q-banded chromosomes of a cell from spontaneous hepatoma, T2, in a male LEC rat, showing a karyotype of 42, XY, −12, +del(10)(q23). The *arrow* indicates an abnormal chromosome

terminal of the long arm, i.e., der(10)t(10;?)(q32;?). One cell had a marker chromosome, although its origin was not identified. The remaining five cells in T1 showed a normal karyotype. In T2, two out of nine cells had a pseudodiploid or a hyperdiploid karyotype; one was monosomic for chromosome 12 and both were partially trisomic for the long arm of chromosome 10 (Fig. 5), the additional chromosome 10 being del(10)(q23) and del(10)(q26) in the two cells, respectively. In T3-A, another partial trisomy for chromosome 10 was observed in two out of eight cells (Fig. 6). The additional chromosome 10 in the two cells had the same deletion within the long arm, i.e., del(10)(q22q26). One of the two cells had a marker chromosome of unknown origin. There was one hypodiploid cell showing a monosomy for chromosome 18, while the remaining five cells had an apparently normal karyotype. In T3-B, three out of five cells had a marker chromosome of unknown origin. In T4, four hepatoma-nodules were analyzed. In T4-A, a small marker chromosome of unknown origin was observed in three out of eight cells (Fig. 7). The remaining five cells in T4-A, all ten cells in T4-B, and all three cells in T4-D showed a normal karyotype. T4-C showed nine normal and two hypodiploid karyotypes, the latter being monosomic for 11 or 19. In T5, one out of 15 cells had a trisomy for chromosome 4, while the remaining 14 cells had a normal karyotype. No abnormal karyotype was found in a total of 18 cells from T6

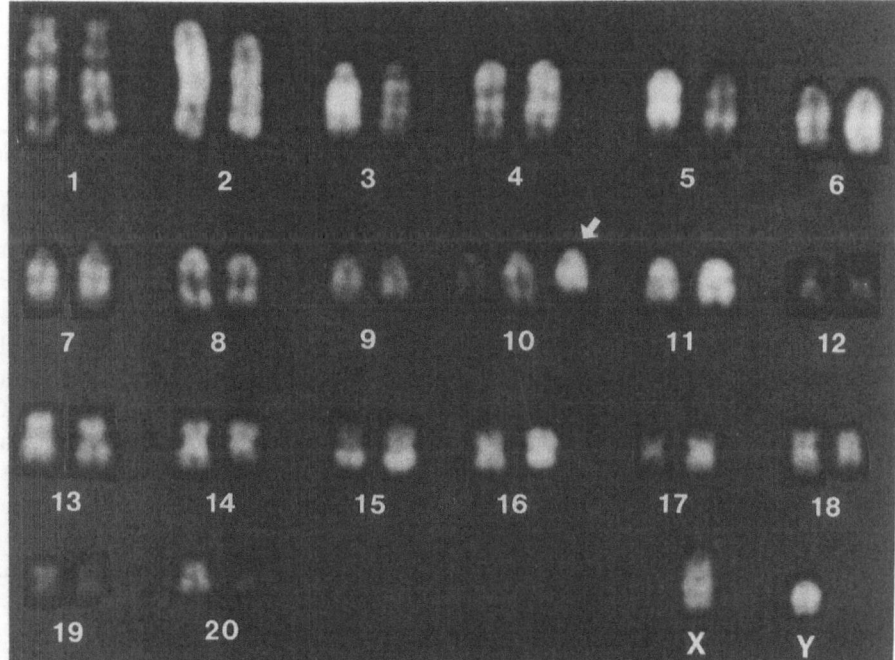

Fig. 6. Q-banded chromosomes of a cell from spontaneous hepatoma, T3-A, in a male LEC rat, showing a karyotype of 43, XY, +del(10)(q22 q26). The *arrow* indicates an abnormal chromosome

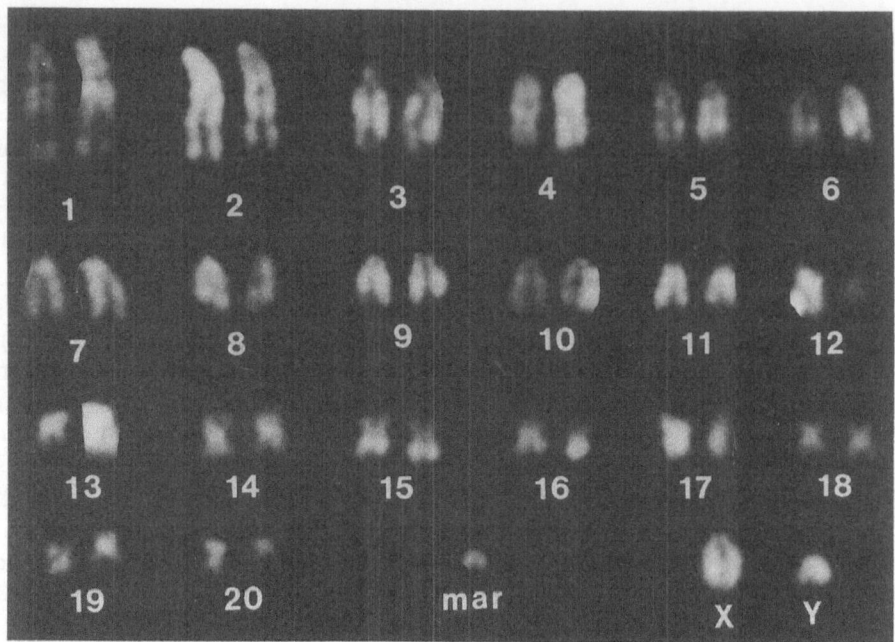

Fig. 7. Q-banded chromosomes of a cell from spontaneous hepatoma, T4-A, in a male LEC rat, showing a karyotype of 43, XY, +mar. *mar*, marker chromosome

and T7. One hypodiploid cell of T7 with 40 chromosomes was not analyzable.

Since karyotypes of spontaneous rat hepatomas have never been described to date, the present data should be noteworthy. The chromosomal numbers of the hepatomas in LEC rats were in the diploid range in all cases, consistent with chemically induced hepatomas reported previously [9,10,17]. Although a normal diploid karyotype predominated in all of the seven cases studied here, five of the seven hepatomas exhibited some chromosomal changes in some cells within each hepatoma nodule. Of particular interest was that a partial or full trisomy for chromosome 10 was observed in some near-diploid or pseudodiploid cells. Certain abnormal karyotypes were shown to be specific for each case of previously reported hepatomas, but no consistent abnormalities common to two or more cases have ever been observed in chemically induced rat hepatomas and their cell lines, even with banding methods [18–22]. In some cases of chemically induced bladder tumors, an abnormality in the long arm of the rat chromosome 10 was reported, although the breakpoints within chromosome 10 were not consistent from case to case [23]. The role played by the extra segment of chromosome 10 and some other minor karyotypic changes as described in the present cases of primary hepatomas is entirely unknown, although these changes may be related to the secondary event

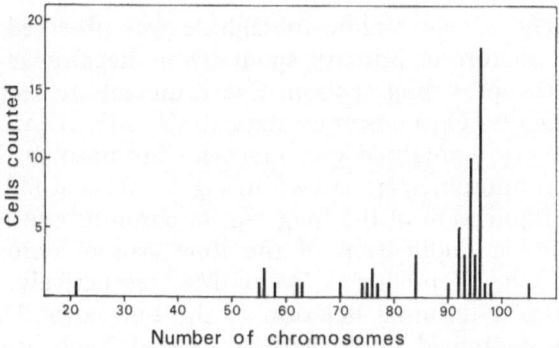

Fig. 8. Frequency distribution of chromosome numbers in 60 metaphases from LSH206G at the seventh passage. (From [12] with permission)

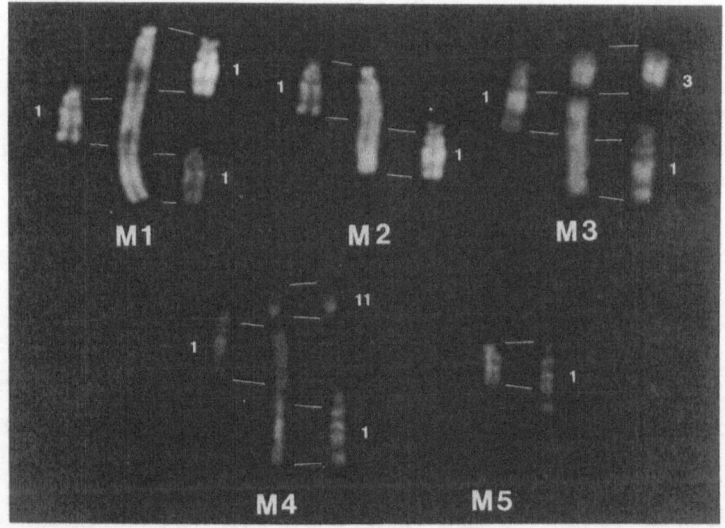

Fig. 9. Origins of specific marker chromosomes, M1–M5, observed in LSH206G. Chromosomes were Q-banded. Normal chromosomes 1, 3, and 11 are compared with banding patterns of marker chromosomes. Structures of marker chromosomes are as follows; M1: dup(1)(q55→q12::q55→q12::q55→p13), M2: dup(1)(q55→q12:: q55→p13), M3: der(3)t(1;1;3)(1q55→1q55::1q55→1q22::3p12→3q43), M4: der(11) t(1;1;11)(1q55→1q12::1q55→1q12::11p12→11q23), M5: del(1)(q41)

during the course of tumor development, but not at the time of tumor initiation.

Karyotypes of a Hepatoma Cell Line LSH206G

Chromosomal analysis was carried out in a total of 60 cells from the spontaneous hepatoma cell line LSH206G at the seventh in vivo passage [12]. Chromosomal numbers were widely distributed from 21 to 105 with a mode of 96 (Fig. 8). No diploid metaphase was observed, as opposed to the karyotype feature of primary spontaneous hepatomas of LEC rats as described in the preceding section. Every metaphase had from three to five specific marker chromosomes, named M1–M5. A metaphase with 21 chromosomes also contained one marker Chromosome, M4. Origins of the marker chromosomes are shown in Fig. 9. M1 and M2 were produced by a tandem-duplication of the long arm of chromosome 1. Translocation between a tandem-duplication of the long arm of chromosome 1 and chromosome 3 or 11 produced M3 or M4, respectively. M5 was chromosome 1 with a terminal deletion of the long arm. Thus, all marker chromosomes contained duplicated or deleted long arm segment(s) of chromosome 1 with variable breakpoints. Detailed analysis of the stemline karyotype was done in six cells with a modal or near-modal number of chromosomes (Table 4). More than two copies of chromosomes were observed in each homologous pair, except for sex chromosomes which were represented by one or two copies. Since each cell had more than three copies of M1–M5 marker chromosomes, in which M4 and M5 were always involved, it is suggested that the development of LSH206G may be monoclonal in origin. A representative full karyotype from the six cells is shown in Fig. 10.

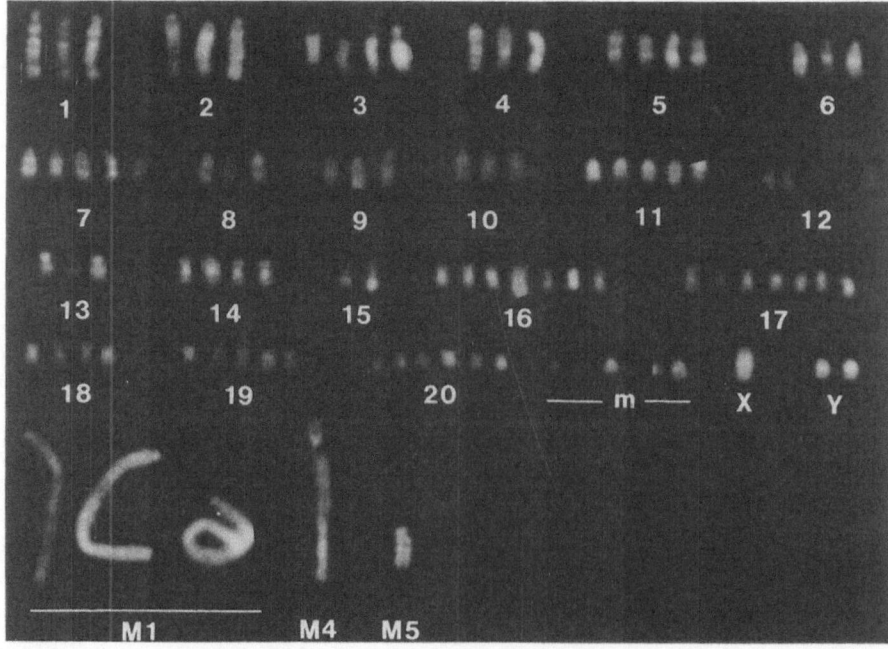

Fig. 10. Q-banded karyotype of a stemline cell, named cell 6, from LSH206G with 96 chromosomes including marker chromosomes M1, M4, M5, and six minute markers (m)

Table 4. Number of chromosomal copies in each homologous pair and marker chromosomes of a hepatoma cell line LSH206G derived from an LEC rat.

Cell	Total no. of chromosomes	1	2	3	4	5	6	7	8	9	10	11	12	13	14	15	16	17	18	19	20	X	Y	M1	M2	M3	M4	M5	Additional markers
														Chromosome no.												Marker no.			
1	97	4	3	4	4	4	4	5	3	3	3	3	4	3	4	4	5	8	4	4	6	2	2	1	2	1	1	1	4
2	94	3	3	2	4	4	5	4	4	4	4	5	4	3	4	4	4	5	3	4	6	2	2	0	3	1	1	1	6
3	96	3	3	3	3	2	2	5	3	3	3	5	5	5	2	4	6	9	3	6	9	1	1	2	0	1	1	1	5
4	96	2	3	4	3	3	4	3	3	4	4	5	4	4	4	4	5	8	5	4	7	1	1	2	2	0	1	1	5
5	97	3	3	4	4	4	4	5	4	3	2	4	2	5	2	3	7	8	4	5	6	2	2	2	1	0	1	1	6
6	96	3	3	4	3	4	3	5	3	3	3	5	5	3	4	2	7	7	4	5	6	1	2	3	0	0	1	1	6

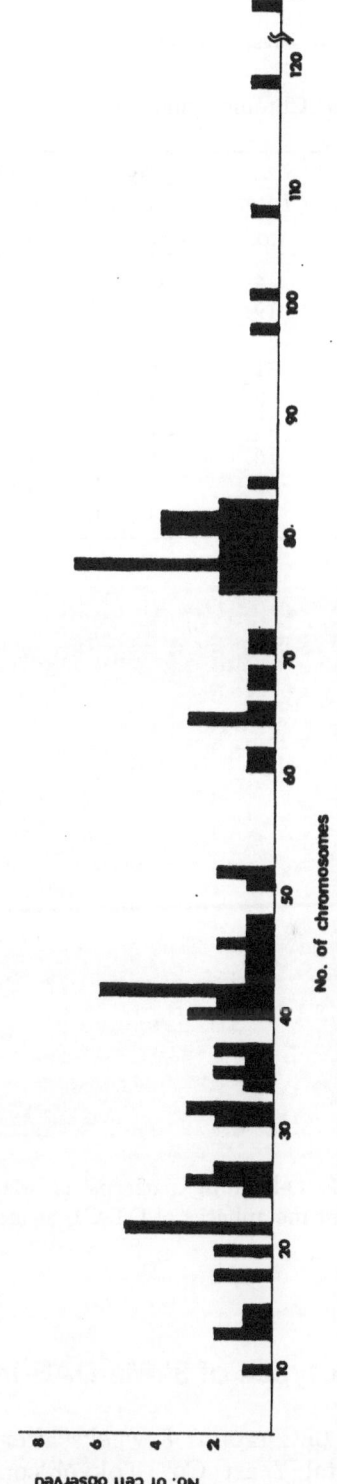

Fig. 11. Frequency distribution of chromosome numbers in 97 metaphases of 3'-Me-DAB-induced hepatoma DT-C1

255

Table 5. Chromosomal analysis of 3'-Me-DAB-induced hepatomas in four LEC rats.

Tumor	Total no.	No. of Cells in 2n range					No. of Cells in the 4n range	No. of Cells with more than 4n
		Cell with chromosome no.						
		≦40	41	42	43	44≦		
DT-A1	4	0	0	4	0	0	0	0
DT-A2	19	2	0	17	0	0	2	0
DT-A3	22	0	1	21	0	0	0	0
DT-B1	31	1	0	30	0	0	1	0
DT-B2	8	0	0	8	0	0	0	0
DT-C1	43	25	2	6	1	9	42	15
DT-C2	16	2	1	13	0	0	3	0
DT-D1	21	0	2	19	0	0	0	0
DT-D2	17	0	0	16	1	0	1	0

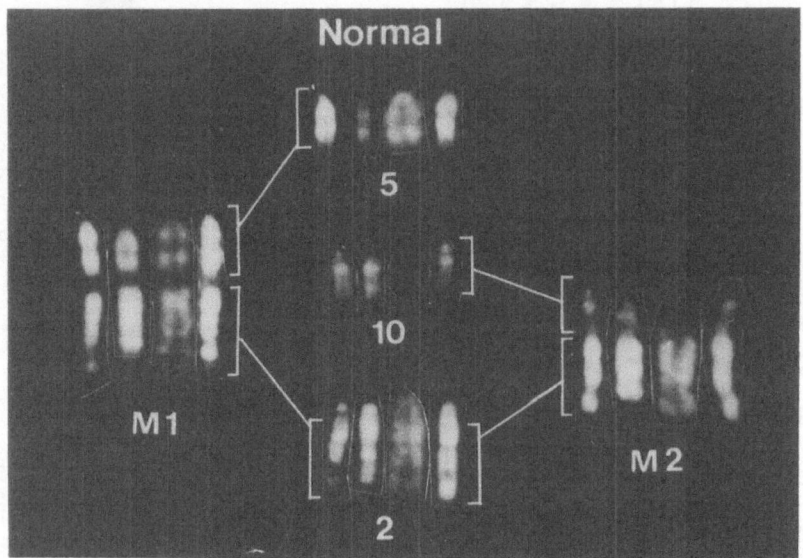

Fig. 12. Q-banding patterns of M1 and M2 marker chromosomes from four different metaphases of DT-C1, as assigned to normal chromosomes 2, 5, and 10

Karyotypes of 3'-Me-DAB-Induced Hepatomas in LEC Rats

Male LEC rats at 8 weeks after birth were fed a laboratory diet (CMF, Oriental Yeast Co., Tokyo) containing 0.03% (w/w) 3'-Me-DAB for 5 weeks, after which the diet was changed to the normal CMF. Of the seven surviving rats, the one animal sacrificed at 8 months had only cholangio-fibrosis without hepatoma. In the other six animals sacrificed at 11–14

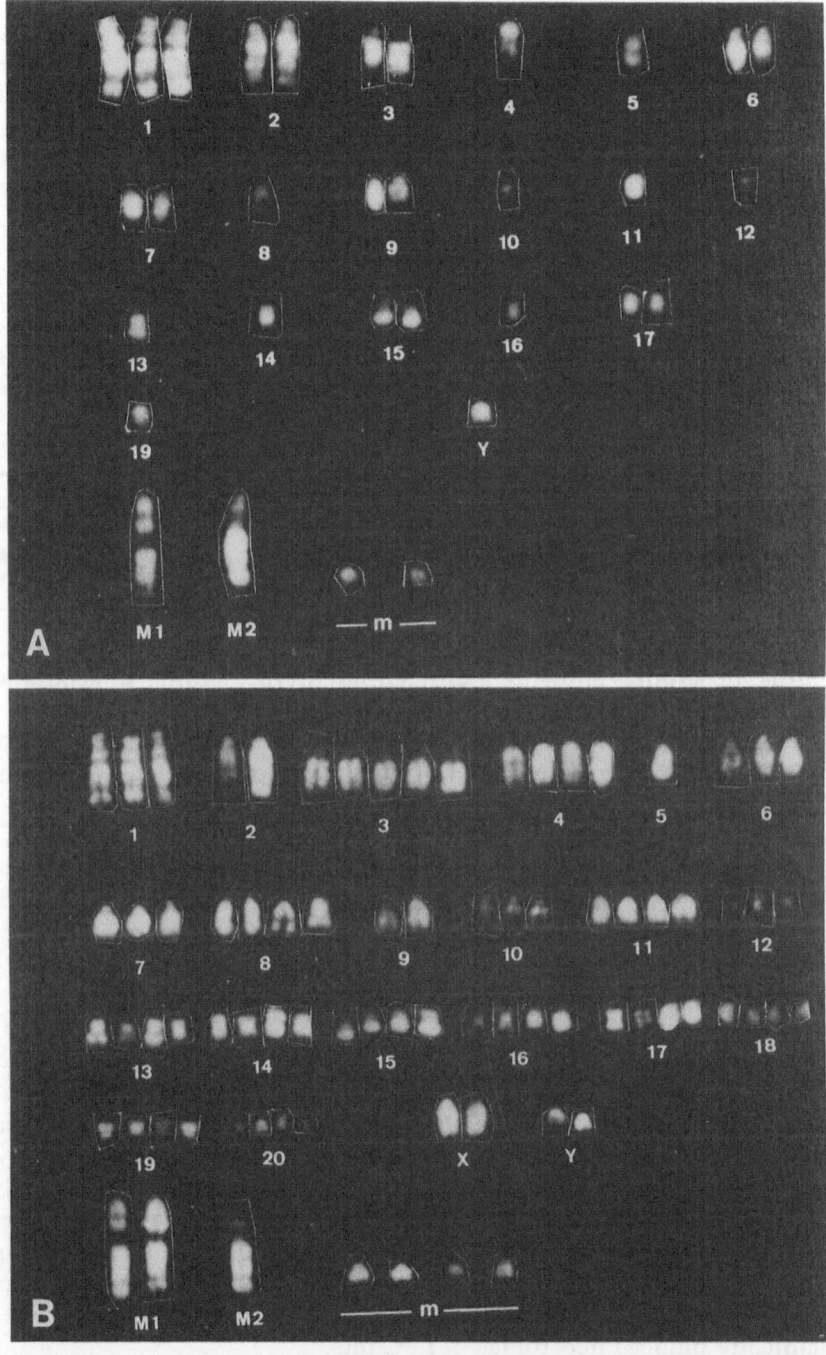

Fig. 13. Q-banded karyotypes of DT-C1. **A** Hypodiploid metaphase with two minute markers and **B** hypotetraploid metaphase with M1 and M2 chromosomes and four minute markers

Table 6. Frequency of marker chromosomes in DT-C1.

Modal no. of chromosomes	M1	M2	m^a	Frequency (%)
2n Range	++	+	+	2.3
	++	−	+	7.0
	+	+	+	11.6
	+	−	+	30.2
	−	+	+	4.7
	−	−	+	4.7
	−	−	−	39.5
4n Range	++	+	+	40.6
	++	−	+	24.3
	+	+	+	5.4
	+	−	+	5.4
	−	−	+	18.9
	−	−	−	5.4

++, Two marker chromosomes; +, one marker chromosome; −, no marker chromosomes;
[a] small markers

months, hepatomas showing a differentiated type, similar to spontaneous hepatomas [11], were observed.

The results of four analyzable cases are summarized in Table 5. Except for DT-C1, all tumors showed a normal karyotype. In DT-C1, the number of chromosomes was widely distributed from 10 to 168 (Fig. 11). Two traceable marker chromosomes, named M1 and M2, were observed in this tumor (Fig. 12). M1 and M2 were produced by translocations of t(2;5) and t(2;10), respectively. Abnormality involving chromosome 2 was reported in other chemically induced tumors in the rat [3] and a common action on chromosomes by different carcinogenic chemicals was suggested [24]. Therefore, it is interesting that a common segment of chromosome 2 was involved in both M1 and M2, although the exact breakpoints were not clear. Figure 13 shows representative karyotypes of DT-C1. As indicated in Table 6, M1 and/or M2 were detected in about 56% of the diploid cells and in 76% of the tetraploid cells. This suggests that M1 and M2 may appear in early stages of tumor development. These two marker chromosomes were not observed in spontaneous primary hepatomas nor in the LSH206G cell line. Changes of the number in the chromosomal copy were detected not only in chromosome 10 but in other chromosomes as well. In order to clarify the relation between cytogenetic abnormalities and hepato-carcinogenesis, further study is needed on more cases of spontaneous and chemically induced hepatomas of LEC rats.

Acknowledgments. We thank Mr. Eikichi Kamimura of the Center for Experimental Plants and Animals of Hokkaido University for his assistance. R.M. was a recipient of a Fellowship for Japanese Junior Scientists from the Japan Society for the Promotion of Science. This work was in part supported by Grants-in-Aid for Scientific Research from the Ministry of Education, Science and Culture, Japan and a fund from Otsuka Pharmaceutical Co., Ltd.

References

1. Rowley JD (1980) Chromosome abnormalities in cancer. Cancer Genet Cytogenet 2:175–198
2. Sandberg AA (1980) The chromosomes in human cancer and leukemia. Elsevier North Holland
3. Sasaki M (1982) Current status of cytogenetic studies in animal tumors with special reference to nonrandom chromosome changes. Cancer Genet Cytogenet 5:153–172
4. Sasaki M (1982) Role of chromosomal mutation in the development of cancer. Cytogenet Cell Genet 33:160–168
5. Mitelman F (1986) Clustering of breakpoints to specific chromosomal regions in human neoplasia. A survey of 5,345 cases. Hereditas 104:113–119
6. Yoshida T (1956) Contributions of the ascites hepatoma to the concept of malignancy of cancer. Ann NY Acad Sci 63:852–881
7. Sasaki M (1971) DNA replication patterns in chromosomes of several transplantable ascites hepatomas of the rat. J Natl Cancer Inst 46:25–35
8. Nowell PC, Morris HP (1969) Chromosomes of "minimal deviation" hepatomas: A further report on diploid tumors. Cancer Res 29:969–970
9. Hori SH, Sasaki M (1969) Glucose 6-phosphate dehydrogenase isoenzyme patterns and chromosomes in primary liver tumors of the rat. Cancer Res 29:880–891
10. Ikeuchi T, Honda T (1971) Cytologic studies of tumors XLVIII. Chromosomes of nine primary rat hepatomas induced by administration of 3'-methyl-4 dimethylaminoazobenzene. Cytologia 36:173–182
11. Masuda R, Yoshida MC, Sasaki M, Dempo K, Mori M (1988) High susceptibility to hepatocellular carcinoma development in LEC rats with hereditary hepatitis. Jpn J Cancer Res 79:828–835
12. Masuda R, Yoshida MC, Sasaki M, Dempo K, Mori M (1988) A transplantable cell line derived from spontaneous hepatocellular carcinoma of the hereditary hepatitis LEC rat. Jpn J Cancer Res 79:250–254
13. Yoshida MC, Ikeuchi T, Sasaki M (1975) Differential staining of parental chromosomes in interspecific cell hybrids with a combined quinacrine and 33258 Hoechst technique. Proc Jpn Acad 51:184–187
14. Seabright M (1971) A rapid banding technique for human chromosomes. Lancet II:971–972
15. Committee for a standardized karyotype of Rattus norvegicus (1973) Standard karyotype of the Norway rat, Rattus norvegicus. Cytogenet Cell Genet 12:199–205
16. Levan G (1974) Nomenclature for G-bands in rat chromosomes. Hereditas 77:37–52
17. Masahito Hitachi P, Yamada K, Takayama S (1974) Diethylnitrosamine-induced chromosome changes in rat liver cells. J Natl Cancer Inst 53:507–516

18. Miller DA, Dev VG, Borek C, Miller OJ (1972) The quinacrine fluorescent and Giemsa banding karyotype of the rat, *Rattus norvegicus*, and banded chromosome analysis of transformed and malignant rat liver cell lines. Cancer Res 32:2375–2382
19. Wolman SR, Phillips TF, Becker FF (1972) Fluorescent banding patterns of rat chromosomes in normal cells and primary hepatocellular carcinomas. Science 175:1267–1269
20. Wolman SR, Cohen TI, Becker FF (1977) Chromosome analysis of hepatocellular carcinoma 7777 and correlation with α-fetoprotein production. Cancer Res 37:2624–2627
21. Becker FF, Wolman SR, Asofsky R, Sell S (1975) Sequential analysis of transplantable hepatocellular carcinomas. Cancer Res 35:3021–3026
22. Holecek BU, Kerler R, Rabes HM (1989) Chromosomal analysis of a diethylnitrosamine-induced tumorigenic and a nontumorigenic rat liver cell line. Cancer Res 49:3024–3028
23. Debiec-Rychter M, Zukowski K, Wang CY (1989) Chromosomal characteristics and malignancy of urothelial cells from carcinogen-treated rats. J Natl Cancer Inst 81:361–367
24. Uenaka H, Ueda N, Maeda S, Sugiyama T (1978) Involvement of chromosome #2 changes in primary leukemia induced in rats by N-nitroso-N-butylurea. J Natl Cancer Inst 60:1399–1404

28 — Drug-Metabolizing Ability and Inducibility of Chromosomal Aberrations and Sister Chromatid Exchanges in LEC Rats Exposed to Cyclophosphamide

Ryuichi Masuda, Syuiti Abe, Michihiro C. Yoshida[1],
Motomichi Sasaki[2], Toshihiro Sugiyama, and Naoyuki Taniguchi[3]

Introduction

The LEC rat strain is a new mutant characterized by the spontaneous development of hepatitis with severe jaundice about 4 months of age [1,2]. Genetic analysis demonstrated that the disease has an autosomal recessive mode of inheritance, being ruled by a single gene named *hts* [3]. Although about 30% of rats die of fulminant hepatitis within 1 week after the onset of jaundice, the remaining animals survive with chronic hepatitis for more than 1 year and develop liver cancer [4].

Another feature of LEC rats is that changes of hepatic enzymes before the onset of hepatitis are quite similar to those observed in rat chemical hepatocarcinogenesis. The enzymatic changes include increased levels of epoxide hydrolase, UDP-glucuronyltransferase, γ-glutamyltranspeptidase and glutathione *S*-transferase, and a decreased level of cytochrome P-450 [5]. Among these enzymes, the cytochrome P-450 content in LEC rats decreased to the level of about one-half of that in LEA rats. It is possible that the lower level of hepatic cytochrome P-450 in LEC rats may affect the metabolism of certain endogenous substances, such as steroids and bile acids, and may accumulate their metabolites which may trigger the spontaneous development of hepatitis.

In the present study, in order to substantiate this possibility, cyclophosphamide (CP), which is known to require metabolic activation to become an ultimate mutagen, was administered to LEC and control LEA rats for comparison of the inducibilty of chromosomal aberrations and/or sister chromatid exchanges (SCEs) in hepatocytes, after partial hepatectomy, and in bone marrow cells between the two rat strains. Mitomycin C (MMC) was used as a positive control, because MMC is

[1] Chromosome Research Unit, Faculty of Science, Hokkaido University, Sapporo, 060 Japan
[2] Sasaki Cancer Institute, Chiyoda-ku, Tokyo, 101 Japan
[3] Department of Biochemistry, Osaka University Medical School, Suita, Osaka, 565 Japan

a well-known direct-acting clastogen which does not require metabolic activation.

Hepatic Cytochrome P-450 Contents and Cytochrome P-450-Catalyzed Monooxygenase Activities in LEA and LEC Rats

Table 1 shows cytochrome P-450 contents and monooxygenase activities in livers of 2-month-old LEA and LEC rats [6]. Activities of pentoxyresorufin O-depentylase (PROD) and ethoxyresorufin O-deethylase (EROD) are known to be due to phenobarbital-inducible forms of cytochrome P-450 and methylcholanthrene-inducible forms of cytochrome P-450, respectively [7,8]. Both cytochrome P-450 contents and PROD activities tended to be lower in females than in males of each strain. The sex difference was especially prominant in LEA rats, showing significantly higher content of cytochrome P-450 ($P < 0.025$) and PROD activity ($P < 0.005$) in males. Comparing the same sex between the two strains, the cytochrome P-450 content and the PROD activity were lower in LEC rats. A statistically significant difference was observed in the cytochrome P-450 content ($P < 0.01$) and in the PROD activity ($P < 0.005$) between LEA and LEC males. The decrease of PROD activity in LEC rats is concordant with our previous report [5]. No sex or strain difference was observed in the EROD activity.

Chromosomal Aberrations in Bone Marrow Cells of Animals Exposed to CP

Table 2 shows chromosomal aberrations observed in bone marrow cells of 2-month-old LEA and LEC rats exposed to CP. Details of the experimental protocol are described in our previous report [6]. In brief, the rats were sacrificed 16 h after intraperitoneal injection of CP, with Colcemid treatment for the final 0.5 h. Bone marrow cells were collected from the femur. Chromosomal preparations were made by the conventional air-drying method, followed by Giemsa staining. A dose-related increase was observed in both the percentage of cells with chromosomal aberrations (aberrant cells) and the frequency of chromosomal aberrations per 100 metaphases. In both LEA and LEC rats, the percentage of aberrant cells in females was lower than that in males at the same dose level (Table 2, Fig. 1). The percentage of aberrant cells tended to be lower in LEC rats when compared to LEA and LEC rats of the same sex and at the same dose level. The mitotic index for each dose was expressed as percentage of mitotic cells among more than 2,000 cells per animal. A dose-dependent decrease in the mitotic index was apparent in both strains of rats.

The observed chromosomal aberrations were chromatid gap (cdg), isochromatid gap (icdg), chromatid break (cdb), isochromatid break (icdb),

Table 1. Cytochrome P-450 contents and cytochrome P-450-catalyzed monooxygenase activities in livers of LEA and LEC rats (From [6] with permission).

Rat strain	Sex	Number of animals	Total content of P-450 (nmol/mg protein) Mean ± SE	Activities of	
				PROD (pmol/min/mg protein) Mean ± SE	EROD (pmol/min/mg protein) Mean ± SE
LEA	F	3	0.42 ± 0.03[a]	3.9 ± 2.8[c]	19.5 ± 2.9
	M	3	0.56 ± 0.02[b]	33.1 ± 2.5[d]	20.4 ± 3.5
LEC	F	3	0.40 ± 0.01	2.3 ± 0.8	20.0 ± 0.5
	M	3	0.43 ± 0.07	4.1 ± 0.4	22.0 ± 1.5

[a] Statistically significant compared with male LEA rats ($P < 0.025$, t-test)
[b] Statistically significant compared with male LEC rats ($P < 0.01$)
[c] Statistically significant copmared with male LEA rats ($P < 0.005$)
[d] Statistically significant compared with male LEC rats ($P < 0.005$)

Table 2. Chromosomal aberrations in bone marrow cells of LEA and LEC rats exposed to cyclophosphamide (CP) (From [6] with permission).

Rat strain	Dose of CP (mg/kg)	Sex	Number of animals	Aberrant cells (%)	Frequency of chromosomal aberrations						Mitotic index (%)
					cdg	icdg	cdb	icdb	frg	cdx	
LEA	0	F	3	4.3 ± 0.9	4.0 ± 1.2	0.3 ± 0.3	0	0	0	0	8.7 ± 1.3
		M	3	5.0 ± 1.2	3.7 ± 0.9	0.3 ± 0.3	0	0	1.0 ± 0.6	0.3 ± 0.3	9.4 ± 1.6
	10	F	3	32.3 ± 4.5	32.3 ± 8.7	9.0 ± 1.2	10.7 ± 1.2	0	6.0 ± 3.8	1.0 ± 0.6	6.8 ± 1.0
		M	3	52.7 ± 1.2	59.3 ± 4.3	10.3 ± 2.4	18.7 ± 2.7	1.0 ± 1.0	16.3 ± 3.2	1.7 ± 0.9	6.0 ± 0.6
	20	F	3	66.3 ± 1.2	91.7 ± 2.6	14.0 ± 7.0	24.7 ± 3.7	1.0 ± 0.6	29.0 ± 10.0	3.3 ± 1.2	4.7 ± 0.5
		M	3	78.0 ± 0.0	143.0 ± 15.6	19.3 ± 3.0	32.7 ± 8.4	1.7 ± 1.2	43.7 ± 15.1	4.3 ± 1.8	2.8 ± 0.1
LEC	0	F	3	4.3 ± 0.7	2.7 ± 0.7	0.7 ± 0.3	0	0	1.0 ± 0.6	0	10.4 ± 0.8
		M	3	2.7 ± 0.3	2.7 ± 0.3	0	0	0	0	0	9.7 ± 0.7
	10	F	3	38.7 ± 3.0	39.3 ± 4.9	5.3 ± 0.7	11.7 ± 3.2	1.3 ± 1.3	12.0 ± 2.0	1.7 ± 0.3	5.3 ± 0.2
		M	3	45.7 ± 1.7	54.3 ± 8.4	9.0 ± 1.0	12.3 ± 0.7	0.3 ± 0.3	15.3 ± 1.8	0.7 ± 0.3	5.7 ± 0.2
	20	F	3	64.0 ± 5.0	90.0 ± 11.3	10.0 ± 1.2	27.0 ± 3.2	0.7 ± 0.7	23.3 ± 3.4	2.0 ± 1.5	3.5 ± 0.7
		M	3	67.3 ± 4.9	124.3 ± 16.3	9.0 ± 2.7	32.7 ± 2.7	0.3 ± 0.3	36.0 ± 11.5	3.3 ± 2.0	2.9 ± 0.3

All values are expressed as mean ± SE. cdg, chromatid gap; icdg, isochromatid gap; cdb, chromatid break; icdb, isochromatid break; frg, fragment; cdx, chromatid exchange

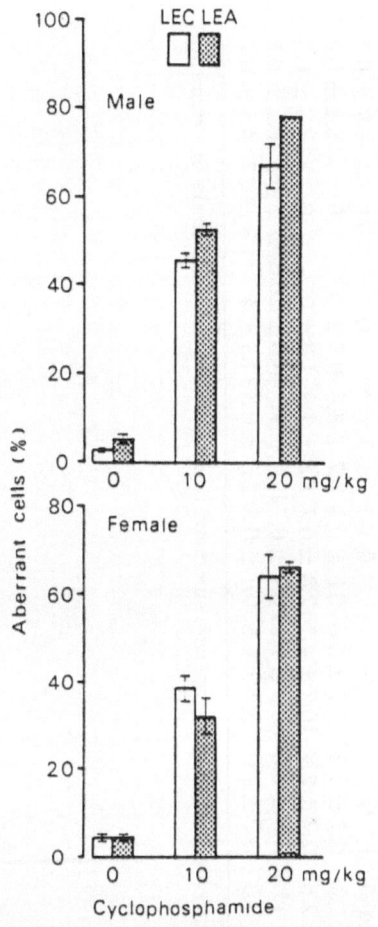

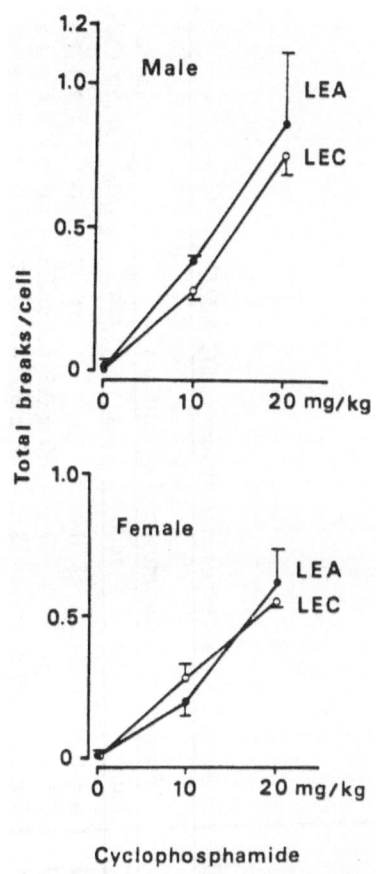

Fig. 1. Percentages of aberrant cells in bone marrow cells of LEA and LEC rats exposed to CP. A significant sex difference in LEA rats was observed at 10 mg CP/kg ($P < 0.025$) and at 20 mg CP/kg ($P < 0.005$). A significant strain difference was observed in males at 10 mg CP/kg ($P < 0.05$)

Fig. 2. Frequencies of total breaks in bone marrow cells of LEA and LEC rats exposed to CP. A significant sex difference was observed in LEA rats at 10 mg CP/kg ($P < 0.025$) and in LEC rats at 20 mg CP/kg ($P < 0.05$). A significant strain difference was observed in males at 10 mg CP/kg ($P < 0.05$). (From [6] with permission)

fragment (frg) and chromatid exchange (cdx). The frequency of each aberration tended to be lower in the females of both strains. Comparing the two strains, the frequency was lower in LEC rats of the same sex and at the same dose level. In order to compare the frequency of chromosomal breaks, a total frequency of cdb, icdb, frg, and cdx was expressed as total breaks (Fig. 2), in which no apparent strain or sex differences were observed.

Table 3. Chromosomal aberrations in bone marrow cells of LEA and LEC rats exposed to Mitomycin C (MMC).

Rat strain	Dose of MMC (mg/kg)	Sex	Number of animals	Aberrant cells (%)	Frequency of chromosomal aberrations							Mitotic index (%)
					cdg	icdg	cdb	icdb	frg	cdx	ring	
LEA	0	F	3	4.3 ± 0.9	4.0 ± 1.2	0.3 ± 0.3	0	0	0	0	0	8.7 ± 1.3
		M	3	5.0 ± 1.2	3.7 ± 0.9	0.3 ± 0.3	0	0	1.0 ± 0.6	0.3 ± 0.3	0	9.4 ± 1.6
	2	F	3	56.0 ± 5.2	69.7 ± 8.4	8.0 ± 1.0	41.0 ± 5.0	0	17.7 ± 3.2	4.0 ± 1.2	0	4.4 ± 0.5
		M	3	56.3 ± 5.9	79.0 ± 9.1	3.7 ± 0.3	49.3 ± 3.7	0.3 ± 0.3	15.7 ± 0.7	3.3 ± 1.3	0	4.8 ± 0.7
	4	F	3	78.7 ± 2.6	66.3 ± 1.8	4.3 ± 0.9	107.0 ± 12.3	1.0 ± 0.6	7.0 ± 2.0	42.0 ± 12.4	0.3 ± 0.3	4.1 ± 0.3
		M	3	79.3 ± 5.0	106.7 ± 14.2	3.7 ± 1.5	129.0 ± 16.5	1.0 ± 0.0	5.0 ± 0.6	42.0 ± 8.6	1.0 ± 1.0	4.1 ± 0.5
LEC	0	F	3	4.3 ± 0.7	2.7 ± 0.7	0.7 ± 0.3	0	0	1.0 ± 0.6	0	0	10.4 ± 0.8
		M	3	2.7 ± 0.3	2.7 ± 0.3	0	0	0	0	0	0	9.7 ± 0.7
	2	F	3	41.0 ± 3.5	34.0 ± 2.1	2.7 ± 1.3	14.7 ± 3.0	0.3 ± 0.3	4.7 ± 3.7	0.7 ± 0.3	0	6.2 ± 0.8
		M	3	48.7 ± 2.4	46.0 ± 2.5	12.7 ± 2.9	10.7 ± 4.7	2.3 ± 0.7	8.3 ± 1.9	1.3 ± 0.9	0	7.3 ± 0.8
	4	F	3	80.3 ± 4.8	90.7 ± 11.7	3.0 ± 0.6	88.3 ± 25.1	0.7 ± 0.7	12.7 ± 9.7	44.0 ± 20.6	0.7 ± 0.3	6.1 ± 0.4
		M	3	76.7 ± 1.8	80.3 ± 3.3	3.0 ± 2.0	72.7 ± 8.6	0.7 ± 0.3	2.3 ± 0.3	34.3 ± 4.7	1.3 ± 0.7	4.1 ± 0.7

All values are expressed as mean ± SE. cdg, chromatid gap; icdg, isochromatid gap; cdb, chromatid break; icdb, isochromatid break; frg, fragment; cdx, chromatid exchange

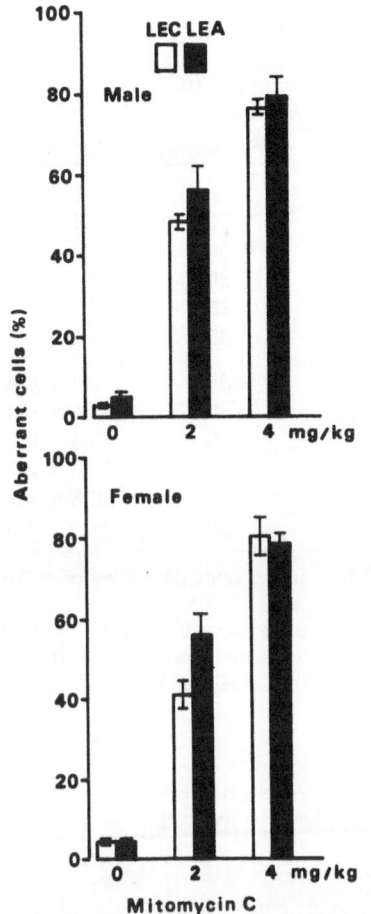

Fig. 3. Percentages of aberrant cells in bone marrow cells of LEA and LEC rats exposed to MMC. No significant sex or strain difference was observed

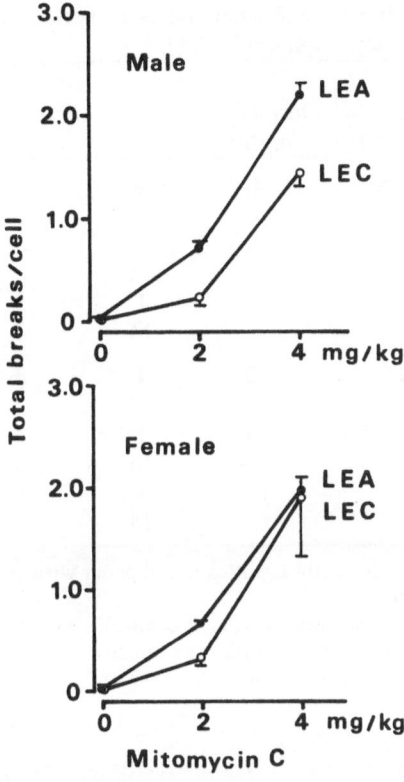

Fig. 4. Frequencies of total breaks in bone marrow cells of LEA and LEC rats exposed to MMC. A significant strain difference was observed at 2 mg MMC/kg in females ($P < 0.01$) and in males ($P < 0.01$), and at 4 mg MMC/kg in males ($P < 0.025$). No significant sex difference was observed in either LEA or LEC rats

Table 3 shows chromosomal aberrations observed in bone marrow cells of both strains of rats exposed to MMC. A dose-related increase was observed in both the percentage of aberrant cells and in the frequency of chromosomal aberrations. The percentage of aberrant cells showed neither significant sex nor strain differences (Fig. 3). Although the frequency of total chromosomal breaks with an additional aberration, ring, in male LEC rats tended to be lower than that in male LEA rats, no clear strain difference was observed in females (Fig. 4). In addition, no significant sex difference was observed in either rat strain.

Table 4. SCE frequencies in bone marrow cells of LEA and LEC rats exposed to cyclophosphamide (CP).

Rat strain	Dose of CP (mg/kg)	Sex	Number of animals	Number of cells observed		SCE/Cell (Mean ± S.E.)
				Total	Per animal	
LEA	0	F	3	90	30	5.6 ± 0.4
		M	3	90	30	5.1 ± 0.2
	5	F	3	90	30	30.8 ± 0.9[a]
		M	3	90	30	32.6 ± 2.1
	10	F	3	90	30	49.7 ± 0.8[b,c]
		M	3	90	30	53.3 ± 0.3[d]
LEC	0	F	3	90	30	5.4 ± 0.4
		M	3	90	30	5.6 ± 0.4
	5	F	3	90	30	26.4 ± 0.6
		M	3	90	30	27.3 ± 2.2
	10	F	3	90	30	38.8 ± 3.2
		M	3	90	30	41.3 ± 1.5

[a] Statistically significant compared with female LEC rats at the same dose level ($P < 0.025$, t-test)
[b] Statistically significant compared with female LEC rats at the same dose level ($P < 0.05$)
[c] Statistically significant compared with male LEA rats at the same dose level ($P < 0.025$)
[d] Statistically significant compared with male LEC rats at the same dose level ($P < 0.005$)

SCEs in Bone Marrow Cells of Animals Exposed to CP

Table 4 shows the frequency of SCEs in bone marrow cells exposed to CP. As described in our previous report [6], agar-coated 5-bromodeoxyuridine (BrdU) tablets were implanted subcutaneously 24 h before sampling. CP was injected intraperitoneally to rats 8 h after tablet implantation. Chromosomal preparations were the same as those for chromosomal aberration analysis. The fluorescence plus Giemsa technique [9] with a slight modification was used for the differentiation of sister chromatids. A dose-related increase was observed in the SCE frequency. Similar to the results of chromosomal aberrations, the SCE frequency in females was lower than in males of both LEA and LEC rats at the same dose level. Comparing the two strains in the same sex and at the same dose level, the SCE frequency was lower in LEC rats.

Table 5 shows the frequency of SCEs induced by MMC. A dose-related increase was apparent in the SCE frequency. In LEA at a dose of 2 mg MMC/kg, the SCE frequency was significantly lower in females ($P < 0.05$). However, no significant strain difference in the SCE frequency was observed in the same sex and at the same dose level.

Table 5. SCE frequencies in bone marrow cells of LEA and LEC rats exposed to Mitomycin C (MMC).

Rat strain	Dose of MMC (mg/kg)	Sex	Number of animals	Number of cells observed		SCE/Cell (Mean ± S.E.)
				Total	Per animal	
LEA	0	F	3	90	30	5.6 ± 0.4
		M	3	90	30	5.1 ± 0.2
	1	F	3	90	30	18.6 ± 1.2
		M	3	90	30	15.0 ± 3.6
	2	F	3	90	30	25.1 ± 0.9[a]
		M	3	90	30	29.9 ± 1.1
LEC	0	F	3	90	30	5.4 ± 0.4
		M	3	90	30	5.6 ± 0.4
	1	F	3	90	30	16.7 ± 0.2
		M	3	90	30	17.0 ± 2.6
	2	F	3	90	30	27.3 ± 0.9
		M	3	90	30	25.6 ± 1.2

[a] Statistically significant compared with male LEA rats at the same dose level ($P < 0.05$, t-test); no significant difference was observed between LEA and LEC rats at the same dose level

Table 6. SCE frequencies in regenerating hepatocytes of LEA and LEC rats exposed to cyclophosphamide (CP).

Rat strain	Dose of CP (mg/kg)	Sex	Number of animals	Number of cells observed		SCE/Cell (Mean ± S.E.)
				Total	Per animal	
LEA	0	F	3	51	17	6.6 ± 0.7[a]
		M	3	34	11	4.2 ± 0.2[b]
	2.5	F	3	40	13	21.7 ± 1.8
		M	3	32	11	18.7 ± 0.4
	5.0	F	3	38	13	32.7 ± 1.3
		M	3	19	6	31.9 ± 2.0
LEC	0	F	3	32	11	5.7 ± 0.4
		M	3	41	14	5.9 ± 0.5
	2.5	F	3	29	10	18.5 ± 0.7
		M	3	47	16	18.2 ± 0.4
	5.0	F	3	29	10	29.1 ± 4.3
		M	3	38	13	34.3 ± 2.3

[a] Statistically significant compared with untreated male LEA rats ($P < 0.05$, t-test)
[b] Statistically significant compared with untreated male LEC rats ($P < 0.05$)

SCEs in Regenerating Hepatocytes of Animals Exposed to CP

The SCE frequency was examined in regenerating hepatocytes of LEA and LEC rats exposed to CP because SCE analysis appeared to be more sensitive and required a smaller number of cells to be analyzed than chromosomal aberration analysis in detecting genotoxic effects of mutagens/carcinogens. Table 6 shows the frequency of SCEs induced by CP in regenerating hepatocytes. Details of the procedures are described in our previous report [6]. In brief, BrdU tablets were implanted sub-cutaneously 12h after 2/3 partial hepatectomy. CP was injected intra-peritoneally 36h after hepatectomy. The regenerating liver was obtained 16h after drug administration, with Colcemid treatment for the final 0.5h. Liver tissues were treated with collagenase to separate hepatocytes for SCE analysis. A dose-related increase in SCE frequency by CP was observed. No significant sex or strain difference in the SCE yield was observed when compared in the same sex and at the same dose level. Although a certain discrepancy existed in the baseline frequency between males and females of LEA rats and between males of the two strains, the reason for this is unknown at present.

Correlation Between Drug-Metabolizing Ability and Chromosomal Damage in LEC Rats

The present study revealed that the cytochrome P-450 content was significantly lower in LEC rats than in LEA rats. This is apparently ascribed to the lower level of PROD in LEC rats. In addition to this strain difference, a sex difference was also observed in that the level of cytochrome P-450 was generally lower in the females of both strains. Furthermore, LEC rats showed a lower frequency of chromosomal aberrations and SCEs in bone marrow cells than LEA rats when exposed to CP, which is known to be metabolically activated by phenobarbital-inducible forms of cytochrome P-450 [10,11], although such a strain difference was not clear in the chromosomal damage induced by direct-acting MMC. Thus, the level of cytochrome P-450 in the liver paralleled the degree of cytogenetic damages in bone marrow cells induced by CP. The sex difference observed in the yield of cytogenetic damages was also in parallel with the level of cytochrome P-450. The observed parallelism, therefore, suggests that the lower level of cytochrome P-450 might result in the reduced production of genotoxic metabolites of CP. If this is the case, phenobarbital admin-istration is expected to increase the susceptibility of LEC rats to the genotoxic effects of CP, particularly since phenobarbital-treated LEA and LEC rats exhibit almost the same maximally induced levels of phenobarbital-inducible forms of cytochrome P-450 and its associated

PROD activity [12]. The observed sex difference may reflect a genetic difference in the hormonal regulation of activities of carcinogen-activating enzymes, as has been suggested in the case of the tryptophan pyrolysates, Trp-P-1 and Trp-P-2, both of which are more carcinogenic in female than in male mice and rats [13].

Species of cytochrome P-450 are classified into two types which are inducible by phenobarbital and methylcholanthrene. Tice et al. [14] reported that the elevation of drug-metabolizing enzymes by phenobarbital treatment increased benzene-induced SCE formation in mice, although the effect was observed only in females. In contrast, Schreck et al. [15] demonstrated that the SCE frequency in mice with phenobarbital treatment was not significantly different from that obtained in the absence of enzyme induction. The present results give a new clue to the above debate.

In regenerating hepatocytes, the frequency of SCEs induced by CP did not show any significant sex or strain difference in LEA and LEC rats, although the liver is a main site of drug-metabolism. Metabolic pathways of carcinogenic mutagens are complex, including both activation and detoxication processes. It has been reported that activities of drug-detoxication enzymes, such as UDP-glucuronyltransferase, epoxide hydrolase, and glutathione S-transferase, in livers of LEC rats before the onset of hepatitis, were observed at high levels, comparable to those seen in azo-dye hepatocarcinogenesis [5]. It should be mentioned that the hepatocytes used in this study were obtained from regenerating livers, which usually show reduced levels of cytochrome P-450 compared to the intact liver [16]. Therefore, the present findings on the induction of SCEs by CP in regenerating livers may not directly reflect cytogenetic effects on the intact liver. Further cytogenetic analysis using mutagens/carcinogens metabolized by different cytochrome P-450 species is necessary to clarify the susceptibility of LEC rats to genotoxic effects.

Acknowledgments. This work was partly supported by Grants-in-Aid for Scientific Research from the Ministry of Education, Science and Culture of Japan, and by a fund from Otsuka Pharmaceutical Co., Ltd. R.M. was a recipient of a Fellowship for Japanese Junior Scientists from the Japan Society for the Promotion of Science.

References

1. Sasaki M, Yoshida MC, Kagami K, Takeichi N, Kobayashi H, Dempo K, Mori M (1985) Spontaneous hepatitis in an inbred strain of Long-Evans rats. Rat News Lett 14:4−6
2. Yoshida MC, Msuda R, Sasaki M, Takeichi N, Kobayashi H, Dempo K, Mori M (1987) New mutation causing hereditary hepatitis in the laboratory rat. J Hered 78:361−365

3. Masuda R, Yoshida MC, Sasaki M, Dempo K, Mori M (1988) Hereditary hepatitis of LEC rats is controlled by a single autosomal recessive gene. Lab Anim 22:166–169
4. Masuda R, Yoshida MC, Sasaki M, Dempo K, Mori M (1988) High susceptibility to hepatocellular carcinoma development in LEC rats with hereditary hepatitis. Jpn J Cancer Res 79:828–835
5. Sugiyama T, Takeichi N, Kobayashi H, Yoshida MC, Sasaki M, Taniguchi N (1988) Metabolic predisposition of a novel mutant (LEC rats) to hereditary hepatitis and hepatoma: Alterations of the drug metabolizing enzymes. Carcinogenesis 9:1569–1572
6. Masuda R, Abe S, Yoshida MC, Sasaki M, Sugiyama T, Taniguchi N (1990) Cytochrome P-450 and chromosome damage by cyclophosphamide in LEC strain rats predisposed to hereditary hepatitis and liver cancer. Mutation Res 244:309–316
7. Lubet RA, Mayer RT, Cameron JW, Nims RW, Burke MD, Wolff T, Guengerich FP (1985) Dealkylation of pentoxyresorufin: A rapid and sensitive assay for measuring induction of cytochrome(s) P-450 by phenobarbital and other xenobiotics in the rat. Arch Biochem Biophys 238:43–48
8. Mayer RT, Jermyn JW, Burke MD, Prough RA (1977) Methoxyresorufin as a substrate for the fluorometric assay of insect microsomal O-dealkylases. Pest Biochem Physiol 7:349–354
9. Perry P, Wolff S (1974) New Giemsa method for the differential staining of sister chromatids. Nature 251:156–158
10. Sladek NE (1971) Metabolism of cyclophosphamide by rat hepatic microsomes. Cancer Res 31:901–908
11. Sladek NE (1972) Therapeutic efficacy of cyclophosphamide as a function of its metabolism. Cancer Res 32:535–542
12. Sugiyama T, Suzuki K, Ookawara T, Kurosawa T, Taniguchi N (1989) Selective expression and induction of cytochrome $P450_{PB}$ and $P450_{MC}$ during the development of hereditary hepatitis and hepatoma of LEC rats. Carcinogenesis 10:2155–2159
13. Degawa M, Hishinuma T, Yoshida H, Hashimoto Y (1987) Species, sex and organ differences in induction of a cytochrome P-450 isozyme responsible for carcinogen activation: Effects of dietary hepatocarcinogenic tryptophan pyrolysate compounds in mice and rats. Carcinogenesis 8:1913–1918
14. Tice RR, Costa DL, Drew RT (1980) Cytogenetic effects of inhaled benzene in murine bone marrow: Induction of sister chromatid exchanges, chromosomal aberrations, and cellular proliferation inhibition in DBA/2 mice. Proc Natl Acad Sci USA 77:2148–2152
15. Schreck RR, Paika IJ, Latt SA (1982) Differences in murine procarcinogen activation enzymes are not accompanied by parallel differences in procarcinogen-induced sister-chromatid exchange. Mutation Res 94:143–153
16. Henderson RT, Kersten KJ (1970) Metabolism of drugs during rat liver regeneration. Biochem Pharm 19:2343–2351

29 — Altered Oncogene Expression in Hepatocellular Carcinomas Developing Spontaneously in LEC Rats

Minako Nagao[1], Yoshinori Fujimoto[1], Yukihito Ishizaka[1], Katsuhiko Enomoto[2], Hidetoshi Takahashi[2], Michio Mori[2], and Takashi Sugimura[1]

Introduction

LEC rats spontaneously suffer hepatitis at around 4 months after birth, enter the chronic phase of hepatitis, and spontaneously develop hepatocellular carcinomas (HCCs) between 1–1.5 years after birth [1]. Although dominant oncogene activation in chemically induced HCCs in rats is generally understood to be relatively rare, for the LEC rat, in which an endogenous causative agent appears to be involved, the situation remains unclear. Ha-*ras* activation has been found with a very high frequency in both chemically induced and spontaneously induced liver carcinomas of B6C3 F_1 mice [2–5], but, with the exception of those induced by aflatoxin B_1 [6,7], any type of activated *ras* was only rarely observed in chemically induced rat liver tumors [4,8,9]. We examined HCCs in LEC rats for Ha-, Ki- and N-*ras* gene mutations. The polymerase chain reaction (PCR) was adopted for amplifying discrete specific DNA fragments [10,11], and the sequences were determined directly.

The mRNA expression of three proto-oncogenes, c-*myc* [12–15], Ha-*ras* [12,14] and c-*raf* (R. Sakai, T. Ushijima, I. Ikeda, et al., unpublished data) [16], which were reported to be markedly increased in rat hepatic tumors induced by various chemical carcinogens, was also examined. We recently established that serine/threonine protein phosphatases, especially type 2A, are involved in malignant cell transformation [17,18]. It was also found that the expression of the type 2A catalytic subunit, mRNA, was increased in most of the HCCs which were induced by food mutagens, 2-amino-3-methylimidazo[4,5-*f*]quinoline (IQ) and 2-amino-3, 8-dimethylimidazo-[4,5-*f*]quinoxaline [19,20]. Therefore, an investigation of the mRNA levels of the protein phosphatase 2A catalytic subunit, *PP-2Aα*, in LEC rat HCCs was also included.

[1] Carcinogenesis Division, National Cancer Center Research Institute, Tokyo, 104 Japan
[2] Department of Pathology, Sapporo Medical College, Sapporo, 060 Japan

273

The *ras* Mutation in HCCs

Spontaneously developed HCCs were obtained from four LEC rats older than 12 months, and DNAs were extracted by the phenol-chloroform method [21]. Desired regions of genomic DNA were amplified by PCR using oligonucleotides primers 1 and 2, as is schematically illustrated in Fig. 1 [21]. Codons 12, 13, and 61 of Ha-*ras*, Ki-*ras*, and N-*ras* were targeted for analysis. In order to obtain single- and double-stranded DNA fragments, the ratios of primer 1 to primer 2 were adjusted to 10:1 and 10:10, respectively. Either primer 1 or 2 was designed to include the intron sequence surrounding exon 1 or 2 of each gene in order to prevent the amplification of pseudogenes. The nucleotide sequences of amplified DNA fragments were determined by direct sequencing utilizing primer 3. In most cases, the direct sequencing bands were clear enough to detect the presence or absence of mutation. Using known amounts of the mutated Ki-*ras* sequence DNA of the rat, the PCR-direct sequencing method was shown to be capable of detecting a mutant allele constituting more than 10% of the total allele (T. Ushijima and M. Nagao, unpublished data). In 5 out of 24 cases in which direct sequencing was not definitive, the results were confirmed by subcloning. Eight independent plasmid clones were sequenced in each of these 5 cases.

In spite of the intensiveness of this study, no mutations were detected in codons 12, 13, or 61 of any *ras* gene in LEC rat HCCs. Thus, *ras* activation does not commonly occur in spontaneously developed HCCs of LEC rats, in agreement with the results for most chemical carcinogen-induced rat HCCs.

Overexpression of c-*myc*

Total RNA from the four LEC rats HCCs, the *ras* genes of which had proved not to be activated, were extracted by the acid guanidinium thiocyanate-phenol-chloroform method. Northern blotting analysis was performed using exon 3 of rat c-*myc* as a probe. The mRNA was detected as a band at 2.3 kb in all of the samples of livers and HCCs. As shown in Table 1, exp. 1, all of the four HCCs expressed remarkably increased levels of c-*myc* mRNAs, the values ranging from 7.2- to 34.0-fold that of a 24-week-old LEA (LEC sibling stock) rat liver. However, the c-*myc* gene in these four HCCs was shown by Southern blotting analysis to be neither rearranged nor amplified. Thus, c-*myc* overexpression in these HCCs is probably not due to any gross structural changes in the c-*myc* gene. Since c-*myc* expression is known to be elevated in association with cell proliferation, it is important to clarify whether the results detected for the four HCCs reflect a consequence or a cause of malignant change.

LEC rats suffer from hepatitis at around 4 months after birth, with single cell necroses occurring immediately prior to the onset of hepatitis [22].

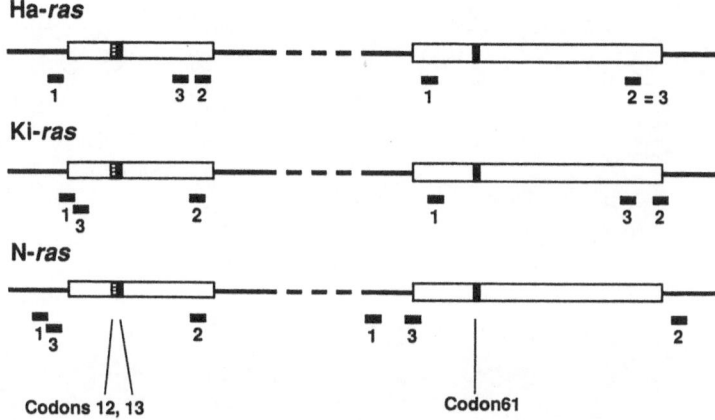

Fig. 1. Schematic illustration of primers used for the polymerase chain reaction in order to analyze mutations of Ha-*ras*, Ki-*ras*, and N-*ras* at codons 12, 13, and 61

Table 1. Relative amounts of c-*myc* mRNA and its relationship with the mitotic index.

Tissue	c-myc *mRNA*	Mitotic index (%)
Experiment 1		
LEA (24 weeks old)	1.0	
LEA (15 weeks old)	0.4	
LEC-HCC-1	27.3	
LEC-HCC-2	31.0	
LEC-HCC-3	34.0	
LEC-HCC-4	7.2	
Experiment 2		
LEA (21 weeks old)	1.0	<0.1
LEA (35 weeks old)	1.0	<0.1
LEC-HCC-5	32.0	0.66
LEC-HCC-6	20.0	0.51
LEC-HCC-7	5.0	1.04
LEC-HN-1	2.0	0.66
LEC-HN-2	1.7	1.19

HCC, hepatocellular carcinoma; *HN*, hyperplastic nodule

Cell proliferation would then be induced for compensation of cell death. Age-dependent changes in c-*myc* expression were, therefore, examined in the livers of LEC and sibling stock LEA rats. The c-*myc* mRNA was high in the livers of both rats 1 day after birth, and then gradually decreased over the next 4 weeks (Fig. 2). During this period, no significant differences in c-*myc* mRNA levels were found between LEC and LEA rats. A

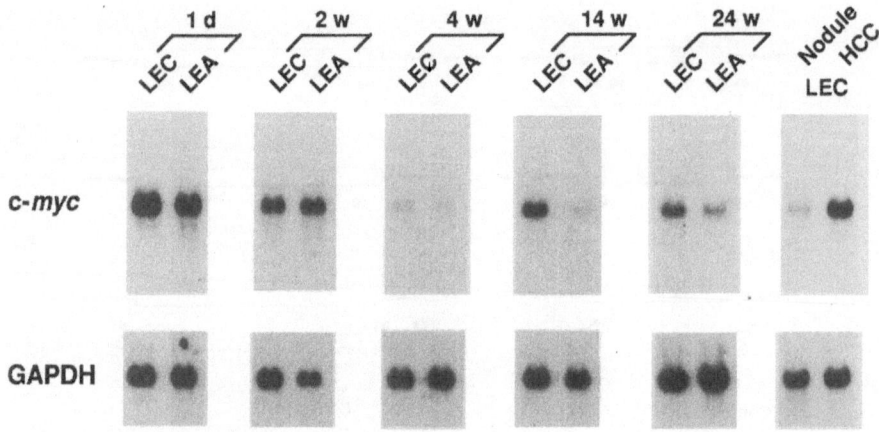

Fig. 2. Time course of c-*myc* mRNA levels in the livers of LEC and LEA rats. The RNAs of the liver of a 24-week-old LEA rat and the HCC of a LEC rat were the same samples used in Table 1, exp 1, LEA (24 weeks old) and LEC-HCC-4, respectively. *d*, day; *w*, weeks; *HCC*, hepatocellular carcinoma

remarkable and specific increase of the c-*myc* mRNA level was noted in the LEC rats at week 14 after birth, when single cell necroses were observed. At week 24, LEC rats in the chronic phase of hepatitis demonstrated only a slight increase in c-*myc* mRNA expression compared with the levels of LEA rats.

Examination of c-*myc* expression in two hyperplastic nodules revealed 1.7- and 2-fold increases in the mRNA level compared to that in the 21- and 35-week-old LEA rat liver (Table 1, exp. 2). Mitotic indexes of the hyperplastic nodules were within the same range as those of the HCCs, and clearly exceeded normal hepatocyte values in the LEA rats. From these results, it is conceivable that overexpression of c-*myc* in HCCs seems to be involved in malignant transformation, and is not simply a reflection of the proliferative status.

Expression of c-*raf*, Ha-*ras*, and PP-2Aα

The relative amounts of c-*raf*, Ha-*ras*, and *PP-2Aα* mRNAs were also determined in total RNAs from each of the four HCCs (HCC 1–4 in Table 1) using v-*raf* BX, BS9, and *PP-2Aα* cDNA, respectively, as probes. The c-*raf* mRNA was detected as a 3.2 kb band in all of the four HCCs, but at levels only up to 2.1-fold that of a 24-week-old LEA rat liver. The increase was not significant, contrary to the results from F344 rat liver tumors induced by partial hepatectomy and *N*-nitrosodiethylamine [16], and those induced by IQ (R. Sakai, T. Ushijima, I. Ikeda, et al., unpublished data).

The Ha-*ras* mRNA was detected as a 1.2 kb band in all of the four HCCs, with the expression level again being up to 2.1-fold that of the 24-week-old LEA rat liver value. Overexpression of Ha-*ras* has been detected in rat liver tumors induced by aflatoxin B_1 and in rat ascites hepatoma lines [12,13], but in the case of LEC HCC, no equivalent significant increase in expression was apparent [21].

The *PP-2Aα* mRNAs were detected as a major band at 2.0 kb and as a minor band at 2.7 kb, but the levels were not at all increased in these four HCCs compared to normal liver, [21]. Thus, in this regard, HCCs of LEC rats are strikingly different from liver tumors induced by IQ [18,19] and MeIQx [20].

Discussion

Since LEC rats accumulate copper in their livers [23], oxygen radicals seem to be involved as a causal factor in HCC development. However, no *ras* gene mutation was detected as is the case in most of the rat liver tumors induced by chemical carcinogens. This study demonstrated a remarkably elevated expression of c-*myc* in 5 out of 7 of the LEC rat spontaneous HCCs (20- to 34-fold), and a moderately elevated expression (5- to 7.2-fold) in 2 of them, although this did not appear to be associated with any structural alteration in the c-*myc* gene. However, since this marked c-*myc* overexpression was not found in hyperplastic nodules where mitotic indexes were within a similar range to that of HCCs, a possible role of overexpressed c-*myc* mRNA in the transformation of premalignant hyperplastic nodule cells to HCC cells is suggested.

This finding and the potential involvement of suppressor genes — suggested to be located on human chromosomes 4, 5, 11, 16, and 17 [24–27] — in hepatocarcinogenesis in LEC rats need to be further elucidated.

Acknowledgments. This work was supported by a Grant-in-Aid for Cancer Research and from the Comprehensive 10-year Strategy for Cancer Control, Ministry of Health and Welfare of Japan.

References

1. Masuda R, Yoshida M, Sasaki M, Dempo K, Mori M (1988) High susceptibility to hepatocellular carcinoma development in LEC rats with hereditary hepatitis. Jpn J Cancer Res 79:828–835
2. Beer DG, Pitot HC (1989) Proto-oncogene activation during chemically induced hepatocarcinogenesis in rodents. Mutat Res 220:1–10

3. Wiseman RW, Stower SJ, Miller EC, Anderson MW, Miller JA (1986) Activating mutations of the c-Ha-*ras* proto-oncogene in chemically induced hepatomas of the male B6C3 F_1 mouse. Proc Natl Acad Sci USA 83:5825–5829

4. Stower SJ, Wiseman RW, Ward JM, Miller EC, Miller JA, Anderson MW, Eva A (1988) Detection of activated proto-oncogene in N-nitrosodiethylamine-induced liver tumors: A comparison between B6C3F_1 mice and Fischer 344 rats. Carcinogenesis 9:271–276

5. Reynolds SH, Stower SJ, Maronpot RR, Anderson MW, Aaronson SA (1986) Detection and identification of activated oncogenes in spontaneously occurring benign and malignant hepatocellular tumors of the B6C3F_1 mouse. Proc Natl Acad Sci USA 83:33–37

6. Sinha S, Webber C, Marshall CJ, Knowles MA, Proctor A, Barrass NC, Neal GE (1988) Activation of *ras* oncogene in aflatoxin-induced rat liver carcinogenesis. Proc Natl Acad Sci USA 85:3673–3677

7. McMahon G, Hanson L, Lee J, Wogan GN (1986) Identification of an activated c-Ki-*ras* oncogene in rat liver tumors induced by aflatoxin B_1. Proc Natl Acad Sci USA 83:9418–9422

8. Watatani M, Perantoni AO, Reed CD, Enomoto T, Wenk ML, Rice JM (1989) Infrequent activation of K-*ras*, H-*ras*, and other oncogenes in hepatocellular neoplasms initiated by methyl (acetoxymethyl)-nitrosamine, a methylating agent, and promoted by phenobarbital in F344 rats. Cancer Res 49:1103–1109

9. Li H, Lee G-H, Cui L, Liu J, Nomura K, Ohtaka K, Kitagawa T (1990) Absence of H-*ras* point mutation at codon 12 in N-methyl-N-nitrosourea-induced hepatocellular neoplasms in the rat. J Cancer Res Clin Oncol 116:331–335

10. Saiki R, Gelfand D, Stoffel S, Sharf S, Higuchi R, Torn G, Mullis K, Erlich H (1988) Primer-directed enzymatic amplification of DNA with a thermostable DNA polymerase. Science 239:487–491

11. Gyllensten UB, Erlich HA (1988) Generation of single-stranded DNA by the polymerase chain reaction and application to direct sequencing of the HLA-DQA locus. Proc Natl Acad Sci USA 85:7652–7656

12. Makino R, Hayashi K, Sato S, Sugimura T (1984) Expressions of the c-Ha-*ras* and c-*myc* genes in rat liver tumors. Biochem Biophys Res Commun 119: 1096–1102

13. Tashiro F, Morimura S, Hayashi K, Makino R, Sugimura T, Kawamura H, Horikoshi N, Nemoto K, Ohtsubo K, Sugimura T, Ueno Y (1986) Expression of the c-Ha-*ras* and c-*myc* genes in aflatoxin B_1-induced hepatocellular carcinomas. Biochem Biophys Res Commun 138:858–864

14. Suchy BK, Sarafoff M, Kerler R, Robes HM (1989) Amplification, rearrangements, and enhanced expression of c-*myc* in chemically induced rat liver tumors in vivo and in vitro. Cancer Res 49:6781–6787

15. Chandar N, Lombardi B, Locker J (1989) c-*myc* gene amplification during hepatocarcinogenesis by a choline-devoid diet. Proc Natl Acad Sci USA 86: 2703–2707

16. Beer DC, Neveu MJ, Paul DL, Rapp PU, Pitot HC (1988) Expression of the c-*raf* proto-oncogene, γ-glutamyltranspeptidase, and gap junction protein in rat liver neoplasms. Cancer Res 48:1610–1617

17. Sakai R, Ikeda I, Kitani H, Fujiki H, Takaku F, Rapp U, Sugimura T, Nagao M (1989) Flat reversion by okadaic acid of *raf* and ret-II transformants. Proc Natl Acad Sci USA 86:9946–9950

18. Nagao M, Sakai R, Kitagawa Y, Ikeda I, Sasaki K, Shima H, Sugimura T (1990) Role of protein phosphatases in malignant transformation. In: Knudson AG, Stanbridge EJ, Sugimura T, Terada M, Watanabe S (eds) Genetic basis for carcinogenesis: Tumor suppressor genes and oncogenes. pp. 177–184, Japan Scientific Society Tokyo/Taylor and Fransis, London
19. Kitagawa Y, Sakai R, Tahira T, Tsuda H, Ito N, Sugimura T, Nagao M (1988) Molecular cloning of phosphoprotein phosphatase 2Aβ cDNA and increased expression of phosphatase 2Aα and 2Aβ in rat liver tumors. Biochem Biophys Res Commun 157:821–827
20. Sasaki K, Shima H, Kitagawa Y, Irino S, Sugimura T, Nagao M (1990) Identification of members of the protein phosphatase 1 gene family in the rat and enhanced expression of protein phosphatase 1a gene in rat hepatocellular carcinomas. Jpn J Cancer Res 81:1272–1280
21. Fujimoto Y, Ishizaka Y, Tahira T, Sone H, Takahashi H, Enomoto K, Mori M, Sugimura T, Nagao M (to be published) Possible involvement of c-myc but not ras genes in hepatocellular carcinomas developing after spontaneous hepatitis in LEC rats. Mol Careinogenesis
22. Yoshida M, Masuda R, Sasaki M, Takeichi N, Kobayashi H, Dempo K, Mori M (1987) New mutation causing hereditary hepatitis in the laboratory rat. J Hered 78:361–365
23. Li Y, Togashi Y, Sato S, Emoto T, Kang J, Takeichi N, Kobayashi H, Kojima Y, Une Y, Uchino J (1991) Spontaneous hepatic copper accumulation in LEC rats with hereditary hepatitis: A model of Wilson's disease. J Clin Invest 87:1858–1861
24. Pasquinelli C, Garreau F, Bougueleret L, Cariani E, Grzeschik KH, Thiers V, Croissant O, Hadchouel M, Tiollais P, Brechot C (1988) Rearrangement of a common cellular DNA domain on chromosome 4 in human primary liver tumors. J Virol 62:629–632
25. Buefow KH, Murray JC, Israel JL, London WT, Smith M, Kew M, Blanquet V, Brechot C, Redeker A, Govindarajah S (1989) Loss of heterozygosity suggests tumor suppressor gene responsible for primary hepatocellular carcinoma. Proc Natl Acad Sci USA 86:8852–8856
26. Tsuda H, Zhang W, Shimosato Y, Yokota J, Terada M, Sugimure T, Miyamura T, Hirohashi S (1990) Allele loss on chromosome 16 associated with progression of human hepatocellular carcinoma. Proc Natl Acad Sci USA 87: 6791–6794
27. Fujimori M, Tokino T, Hino O, Kitagawa T, Imamura T, Okamoto E, Mitsunobu M, Ishikawa T, Nakagama H, Harada H, Yagura M, Matsubara K, Nakamura Y (1991) Allelotype study of primary hepatocellular carcinoma. Cancer Res 51:89–93

2. Pathology

30 — Progress from Chronic Hepatitis to Liver Cancer in Long-Surviving LEC Rats

Tsutomu Namieno[1,2], Noritoshi Takeichi[1], Motomichi Sasaki[3], Kimimaro Dempo[4], Michio Mori[4], Jun-ichi Uchino[2], and Hiroshi Kobayashi[1]

Introduction

In our previous papers, we reported on the clinical and pathological characteristics [1], pathogenesis [2], and combined immunodeficiency of spontaneous hepatitis in LEC rats.

One of the hepadna viruses, the woodchuck hepatitis virus (WHV), is known to cause persistent infection in woodchucks (*Marmota monax*), and WHV-positive woodchucks have shown a high incidence of liver cell cancer [3]. However, it has not been well confirmed whether or not viruses play a role in the incidence of hepatitis in LEC rats [2].

This report focuses on the results of hematological, biochemical, and histopathological tests for the investigation of the transient course from hepatitis to liver cancer in long-surviving LEC rats.

Materials and Methods

Rats

We used LEC rats, aged 4–5 months or older, with acute hepatitis and which had a long survival time. They had been selected from the Long-Evans rats isolated at the Center for Experimental Plants and Animals, Hokkaido University. The LEC rats used in this study ranged from the 33rd to the 38th generations. Age-matched LEA rats were used as control.

---

[1] Laboratory of Pathology, Cancer Institute, [2] First Department of Surgery, School of Medicine, Hokkaido University, Sapporo, 060 Japan and
[3] Sasaki Cancer Institute, Chiyoda-ku, Tokyo, 101 Japan
[4] Department of Pathology, Sapporo Medical College, Sapporo, 060 Japan

Qualitative Chemical Urinalysis

A Multistix III (Miles-Sankyo Co., Ltd. Tokyo) was used for testing bilirubin, protein, and other substances in the urine.

Hematological Tests

The left or right jugular vein of each rat was punctured with a 23G needle, and 4–5 ml of peripheral blood was removed; approximately 1 ml of this blood was divided into containers in which EDTA-2K salt had been placed, and was used for hemocytometry. The remaining blood was centrifuged (2,000 rpm for 30 min), and the serum was separated out and used for biochemical tests.

Hemocytometry and other pertinent tests were carried out using an automatic cell counter (Sysmex Toa Medical Electronics Co. E4000: resistance-type, Tokyo). Reticulocyte (Ret) counts were calculated by microscopic examination using the new methylene blue stain method.

Biochemical Tests

The serum samples were taken as described above. Various tests were carried out by the following procedures: the stable diazonium salt method for total bilirubin; the ultraviolet absorption method for glutamic oxaloacetic transaminase (GOT), glutamic pyruvic transaminase (GPT), and lactate dehydrogenase (LDH); the P-nitrophenyl phosphoric acid method for alkaline phosphatase (ALP); the Jaffe method for creatinine (BUN); the BCG method for albumin (Alb), and the enzyme method for total cholesterol (T. chol). The TBA-60R (Toshiba Medical Co., Ltd.) was used for these measurements. Serum protein fractions were measured by cellulose acetate membrane electorphoresis (ADC-800, Kayagaki Co, Tokyo) [1].

Using the LEC and LEA rats (average age: 6 months), we measured the retention rate of indocyanin green ($ICGR_{15}$) in the blood for 15 min. This procedure was carried out in the following manner: 25 mg indocyanin green (Daiichi Pharmaceuticals Co., Ltd., Tokyo) was dissolved in 5 ml of Japan Pharmacopoeia distilled water attached for injection. The solution was injected into the caudal vein of the rats at a dose of 0.1 ml/100g body weight (5 ml/kg body weight). After 15 min of intravenous infusion, a blood sample, taken from the jugular vein, was centrifuged (3,000 rpm for 10 min) together with a blind-test blood sample, taken from the jugular vein prior to the administration of the indocyanin green solution, to obtain the test serum. A calibration curve was obtained by graduated dilution of the indocyanin green solution which was required to prepare standard solutions of 0.05 mg/dl – 1.5 mg/dl. We measured the absorption rate of the test serum and standard samples at an absorption wave length of 805 nm using the Hitachi Model 220A spectrophotometer in order to determine the ICG concentration (mg/dl) in the serum.

Immunological Tests

Measurement of Serum IgG

Using the serum from the LEC and LEA rats (average age: 10 months), we measured serum IgG and IgM by the single radial immunodiffusion assay method, as previously mentioned [1].

Measurement of Blastogenesis

Splenic cells were taken from the LEC and LEA rats (average age: 10 months) and were adjusted to 5×10^6 cells/ml. Concentrations of phytohemaglutinin-P (PHA-P) (Difco, Detroit), concanavalin A (Con A) (Difco, Detroit), and lipopolysaccharide (LPS) (Sigma Chemical Co. St Louis, USA) were adjusted in advance to 200 mg/ml, 100 mg/ml, and 2 mg/ml, respectively, and were subjected to graduated dilution to obtain 3 concentrations of these mitogens. A 100 µl of the splenic cell suspension and 100 µl each of the 3 concentrations of PHA-P, Con A, and LPS were placed in a 96-well flat bottom microplate (Corning, New York). A control was prepared: 100 µl of splenic cell suspension was added to 100 µl of complete medium of RPMI1640 supplemented with 10% newborn calf serum (FCS) (GIBCO, Rhode Island, USA), 1 M Hepes (0.01 ml/ml), 100-fold diluted sodium pyruvate (0.01 ml/ml), 100-fold diluted nonessential aminoacid (0.01 ml/ml) and 2-mercaptoethanol (5×10^{-4} ml/ml), (in triplicate). This microplate was placed in stationary culture for 3 days in an incubator at 37°C and 5% CO_2. Triitiated thymidine (^{3}H-TdR) (Amersham International plc Buckinghamshire, UK), 0.5 µl Ci (20 µl/well), was added 18 h before harvesting. Measurement of radioactivity by a liquid scintillation counter revealed the uptake rate of ^{3}H-TdR.

In the evaluation of blastogenic response, a twofold increase of the ^{3}H-TdR uptake rate (cpm) was considered as a significant difference; the rate of 1.5, a figure converted to the stimulation index, was likewise considered significant.

Histopathological Examinations

LEC rats were sacrificed at various clinical stages for gross post-mortem examination. The liver tissues received hematoxylin and eosin staining after being fixed with Carnoy's solution or Bouin's solution. Immunohistological staining was also carried out after the tissues were fixed with a mixed solution of glutaraldehyde and formalin.

Immunohistological studies (ABC method) were carried out for anti-glutathione S-transferase placental form (GST-p) antibodies by the method of Sato et al. [4]; and for anti-α-fetoprotein (AFP) antibodies by the method of Dempo et al. [5].

Table 1. Comparison of hematological data in long-surviving LEC[a] and age-matched LEA rats.

Items	LEC		LEA	P-value[c]
	γ-Globulin(+)[b]	γ-Globulin(−)		
WBC (/mm³)	11684 ± 3872[d] (26)[e]	10605 ± 3136 (20)[e]	10138 ± 2681 (16)[e]	N.S.
RBC (×10⁴/mm³)	652.0 ± 111.2 (26)	706.0 ± 66.8 (20)	799.6 ± 53.9 (16)	<0.001
Pt (×10⁴/mm³)	65.2 ± 21.1 (26)	62.3 ± 18.2 (20)	93.7 ± 12.8 (16)	<0.001
Hb (g/dl)	12.0 ± 1.6 (26)	12.8 ± 0.8 (20)	14.2 ± 1.6 (16)	<0.005
Ht (%)	32.1 ± 6.1 (26)	34.7 ± 3.6 (20)	44.2 ± 1.6 (16)	<0.001
Ret (‰)	22.8 ± 8.6 (11)	22.4 ± 8.3 (11)	14.0 ± 3.0 (15)	<0.025

[a] These LEC rats survived for over 8 months (mean age 10 months)
[b] The γ-globulin(+) means positive of the γ-globulin fraction of serum protein by a cellulose-acetate electrophoresis
[c] by Student's t-test
[d] Mean ± standard deviation
[e] Numbers in the parentheses indicate the number of rats used
N.S., not significant

Statistical Analysis

The results were expressed as mean values ± standard deviation, and Student's *t*-test was performed.

Results

The serum protein fractions of the LEC rats were examined by cellulose acetate membrane electrophoresis. Those in which the γ-globulin fraction was detectable by the densitometer were classified as the γ-globulin(+) group (56 animals); those in which the γ-globulin fraction was undetectable by the densitometer were classified as the γ-globulin(−) group (40 animals). The γ-globulin of the LEA rats was positive in all cases.

Qualitative Chemical Urinalysis

Ninety-three of the 97 LEC rats (97%) were positive for urinary protein (1+−2+), and 41 (42%) were positive for urinary bilirubin (1+). The control LEA rats (*n* = 50) showed normal values in both tests.

Hematological Tests (Table 1)

Although WBC was not significantly different between the LEC and LEA rats, RBC, Plt, Hb, and Hct of the LEC rats were lower than those of

Table 2. Comparison of biochemical data in long-surviving LEC rats[a] and age-matched LEA rats.

Items	LEC γ-Globulin(+)[b]	LEC γ-Globulin(−)[b]	LEA	P-value[c]
T. Bil (mg/dl)	0.31 ± 0.09[d] (27)[e]	0.27 ± 0.08 (21)[e]	0.31 ± 0.10 (17)[e]	N.S.
SGOT (K.U)	249 ± 75 (56)	241 ± 52 (40)	136 ± 36 (17)	<0.001
SGPT (K.U)	141 ± 65 (56)	137 ± 46 (40)	42 ± 5 (17)	<0.001
LDH (Wrob. U)	3049 ± 1947 (52)	3050 ± 1616 (38)	1637 ± 876 (17)	<0.001
Alp (K.A.U)	34.8 ± 9.9 (53)	32.8 ± 8.3 (38)	11.1 ± 2.3 (17)	<0.001
T.Chol (mg/dl)	42.0 ± 14.8 (48)	40.8 ± 14.6 (36)	69.4 ± 10.2 (17)	<0.001
Crt (mg/dl)	0.90 ± 0.20 (47)	0.85 ± 0.20 (38)	0.49 ± 0.03 (17)	<0.001
BUN (mg/dl)	26.5 ± 2.5 (45)	26.7 ± 2.1 (34)	21.0 ± 1.8 (17)	<0.001
Alb (mg/dl)	2.6 ± 0.3 (50)	2.7 ± 0.2 (34)	3.9 ± 0.3 (17)	<0.001

[a] These LEC rats survived for over 8 months (mean age 10 months)
[b] The γ-globulin(+) means positive of the γ-globulin fraction of serum protein by cellulose. acetate electrophoresis
[c] by Student's *t*-test
[d] Mean ± standard deviation
[e] Numbers in the parentheses indicate the number of rats used
N.S., not significant

Table 3. Comparison of $ICGR_{15}$, SGPT, and T.Bil in LEC and LEA rats[a].

Items	LEC (n = 35)	LEA (n = 7)	P-value[b]
$ICGR_{15}$ (mg/dl)	1.25 ± 1.56[c]	0.50 ± 0.16	<0.01
SGPT (K.U)	221.7 ± 140.4	40.7 ± 8.0	<0.001
T. Bil (mg/dl)	0.45 ± 0.19	0.29 ± 0.03	<0.001

[a] All the LEC rats survived from acute hepatitis (systemic jaundice) (mean age 6 months). LEA rats were age-matched
[b] By Student's t-test
[c] Mean ± standard deviation

Table 4. Comparison of serum IgG and IgM levels in long-surviving LEC and LEA rats[a].

	LEC			
Items	γ-Globulin(+)	γ-Globulin(−)	LEA	P-value[c]
IgG (mg/dl)	3.0 ± 1.0[d] (16)[e]	3.0 ± 1.0 (13)[e]	17.2 ± 2.7 (12)[e]	<0.001
IgM (mm²)	390 ± 104 (16)	425 ± 230 (13)	376 ± 78 (12)	N.S.

[a] These LEC rats survived for over 8 months (mean age 10 months); LEA rats were age-matched
[b] The γ-globulin(+) means positive of the γ-globulin fraction of serum protein by a cellulose.acetate electrophoresis
[c] by Student's t-test
[d] Mean ± standard deviation
[e] Numbers in the parentheses indicate the number of rats used
N.S., not significant

the LEA rats and Rct counts of the LEC rats were slightly increased. However, there were no significant differences of these results between the γ-globulin(+) and γ-globulin(−) groups in the LEC rats.

The above results show that the LEC rats had a higher frequency of anemia complication, and that the increase in Ret counts may be a compensation for this anemia.

Biochemical Tests (Table 2)

Although the values of SGOT, SGPT, LDH, Alp, Crt, and BUN of the LEC rats were significantly higher than those of the LEA rats, the values of T.chol and Alb of the LEC rats were lower than those of the LEA rats, while there were no significant differences in these results between the γ-globulin(+) and γ-globulin(−) groups in the LEC rats. The $ICGR_{15}$ values of the LEC rats were higher than that of the LEA rats (Table 3).

Immunological Tests

Serum IgG test (mg/dl)

Identical values were obtained from the γ-globulin(+) group (n = 16) and the γ-globulin(−) group (n = 13), and these values were significantly lower (P < 0.01) than those of the LEA rats (n = 12) (Table 4).

Serum IgM test (mm²)

No significant differences were observed among the γ-globulin(+) group (n = 16), the γ-globulin(−) group (n = 13), and the LEA rats (n = 12) (Table 4).

Blastogenic response

In the splenic cells of LEC rats which had received a complete medium instead of mitogens, the γ-globulin(+) group (n = 5) and the γ-globulin(−) group (n = 5) of the LEC rats did not show any difference in the ^{3}H-TdR uptake rate of the splenic cells. However, the ^{3}H-TdR uptake of the splenic cells of the LEA rats (n = 5) was about threefold that of the LEC rats. These results show that the splenic cells of the LEC rats had a low blastogenic capacity when mitogens were not present. We examined the ^{3}H-TdR uptake of the splenic cells in relation to the various mitogens: the LEC rats showed significantly low values which all concentrations compared to the LEA rats. However, when these values were converted to a ratio with the control values, i.e., the stimulation index (S.I.), the results were as follows: in the S.I. for PHA-P, no significant difference was observed between the γ-globulin(+) groups of the LEC and LEA rats, but the γ-globulin(−) groups showed lower values than the other two groups; in the S.I. for Con A, the LEC rats showed significantly higher values than the LEA rats at two concentrations of 50 and 100 mg/ml; in the S.I. for LPS, no difference was observed between the LEC and LEA rats (Table 5).

Pathological Study

Gross examination

In the LEC rats which underwent acute hepatitis between 4–5 months of age, it was not detected any gross abnormalities in the liver between the age of 6–10 months. Around the age of 1 year, however, the abdomen began to swell and tumors were detected by palpation in a few cases. Under laparotomy, the entire liver appeared swollen, and lost its surface luster; microgranular changes were also observed. These changes were not attributable to differences in the hepatic lobes, and there were few signs of malignancy which presented as red color and soft texture compared to other areas that seemed to be normal.

Table 5. Blastogenic responses[a] of spleen cells to PHA-P, Con A, and LPS[b] in long-surviving LEC and age-matched LEA rats[c].

Mitogen	Concentration (mg/ml)	LEC (+)[d]	LEC (−)[d]	LEA
PHA-P	200	30492 ± 11733 (8.0 ± 3.1)[e]	14556 ± 1555 (3.5 ± 0.4)	101276 ± 14149 (7.4 ± 1.0)
	100	19697 ± 4373 (5.1 ± 1.1)	9656 ± 1236 (2.3 ± 0.3)	65517 ± 4628 (4.8 ± 0.3)
	50	12903 ± 2438 (3.4 ± 0.6)	5988 ± 1471 (1.4 ± 0.4)	55729 ± 2981 (4.0 ± 0.2)
Con A	100	73441 ± 7165 (19.2 ± 1.9)	72552 ± 20883 (17.4 ± 5.0)	143015 ± 12160 (10.4 ± 0.9)
	50	48409 ± 4634 (12.6 ± 1.2)	38710 ± 16070 (9.3 ± 3.9)	90888 ± 15295 (6.6 ± 1.1)
	25	10178 ± 6383 (2.7 ± 1.7)	9227 ± 6344 (2.2 ± 1.5)	36109 ± 14752 (2.6 ± 1.1)
LPS	2	3973 ± 1379 (1.04 ± 0.36)	3181 ± 66 (0.76 ± 0.02)	15085 ± 1989 (1.09 ± 0.14)
	1	3709 ± 967 (0.97 ± 0.25)	2549 ±110 (0.61 ± 0.03)	11116 ± 2188 (0.81 ± 0.16)
	0.5	2067 ± 475 (0.54 ± 0.12)	1698 ± 103 (0.41 ± 0.02)	7755 ± 3242 (0.56 ± 0.24)
Control		3828 ± 2208	4166 ± 2597	13779 ± 1102

[a] Blastogenic response was measured by uptake (cpm) of ^{3}H-thymidine

[b] *PHA-P*, Phytohemmaglutinin-P; *Con A*, Concanavalin A; *LPS*, lipopolisaccharide

[c] The mean age of LEC and LEA rats used was 10 months (range: 8–12 months)

[d] By cellulose.acetate electrophoresis, the γ-globulin fraction of serum protein was positive in LEC(+) and negative in LEC(−)

[e] Parentheses indicate Stimulation Index (experiment cpm/control cpm)

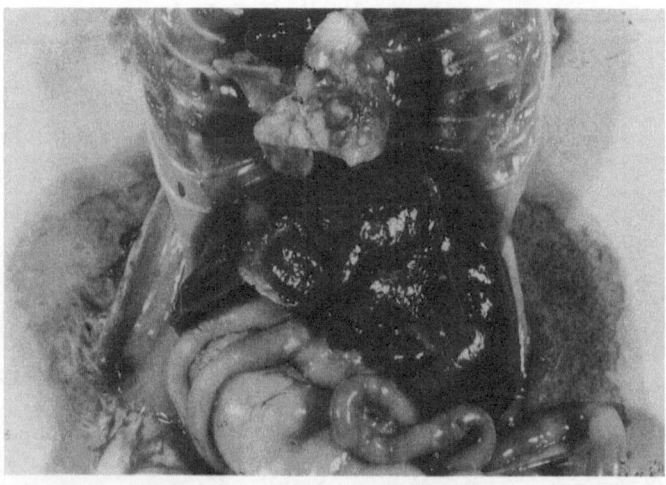

Fig. 1. Macroscopic findings in the LEC rat with spontaneous liver cancer. The liver was markedly enlarged, especially the left lateral lobe, and its surface was rough and granular. In the liver, the white-colored cancerous lesions were detected with metastatic lung tumors. Mesenteric lymph nodes were also swollen

Eighteen months later, the liver showed more pronounced diffuse swelling, which made it possible to clearly recognize the tumors by abdominal palpation (in about 55% of the cases); some of the tumors grew as large as 8 cm or more in diameter. The surface of the liver which showed pronounced diffuse swelling was losing its luster and showed extensive microgranular changes including nodular swollen areas. There were some isolated areas, however, which had retained the color considered to be normal for liver tissue. Macroscopical examination suggested that this microgranular morphology might have been caused by fibrotic changes. Scattered white or grayish-white lesions were also present in this area, and were identified as liver cancer.

Although metastatic complications were not frequent, metastatic sites were mainly in the lungs. The mesenteric lymph nodes also showed piled swelling to be 2 cm or more in diameter (Fig. 1).

Histopathological findings

1. Liver tissue features in the stage of choronic hepatitis: The LEC rats which underwent remission after developing acute hepatitis and those rats which went through the acute hepatitis stage without exhibiting jaundice survived for long periods of time, with a small number of exceptions which had recurrences after 6 months. In the long survived rats, sloughed liver cells as well as cholangiolar cells (oval cells) in the marginal zone of the hepatic lobule adjacent to giant liver cells were observed; small regenerative liver cells with round nuclei were observed contiguous to the oval cells (Fig. 2). In some cases, clusters of liver cells with basophilic cytoplasm and small round nuclei were observed in the marginal zone of the hepatic lobule.

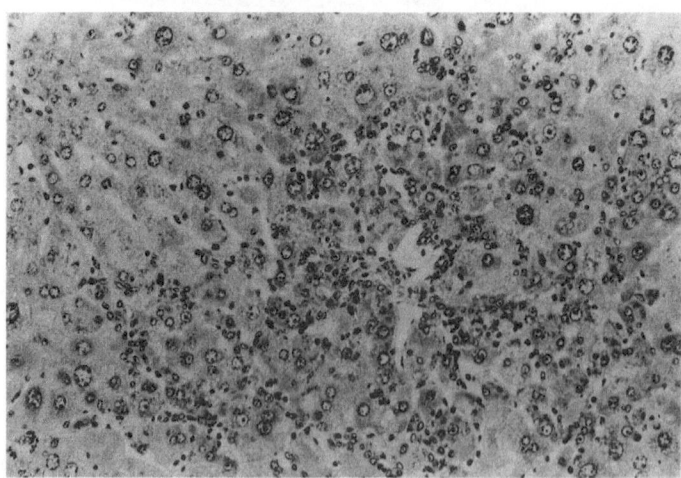

Fig. 2. Chronic hepatitis. Oval cells and small hepatocytes were observed with necrotic and giant hepatocytes. H and E, × 170

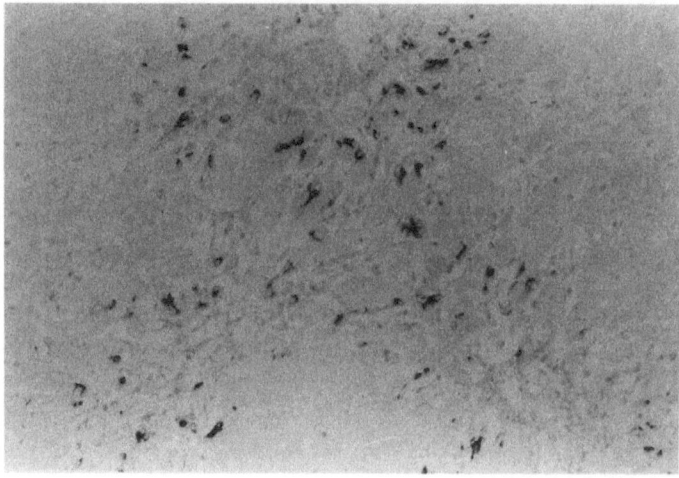

Fig. 3. AFP-producing cells. Dark staining cells were AFP-positive cells. ABC method, × 170

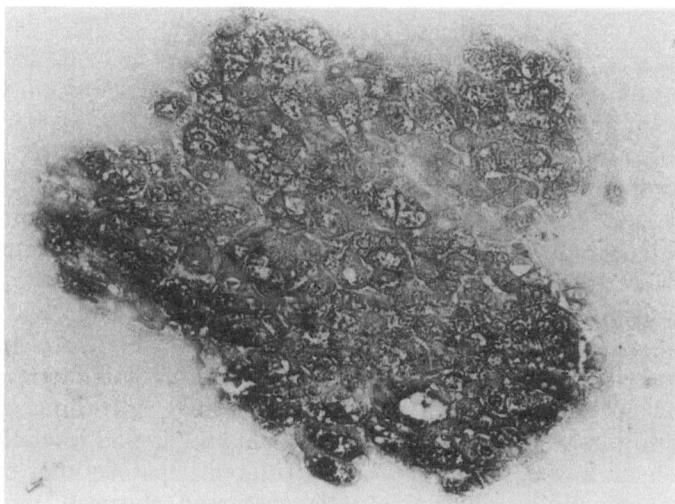

Fig. 4. GST-p positive cells. Hyperplastic foci were detectable. ABC method, × 170

2. AFP-producing cells: A study of AFP production in liver tissue revealed AFP-positive cells (Fig. 3). The cells are considered to correspond with the transitional cells observed in the course of carcinogenesis by azo-dye.
3. Hyperplastic foci: A study to determine the presence of GST-p in the LEC rats aged 6 months or more revealed positive staining of the small liver cell clusters (Fig. 4).

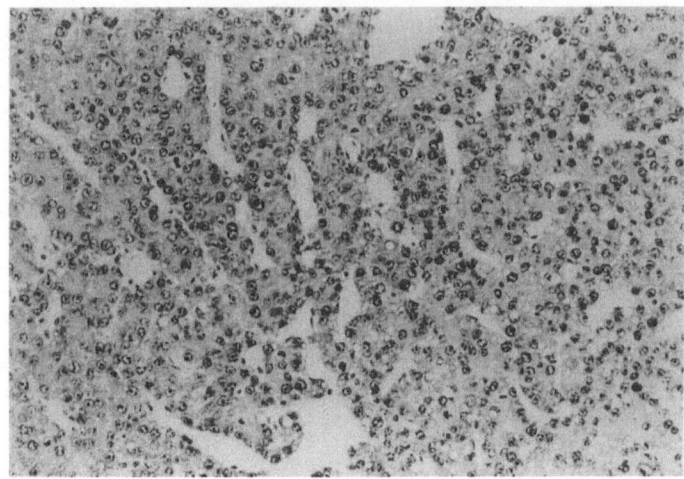

Fig. 5. Hepatocellular carcinoma. Trabecular hepatocellular carcinoma cells which had a relatively low grade of atypia and were well differentiated were observed. (H and E, × 170)

4. Hyperplastic nodules: The liver tissues of the LEC rats aged around 12 months revealed hyperplastic nodules. The cell clusters with clear cytoplasm and small round nuclei caused compression against the liver cells surrounding the cluster periphery.

5. Microscopic findings of hepatocellular carcinoma (HCC): Around 18 months after birth, the LEC rats showed liver cancer, which was confirmed by gross and pathological examinations. Virtually most of the cancers were highly differentiated trabecular hepatocellular carcinoma (Edmondson classification: I-II) (Fig. 5). Furthermore, the LEC rats showed cholangiofibrosis, which affected extensive areas of the liver in some cases. With marked hyperplasia of fibrous connective tissue in the background, the duct structure presented in various sizes. The heteromorphism of the cells seemed to be bile duct epithelial cells.

6. Electron microscopy of highly differentiated hepatocellular carcinoma: The hepatocellular carcinoma cells possessed glycogen, peroxisomes, and other substances. There were variations in the size of mitochondria, and the granular endoplasmic reticulum was well developed (Fig. 6).

Discussion

The LEC rats not only develop a high rate of spontaneous acute hepatitis, but also present a variety of pathological states, such as the development of complications of anemia [1] and combined immunodeficiency [6] prior to developing acute hepatitis.

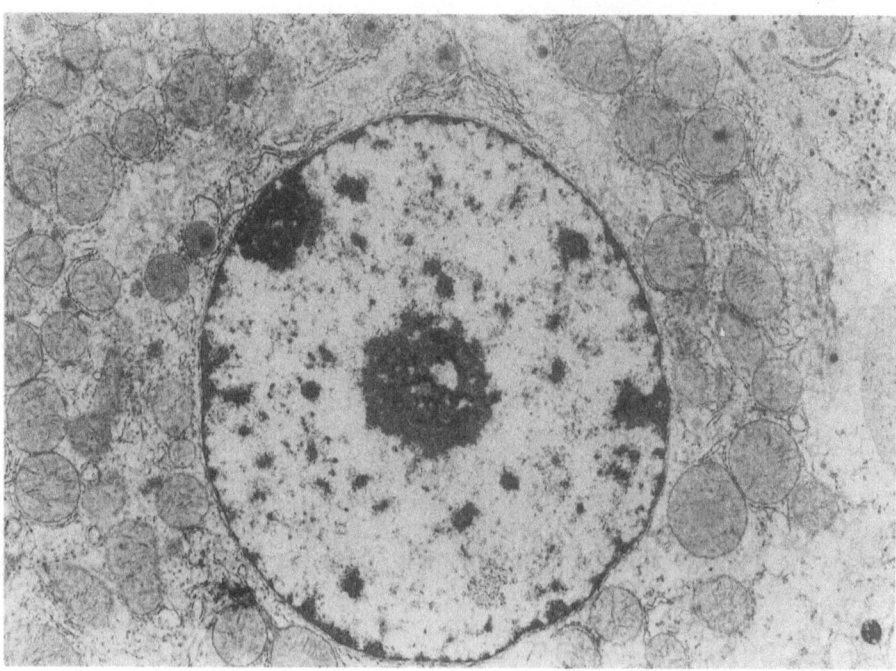

Fig. 6. Electromicrograph of a hepatocellular carcinoma cell. Mitochondria were various in size; the rough-surfaced endoplasmic reticulum was well developed, and peroxysome and glycogen were also observed, × 7000

By long-term follow-up of the LEC rats which have suffered from acute hepatitis, we can easily identify the occurrence of anemia in the bulbar conjunctiva. RBC, Hb, and Hct were low in the LEC rats compared to those in the control LEA rats. Moreover, the LEC rats showed high Ret counts compared to the LEA rats: this is considered to be a compensation for the anemia. Based on the average red blood cell parameter values (MCV, MCH, MCHC) and the stain pictures of the smear (data not shown), we suggest that this may be hypovolemic and hypochromic anemia. The cause of this anemia is not known. Since total blood bilirubin is within normal range, we can hardly assume that the anemia of the LEC rats is hemolytic. Although the LEC rats showed significant decreases in the RBC and Plt, there was no difference in the WBC between the two strains. However, the LEC rats were in a state of immunosuppression [6] and were considered to be susceptible to bacterial infection. Accordingly, we assume that the WBC might have been affected by increased reactivity due to bacterial infection. If we suppose that bone marrow functions were normal due to the increase in the Ret count, we can justify the increase in the WBC. If this hypothesis is correct, the long-surviving LEC rats would have a relative pancytopenia compared to the LEA rats, which will resemble the clinicobiochemical state of human liver cirrhosis. The values of SGOT, SGPT, LDH, and ALP of the LEC rats were higher than those of the LEA rats, which clearly indicates the presence of some liver disorder. The decrease in T. Chol was also considered to be a sign of persistent chronic liver disorder in the LEC rats. It is known that the normalization of $ICGR_{15}$ in the blood becomes more rapid in remission of acute hepatitis, but the $ICGR_{15}$ of the LEC rats, at an average age of 6 months and which had experienced acute hepatitis at the age of 4–5 months, was higher than that of the same-aged LEA rats. This finding showed a correlation with the elevated levels of SGOT and T. Bil, which supports the assumption that the LEC rats bear persistent liver disorders after recovering from acute hepatitis.

We have reported that the LEC rats are likely to suffer from liver disorders at around the age of 2 months and develop acute hepatitis at 4–5 months [1]. The LEC rats which have survived the acute hepatitis will show liver cell necrosis and small regenerative liver cells; these histological findings are identical to those of human chronic hepatitis. Oval cells, i.e. AFP-production-positive cells, identified in the liver tissue of LEC rats, are considered to be cholangiolar cells, the precursors of small regenerative liver cells. In accordance with the advancing age of the LEC rats, a GST-p stain showed hyperplastic foci in the liver tissue, which then underwent the transition to hyperplastic nodules. This transition in the LEC rats eventually resulted in hepatocellular carcinoma. This course is similar to the onset of liver cancer induced by carcinogens such as azo-dyes [5,7–11]. Concerning the frequency of concurrent liver cancer in the LEC rats, Masuda et al. [12] reported a frequency of 90% or more. The biochemical findings of liver disorders in the LEC rats matched very well with histological findings. However, it has not yet been possible to obtain findings similar to human liver cirrhosis which would confirm the hematological assumption of relative pancytopenia. There have been numerous reports of artificially prepared liver cirrhosis models in rats, but these models cannot meet our experimental protocols. The question is whether or not the pathological state of liver cirrhosis occurs spontaneously in rats. There were sex differences in the incidence of liver cancer in the LEC rats, and the complication of cholangiofibrosis was always present in its background. Accordingly, these findings indicate that the cholangiofibrosis observed with a high frequency in liver cancer of the LEC rats may resemble human liver cirrhosis.

The ^{3}H-TDR uptake capacity of the splenic cells in the LEC rats was clearly reduced compared to that of the LEA rats. However, when mitogens were added, the S.I. of the LEC rats with respect to PHA-P was elevated in the same way as that of the LEA rats, with the exception of the γ-globulin(−) group. These facts seem to support the finding that proliferation of isolated liver cells is extremely poor, even under optimum conditions (data not shown).

According to the immunological studies of the LEC rats surviving over a long term, identical IgG values were obtained from both the γ-globulin(−) and γ-globulin(+) groups of the LEC rats, and these values were also significantly low compared to those of the LEA rats. We have not yet clarified why IgG values were identical in the two groups of LEC rats. Although the main fraction of γ-globulin is IgG, it is distributed up to β and α_2. The IgG of the γ-globulin(−) group is considered to be distributed mainly in fractions other than the γ-globulin fraction. This leads us to infer the presence of qualitative abnormalities in IgG in the LEC rats. However, when Matsumoto et al. [13] prepared (LEC × LEA) F_1 × LEC backcross (BCI) rats and investigated the Ig content in the blood of the BCI rats prior to the development of hepatitis according to subclass by the Ouchterlony method, they found no correlation between the development of hepatitis in the BCI rats and the content of IgG1 and IgG2a in the blood. Nevertheless, they do not deny the possibility that immune disorders may play a role in the transition from chronic liver disorders to liver cancers in LEC rats.

The fact that LEC rats possess a hereditary background of autosomal recessive inheritance has been previously reported [2]. The presence of metabolic abnormalities in the rats with this type of hereditary background should be taken into considereation. It has been pointed out that soon after birth LEC rats show abnormalities in metabolic enzymes by detoxification of drugs, such as cytochrome P-450, epoxide hydrolase, and γ-glutathione-S-transpeptidase [14]. LEC rats showed complications of chronic hepatitis and immunological abnormalities, and their terminal features included the complication of HCC. We suggest the possiblity that these progressive pathological states could be based upon metabolic abnormalities stipulated by autosomal recessive inheritance. The hepatic lesions in LEC rats follow the course of acute hepatitis-chronic hepatitis-liver cancer. In this respect, this animal model will provide valuable information for elucidating the pathology of the courses of acute hepatitis-fulminant hepatitis or chronic hepatitis-liver cirrhosis-liver cancer in humans.

Conclusions

1. In liver enzyme tests, significantly increased level of SGOT, SGPT, LDH, and ALP were seen in LEC rats, whereas total cholesterol and albumin showed decreases; $ICGR_{15}$ in the 6-month-old LEC rats showed a significant increase. These biochemical findings indicated the presence of chronic hepatitis in the LEC rats.
2. Pathological examination of liver tissue of the long-surviving LEC rats showed small limited areas of liver cell necrosis and regenerative small liver cells, indicating the presence of chronic hepatitis.

3. Oval cells, hyperplastic foci, and hyperplastic nodules, identified with those observed after the administration of chemical carcinogenic substances, were noticed in the transient course to liver cancer in LEC rats.
4. The liver cancer observed in the LEC rats was mostly a trabecular, highly differentiated hepatocellular carcinoma; additionally, there was a high degree of concurrent cholangiofibrosis.

These findings support the proposal that chronic hepatitis tends to take a transitional course to liver cancer in the long-surviving LEC rats.

Acknowledgment. This work was supported in part by grants from the Ministry of Education, Science and Culture of Japan.

References

1. Namieno T, Takeichi N, Sasaki M, Dempo K, Mori M, Uchino J, Kobayashi H (to be published) Clinical and pathological characteristics in Long-Evans Cinnamon (LEC) rats with spontaneous development of hepatitis
2. Namieno T, Takeichi N, Sasaki M, Dempo K, Mori M, Uchino J, Kobayashi H (to be published) Pathogenesis of spontaneous hepatitis in Long-Evans Cinnamon (LEC) rats
3. Summers J, Smolec JM, Smyder R (1978) A virus similar to human hepatitis B virus associated with hepatitis and hepatoma in woodchuck Proc Natl Acad Sci USA 75:4533–4537
4. Sato K, Kitahara A, Sone Y (1985) Purification, induction and distribution of placental glutathione transferase: A new marker enzyme for preneoplastic cells in the rat chemical carcinogenesis. Proc Natl Acad Sci USA 82:3964–3968
5. Dempo K, Chisaka N, Yoshida Y (1975) Immunofluorescent study on alpha-fetoprotein producing cells in the early stage of 3'-methyl-4-dimethyl-aminoazobenzene carcinogenesis. Cancer Res 35:1282–1287
6. Namieno T, Takeichi N, Sasaki M, Dempo K, Mori M, Uchino J, Kobayashi H (to be published) Combined immunodeficiency in Long-Evans Cinnamon (LEC) rats with spontaneous hepatitis
7. Dempo K, Sasaki M, Kaku T (1983) Immunohistochemical studies on α-fetoprotein and albumin containing cells in the liver oncogenesis and early stage of 3'-Me-DAB hepatocarcinogenesis. Ann NY Acad Sci 417:195–202
8. Onoe T, Dempo K, Kaneko A (1973) Significance of α-fetoprotein appearance in the early stage of azo-dye carcinogenesis. Jpn J Cancer Res 14(monogram):233–247
9. Onoe T, Kaneko A, Dempo K (1975) α-fetoprotein and early histological changes of hepatic tissue in DAB-hepato-carcinogenesis. Ann NY Acad Sci 259:167–180
10. Sell S, Leffert HL (1982) An evaluation of cellular lineages in the pathogenesis of experimental hepatocellular carcinoma. Hepatology 2:77–86
11. Mori M, Kaku T, Dempo K (1980) Histochemical investigation of precancerous lesions induced by 3'-Me-DAB in rat liver. Jpn J Cancer Res 25(monogram):103–114

12. Masuda R, Yoshida MC, Sasaki M (1988) High susceptibility to hepatocellular carcinoma development in LEC rats with hereditary hepatitis. Jpn J Cancer Res 79:828–835
13. Matsumoto K, Takeichi N, Izumi K, Yoshida MC, Sasaki M, Ootsuka H (1987) Genetic study for IgG polymorphism and hepatitis in spontaneously hepatitic rat (LEC). Proc Jpn Soc Immunol 17:805
14. Sugiyama T, Takeichi N, Kobayashi H (1988) Metabolic predisposition of a novel mutant (LEC rats) to hereditary hepatitis and hepatoma: Alterations of the drug metabolizing enzymes. Carcinogenesis 9:1569–1572

31 — Neoplastic and Non-Neoplastic Lesions in Aging LEC/Otk Rats

Kazuya Kawano, Tsukasa Hirashima, Shigehito Mori, Sumio Bando, Kenichi Yonemoto, Fumiko Abe, and Takashi Natori[1]

Introduction

We have previously reported that the SPF-conditioned LEC/Otk rat has characteristic pathological features. (1) Jaundice develops in almost all rats with increase in the plasma glutamic pyruvic transaminase (P-GPT) level. (2) The animals show episodes of jaundice, a high P-GPT level, and liver cell necrosis, but only slight inflammatory cell infiltration. (3) The liver cells show characteristic microvesicular fatty changes. (4) The P-GPT level shows increases, first at 18 weeks and then at 25 weeks of age. (5) The rats show immunological disorders, such as deficiency of immunoglobulins, especially IgG_1, and of helper T cells [1].

It was reported by others that hepatomas arise in a high frequency in the aged LEC rats (living for more than 18 months) [2]. We have also observed many hyperplastic nodules in the liver of LEC/Otk rats after 6 months of age. The present report describes neoplastic or tumor-like lesions which occurred in the liver or in other organs of aged LEC/Otk rats.

Materials and Methods

Animals

The LEC/Otk rat, that was established at F_{40} from the original LEC line of Hokkaido University in specific-pathogen free (SPF) conditions, were used. LETO and LEA/Otk rats were used as control animals. Rats were maintained in our SPF facility as described previously [1].

A total of 58 LEC/Otk rats were subjected to a long-term period of observation, at most up to 85 weeks of age. All rats were necropsied, and the organs were carefully examined for gross pathological lesions,

[1] Tokushima Research Institute, Otsuka Pharmaceutical Co., Ltd., Tokushima, 771-01 Japan

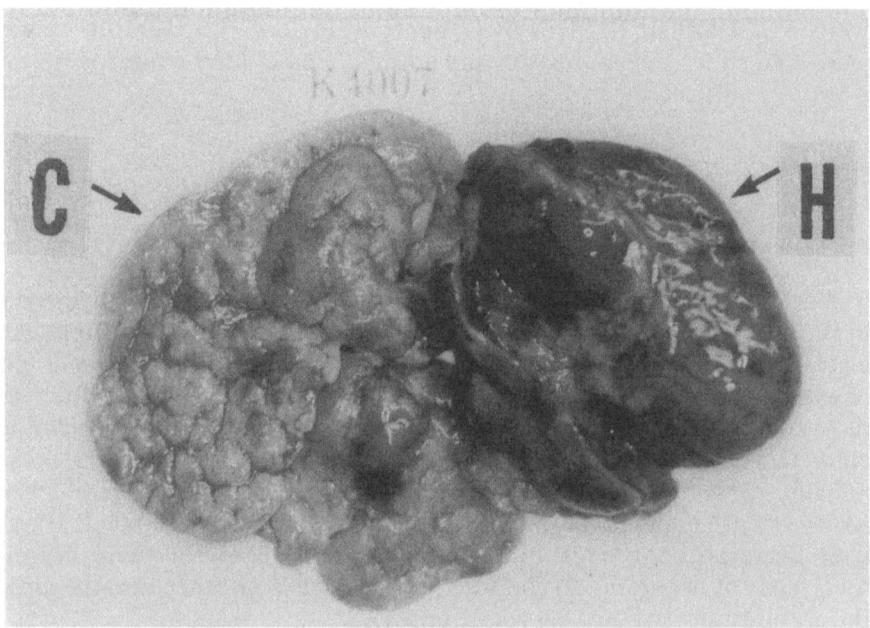

Fig. 1. The gross appearance of liver neoplastic changes consisting of reddish soft tumors (*H*) and hard whitish nodules (*C*) that occupied almost the entire surface of the liver in LEC/Otk rats

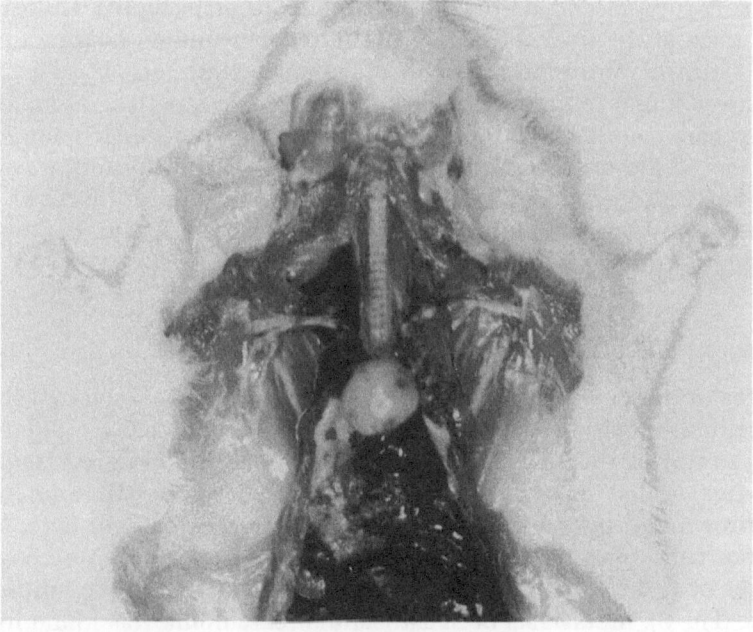

Fig. 2. The gross appearance of the thymus of a LEC/Otk rat with an enlargement to 10–15 mm in size

weighed, and then fixed in 10% neutralized formalin. Paraffin sections were stained with hematoxylin and eosin (H and E) by the routine method.

Results

Clinical Course

It was found that jaundice in the LEC/Otk rats develops with increases in the P-GPT level at approximately 4 months of age, and that histopathologically the livers show submassive necrosis and microvascular fatty changes. Less than 30% of these rats died within a week. Rats that recovered survived for more than 1 year with increase in body weight, and enlargement of livers which were palpable. Rats died at 68 weeks (1 female), 73 weeks (1 female), 80 weeks (1 male), 82 weeks (1 female), and 83 weeks (1 male) after birth. The causes of death included massive liver necrosis, congestion of liver by obstruction of the vena hepatica, metastasis of hepatoma to the lung, or metastasis of other tumors such as theca cell tumor.

Macroscopic Findings

All the rats were sacrificed and necropsied between 83–85 weeks of age. The major finding at a necropsy was neoplastic changes consisting of reddish soft tumors and hard whitish nodules that occupied almost the entire surface of the liver (Fig. 1). Multiple reddish tumors ranging in size from 10–20 mm were found in both male and female rats. Hard whitish nodules were found in more extended area in female rats than in males. In all cases, para-pancreatic lymphonodes (2–4 mm) of reddish color were found. One of the characteristic findings was that the thymus was well preserved at this age (83–85 weeks), whereas in the control LETO or LEA rats, the thymus was involuted and replaced with fatty tissue. In one case (male), the thymus was enlarged to 10–15 mm (Fig. 2).

Microscopic Findings

Incidences of tumor occurrence in the LEC/Otk rats are shown in Table 1. Hepatocellular carcinomas were found in 96.9% (male, 32/33) and 100% (female, 25/25) of the LEC/Otk rats. The tumor cells closely resembled normal liver cells, having a round nucleus with a small amount of chromatin containing a distinctive nucleolus and an abundant cytoplasm. The tumor cells appeared to be arranged in a trabecular structure covered by a layer of endothelial cells which were circumscribed by a sinusoidal structure (Fig. 3). Metastasis of hepatocellular carcinoma was found in one case (lung metastasis).

Table 1. Incidence of tumor in 33 male and 25 female aging LEC/Otk rats.

Tumor	Male (%)	Female (%)
Liver		
Hepatocellular carcinoma	32 (96.9)	25 (100)
Cholangiocarcinoma	16 (48.4)	19 (76.0)
Adenoma	16 (48.4)	22 (88.0)
Cystadenocarcinoma	1 (3.0)	7 (28.0)
Cholangioma	1 (3.0)	3 (12.0)
Kidney		
Renal cell carcinoma	0	1 (4.0)
Adenoma	0	1 (4.0)
Pituitary		
Adenoma	3 (9.0)	10 (40.0)
Adrenal		
Pheochromocytoma	1 (3.0)	2 (8.0)
Adenoma	2 (6.0)	1 (4.0)
Ovary		
Granulosa cell tumor		2 (8.0)
Theca cell tumor (thecoma)		1 (4.0)
Thymus		
Thymoma	1 (3.0)	0
Leukemia	1 (3.0)	0
Skin		
Fibroadenoma	1 (3.0)	0

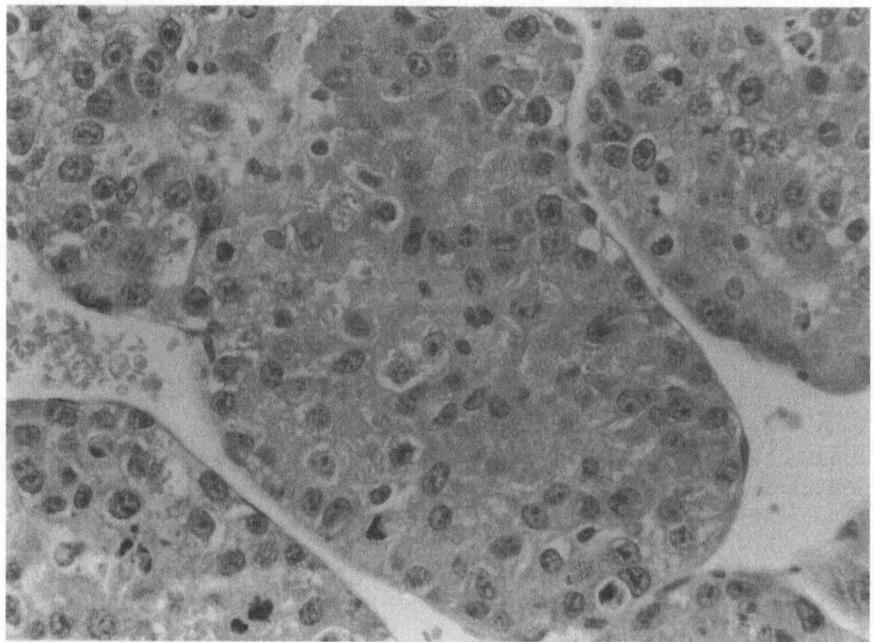

Fig. 3. The microscopic appearance of a reddish soft tumor showing a well-differentiated type of hepatocellular carcinoma. The tumor cells appeared to be arranged in a trabecular structure covered by a layer of endothelial cells circumscribed by a sinusoidal structure. H and E, × 100

Cholangiogenic tumors such as cholangiocarcinoma and adenoma were found in a higher frequency in female rats. Cystadenocarcinoma and cholanginomas were found with less frequency, (3%–28%) although again females had more tumors than males.

Other neoplastic changes such as renal cell tumor, pheochromocytoma, granulosa cell tumor, theca cell tumor (thecoma), fibroadenoma, leukemia, pituitary adenoma, and thymoma were observed with a low frequency. A widespread dissemination to the liver, spleen, kidney, peritoneum, and uterus was found in one case of thecoma. Tumor-like thymus enlargements (1 male and 2 females) were observed. The enlarged thymus consisted of packed small lymphocytes and epithelial cells constructing the normal architecture. Few Hassall's bodies were seen. In the control animals, thymuses at this age were involuted and replaced with fatty tissue. No neoplastic changes were observed in the control strains, LETO and LEA/Otk.

Other non-neoplastic changes are listed in Table 2. Nodular hyperplasia of pale cells in the marginal area was revealed between the zona glomerulosa and zona fasiculata (Fig. 4). Para-pancreatic lymphonodes were swollen and contained an increased number of lymph follicles. Many hemosiderin-bearing macrophages in the sinus of the medulla, erythrocytes, histocytes, mast cells, and plasma cells were observed.

Discussion

The oncogenic mechanisms of hepatocellular carcinoma in the LEC/Otk rats are not yet established. However, it is strongly suggested that the oncogenic process of the LEC rats is very much like, if not identical to, that of chemically induced hepatomas (i.e., 3'-methyl-4-dimethyl-

Table 2. Non-neoplastic lesions in 33 male and 25 female aging LEC/Otk rats.

Lesion	Male (%)	Female (%)
Liver		
Primary biliary cirrhosis	1 (3.0)	0
Cholangiofibrosis	10 (30.3)	2 (8.0)
Adrenal		
Nodular hyperplasia of adrenal cortex	26 (78.7)	18 (72)
Eosinophilic foci of adrenal cortex	5 (15.1)	13 (52)
Thymus		
Hypertrophy	1 (3.0)	2 (6.0)
Lymph Node		
Hypertrophy, hemorrhage	33 (100)	25 (100)
Spleen		
Hypertrophy of white pulp	33 (100)	25 (100)
Extramedullary hematopoiesis	33 (100)	25 (100)

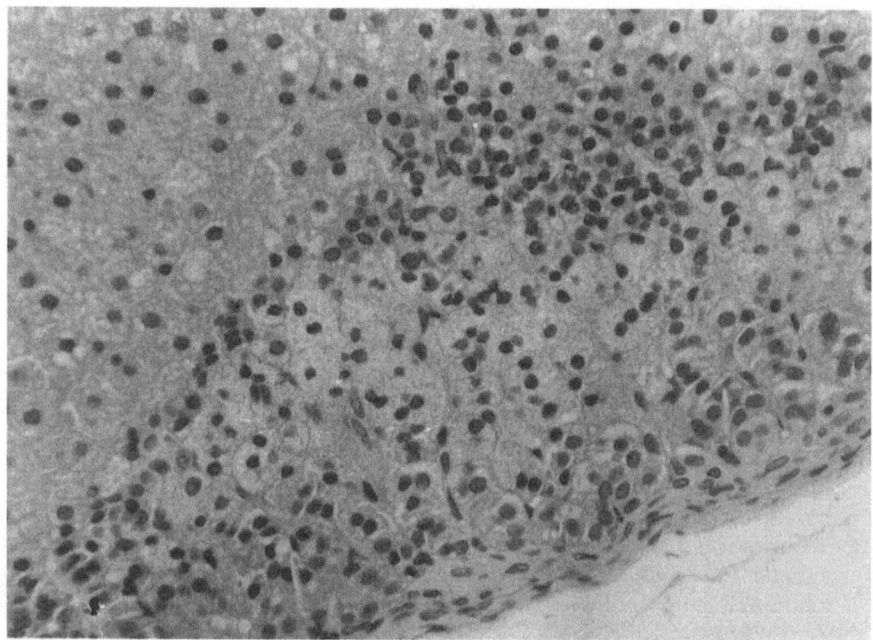

Fig. 4. A histological section of adrenal glands of a LEC/Otk rat. There is nodular hyperplasia of pale cells in the marginal area between the zona glomerulosa and zona fasiculata. H and E, × 100

aminobenzene-hepatomas [DAB-hepatomas]). The assumption is based on the following evidence: (1) oval cells and small hepatocytes that arc reported to appear in the early stages of chemically induced carcinogenesis accumulated in the Glisson sheath area of LEC livers which had recovered from the acute phase of hepatic injury, (2) alpha-fetoproteins (AFPs) were identified immunohistochemically in cells and the levels of blood AFP content increase to 4,000 ng/ml [3], (3) after the stage of oval cells, atypical cells with clear cytoplasm and small nuclei appeared, expanding in the hepatocytes with giant nuclei. These cells were positively stained with placental glutathione S-transferase (P-GST) and γ-glutamyltranspeptidase (γ-GTP), characteristics that resemble those of hyperplastic foci appearing in the process of chemically induced carcinogenesis [4]. It was reported that these hyperplastic foci increase in number and size with age. After 1 year, the foci became visible macroscopically. Histopathologically, they were hyperplastic nodules without any cellular and structural atypism. After 75 weeks of age, large reddish tumors appeared. These were of microscopically well-differentiated hepatocellular carcinoma with a trabecular structure. It was reported that spontaneous hepatocellular carcinomas arise in Map:SD rats (1.4%) [5], Crl:SD rats (2.9%) [5], Om rats

(1%) [6] and WAG/Rij rats (1%) [7], although the incidences are extremely lower than that in LEC rats.

It is noteworthy that enlarged thymuses were found even in a few cases of 85-week-old rats, which is unusual in inbred rats. Although we have no direct evidence, we speculate that the pathologic changes might be related to an immunological disorder, such as CD4 cell deficiency in the thymus [8,9].

References

1. Kawano K, Hirashima T, Mori S, Bando S, Yonemoto K, Abe F, Goto H Natori T (1991) Pathology and laboratory findings in LEC/Otk rats that spontaneously develop hepatic injury. J Gastroenterol Hepatol 6:53–58
2. Masuda R, Yoshida MC, Sasaki M, Dempo K, Mori M (1988) High susceptibility to hepatocellular carcinoma development in LEC rats with hereditary hepatitis. Jpn J Cancer Res 79:828–835
3. Takahashi H, Oyamada M, Fujimoto Y, Satoh MI, Hattori A, Dempo K, Mori M, Tanaka T, Watabe H, Masuda R, Yoshida MC (1988) Elevation of serum alfa-fetoprotein and proliferation of oval cells in the livers of LEC rats. Jpn. J Cancer Res 79:821–827
4. Oyamada M, Dempo K, Fujimoto Y, Takahashi H, Satoh M, Mori M, Masuda R, Yoshidà MC, Satoh K, Satoh K (1988) Spontaneous occurrence of placental glutathione S-transferase-positive foci in the livers of LEC rats. Jpn. J Cancer Res 79:5–8
5. Anver MR, Cohen BJ, Lattuada CP, Foster SJ (1982) Age-associated lesions in barrier-reared male Sprague-Dawley rats: A comparison between Hap: (SD) and Cri: COBS[R] CD[R](SD) stocks. Exp Aging Res 8:3–24
6. Goodman DG, Ward JM, Squire RA, Paxton MB, Reichardt WD, Chu KC, Linhart MS (1980) Neoplastic and nonneoplastic lesion in aging Osborne-Mendel rats. Toxicol Appl Pharmacol: 55:433–447
7. Burek JD (1978) Pathology of aging rats. CRC, Florida
8. Yamada T, Natori T, Izumi K, Sakai T, Agui T, Matsumoto K (to be published) Inheritance of T helper immunodeficiency (thid) in LEC Mutant Rats. Immunogenetics
9. Agui T, Oka M, Yamada T, Sakai T, Izumi K, Ishida Y, Himeno K, Matsumoto K (to be published) Muturational arrest from CD4$^+$8$^+$ to CD4$^+$8$^-$ thymocytes in a mutant strain (LEC) of rat. J Exp Med

32 — The Multistep Nature of Spontaneous Liver Cancer Development in the LEC Rat: Analysis of Incidence and Phenotype of Preneoplastic and Neoplastic Liver Lesions

KATSUHIKO ENOMOTO, MASAKUNI SAWAKI, HIDETOSHI TAKAHASHI, YASUO NAKAJIMA, KIMIMARO DEMPO, and MICHIO MORI[1]

Introduction

The LEC rat has been established and characterized as a new mutant strain which spontaneously develops hepatitis and liver cancer at an extremely high incidence. The LEC rat manifests severe hereditary hepatitis with systemic jaundice and hemorrhagic tendency at around 4 months after birth. About 30%−40% of the rats die during the period of hepatitis because of submassive or massive necrosis of hepatocytes. The remaining rats recover from severe hepatitis and survive more than 1 year. Histopathological examination of the livers of the long-survived LEC rats shows development of preneoplastic and neoplastic lesions at a high incidence with continued hepatocyte death and regeneration (prolonged hepatitis) [1,2].

The process of liver cancer development has been extensively studied using a chemically induced liver carcinogenesis model in which several histochemical markers are used for liver lesions [3,4]. The results of these studies have revealed that the various enzyme-altered preneoplastic liver lesions, such as hyperplastic foci and nodules, appear before development of the liver cancer. This evidence suggests a multistep nature of liver cancer development, a concept which was originally demonstrated in experimental skin carcinogenesis [5].

The rat is the most widely used animal for studies of chemically induced liver carcinogenesis. However, there are only a few reports of spontaneously occurring liver tumors in rat [6−9] and little is known about the process of spontaneously occurring liver tumors.

Thus, in the present study, in order to determine whether or not the process of spontaneous liver carcinogenesis is also multistep, we examined the incidence of enzyme-altered foci, hyperplastic nodules, and hepatocellular carcinomas (HCCs) in both male and female LEC rats after recovery from hepatitis. In addition, we analyzed several markers for liver

[1] Department of Pathology, Sapporo Medical College, Sapporo, 060 Japan

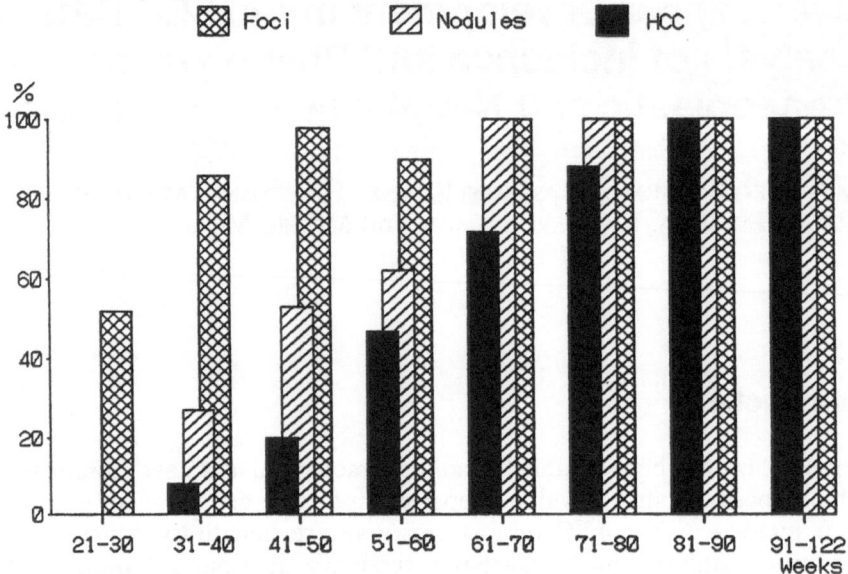

Fig. 1. Incidence of preneoplastic and neoplastic liver lesions in LEC rats examined between 20 and 122 weeks of age

carcinogenesis in order to clarify the phenotypic characteristics of the spontaneously occurring preneoplastic and neoplastic liver lesions.

Histology and Incidence of Preneoplastic and Neoplastic Liver Lesions

A total of 168 LEC rats (♂:90, ♀:78) were examined at different times up to 112 weeks after recovery from severe jaundice. After ether anesthesia, rats were sacrificed and the livers were removed for histological and histo-chemical examinations.

After recovery from severe hepatitis, the sporadic necrosis of hepatocytes with oval cell proliferation and the megalocytotic change of hepatocytes were continuously observed in the livers of the LEC rats. Focal hepatic lesions consisting of clear or basophilic small hepatocytes emerged spontaneously. Some of the foci were hardly detectable without histo-chemical staining because of the continuous liver damage and regenera-tion. Nodular lesions which compressed the surrounding tissues also appeared at around 8 months and HCCs developed thereafter. Figure 1 shows the incidences of enzyme-altered foci, nodular lesions, and HCCs in the LEC rat livers during the study period. As previously reported [10], enzyme-altered foci appeared in the livers immediately after recovery from severe hepatitis. From the 31st week, nodular lesions and hepatocellular

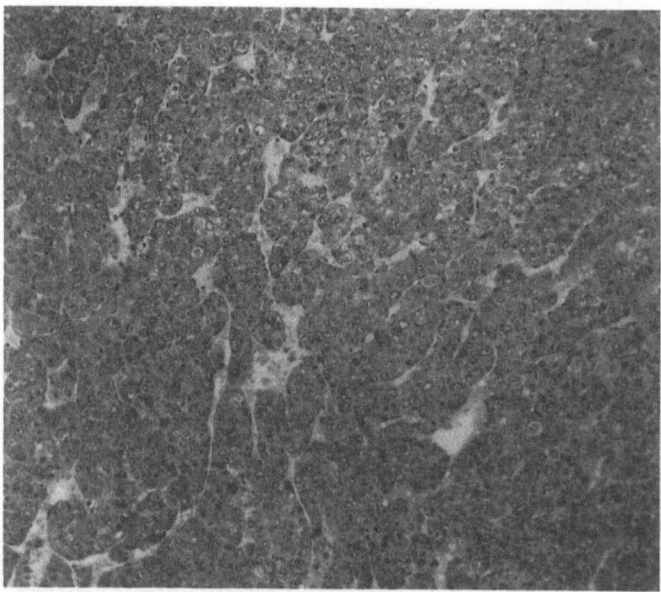

Fig. 2. Histological appearance of spontaneously occurring hepatocellular carcinoma showing a well-differentiated trabecular pattern

carcinomas were observed and the incidence of these lesions increased as a function of time. After 81 weeks, all of the examined LEC rats had one or more HCCs. The majority of carcinomas were of a histologically well-differentiated type showing a trabecular pattern (Fig. 2). Sex differences in the occurrence of liver lesions was also examined. Figure 3 clearly shows that the appearance of liver lesions occurred earlier in male rats compared to female rats.

Spontaneously occurring liver tumors in rats are relatively rare compared to those in mice. Goodmann et al. [7] reported that the incidence of spontaneous liver nodules and HCCs in aged male Fischer 344 rats was only 1.3% and 0.39%, respectively. Recently, it has been shown that the incidence of spontaneous liver neoplasms is low in spite of the high incidence of altered hepatocellular foci in aged Fischer 344 rats [9]. However, the results of this study showed 100% occurrence of liver cancer in aged LEC rats. Time-course analysis of liver lesions clearly demonstrated sequential development of each lesion, i.e., foci initially appeared during the recovery period of severe hereditary hepatitis, after which hyperplastic nodules and HCCs developed in an age-associated manner (Fig. 1). It is of importance to note that such a sequential development of liver lesions is similar to that reported in chemically induced liver carcinogenesis. Other reports [6–9] on spontaneously occurring liver tumors have failed to show such a clear sequence because of the low incidence of liver lesions for analysis. Thus, our results clearly suggest a

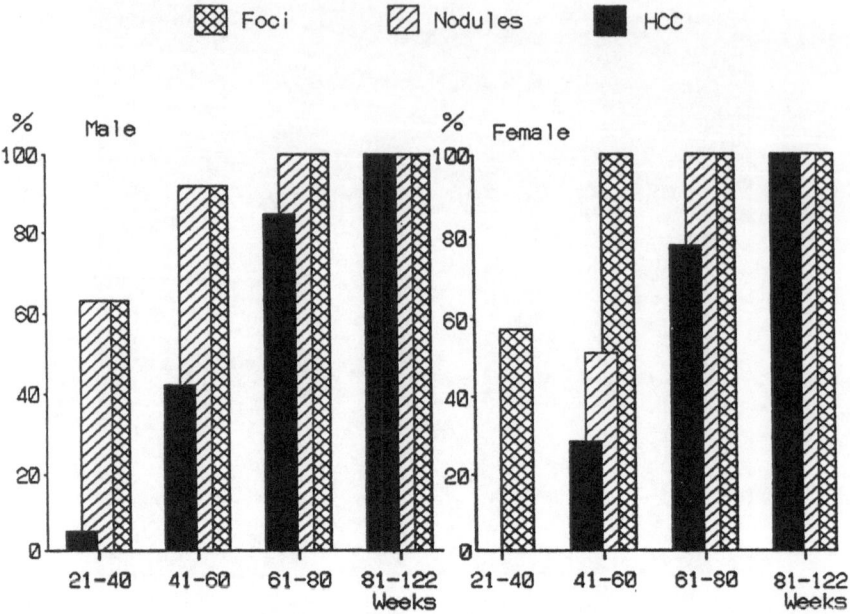

Fig. 3. Incidence of liver lesions in male and female LEC rats. Ninety male and 78 female rats were examined

multistep nature of spontaneous liver carcinogenesis in the LEC rat. Our results also indicate that spontaneous liver lesions occurred earlier and more frequently in male LEC rats than in female rats. This suggests the importance of the hormonal environment in the promotion stage of spontaneous liver carcinogenesis. Time-course analysis also showed that the appearence of preneoplastic and neoplastic liver lesions was seen only after the occurrence of spontaneous hepatitis. This strongly suggests a close correlation of liver damage to the genesis of liver cancer.

Phenotypic Alteration of LEC Rat Liver Lesions

It would be interesting to know whether the phenotypic characteristics of spontaneous preneoplastic and neoplastic lesions are identical to those appearing during chemically induced liver carcinogenesis. In studying chemically induced liver carcinogenesis, various histochemical markers have been used for analyzing liver lesions. From among these markers, we examined 3 negative and 2 positive markers for the staining of spon- taneous liver lesions.

Glucose-6-phosphatase (G6P), adenosine triphosphatase (ATP), and non- specific esterase (ES) were used as negative markers, and gamma- glutamyltransferase (GGT) and glutathione S-transferase placental form

Table 1. Histochemical and immunohistochemical analysis of spontaneous liver lesions during liver carcinogenesis of LEC rats.

	Foci	Nodules	Carcinomas
G6Pase	↓	↓	↓
ATPase	↓	↓	↓
ES	↓	↓	↓
GST-P	↑	↑	↑
GGT	↑	↑	↑

↓ :Activity decreased ↑ :Activity increased

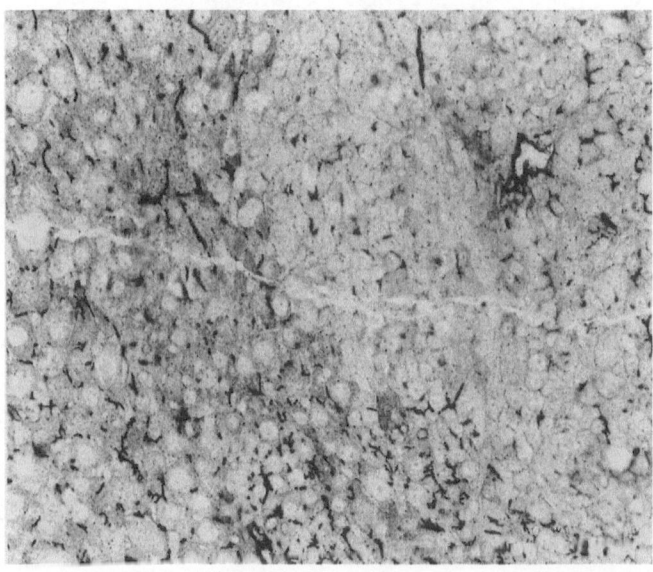

Fig. 4. ATPase-negative spontaneously occurring liver foci appeared after the occurrence of spontaneous hepatitis

(GST-P) were used as positive markers. As summarized in Table 1, the 3 negative markers (G6P, ATP, and ES) showed decreased activity in spontaneous liver lesions (Fig. 4). Thus, the decrease in activity of these enzymes in preneoplastic and neoplastic lesions seems to be a common phenotypic change in both spontaneous and chemically induced liver lesions.

On the other hand, GGT and GST-P are the most commonly used positive markers for analyzing chemically induced liver carcinogenesis. In order to examine the relation between the 2 positive markers in the spontaneous preneoplastic and neoplastic liver lesions of LEC rats, serial sections were stained for GGT, GST-P, and hematoxylin and eosin (H and E). Positive staining of GGT was observed not only in the preneoplastic

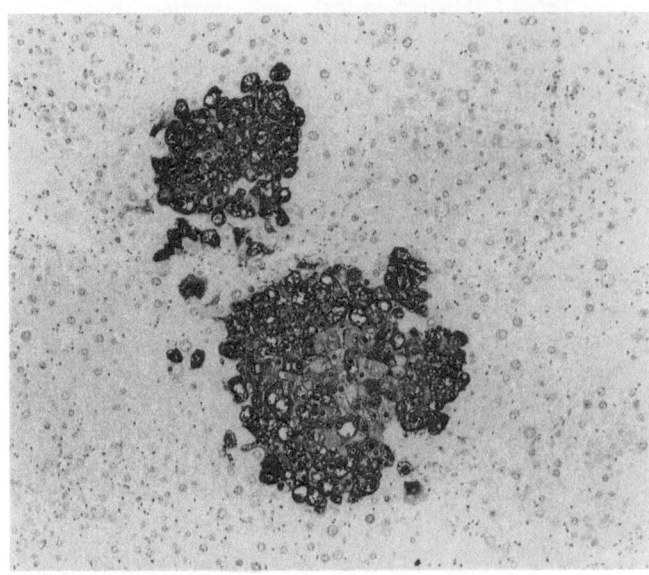

Fig. 5. GST-P-positive spontaneously occurring liver foci

Table 2. Expression of GST-P and GGT in spontaneous liver lesions of male LEC rats.

		No. of lesions examined		
		Foci(%)	*Nodules(%)*	*Carcinomas(%)*
GST-P(+)	GGT(+)	179(85.6)	36(58.1)	19(32.2)
	GGT(−)	30(14.4)	14(22.6)	20(33.9)
GST-P(−)	GGT(+)	N.D.	3(4.8)	6(10.2)
	GGT(−)	N.D.	9(14.5)	1(23.7)

N.D.: Not determined

and neoplastic lesions but also in the hepatocytes of periportal areas (zone 1). Therefore, a simple GGT staining is not suitable for estimation of the liver foci in LEC rats unless it is used in combination with other markers. In contrast to GGT, GST-P appeared to be a more reliable marker when checked by contiguous H and E-stained sections (Fig. 5). Serial section analysis on GGT positivity in GST-P-positive liver foci showed that approximately 85.6% of the GST-P-positive foci were also GGT positive in male LEC rats. However, nodules and carcinomas showed a lower percentage of GGT positivity in GST-P-positive lesions. Since nodules and carcinomas were easily identified by H and E staining, a more detailed analysis of these markers was performed on these lesions (Table 2). In male LEC rats, the majority of nodules (86%) and carcinomas (76%) were either positive for one or both of these markers. The staining diversity became more prominent in carcinomas. These results show that the phenotypic alterations in the liver lesions of LEC rats are essentially the same as those seen in chemically induced liver carcinogenesis.

Although the mechanisms of spontaneous development of HCC are still unknown, we found that the LEC rat hepatocytes were highly sensitive to the initiating effects of diethylnitrosamine compared with the control LEA and Fischer 344 rat hepatocytes [11]. This evidence leads to the possibility that hepatocytes is LEC rat liver are easily initiated by a small amount of environmental carcinogens, so that the number of initiated hepatocytes is high enough to progress to a further carcinogenic process. It has been reported that a high proliferative response to growth stimuli is an important characteristic of the hepatocytes in spontaneous liver foci [12]. In LEC rat liver, strong growth stimuli are present under the condition of continuous loss of hepatocytes in association with chronic spontaneous hepatitis. Thus, pre-existing initiated hepatocytes in LEC rat liver may preferentially respond to such growth stimuli and undergo further steps of neoplastic development. This hypothesis is also supported by the results of incidence analyses of liver lesions which indicate an intimate correlation between the occurrence of hepatitis and the development of liver lesions.

Acknowledgments. We thank Ms. K. Kagami and Ms. N. Kawano for their careful breeding of LEC rats. This work was supported by a Grant-in-Aid for Scientific Research from the Ministry of Education, Science and Culture and the Ministry of Health and Welfare, Japan.

References

1. Masuda R, Yoshida MC, Sasaki M, Dempo K, Mori M (1988) High susceptibility to hepatocellular carcinoma development in LEC rats with hereditary hepatitis. Jpn J Cancer Res (Gann) 79:828–835
2. Enomoto K, Takahashi H, Sawaki M, Sawada N, Ikeda T, Hattori A, Mori M (1989) High incidence of spontaneous hepatocellular carcinoma in a new mutant rat of hereditary hepatitis. Proc Am Assoc Cancer Res 30:194
3. Ogawa K, Solt D, Farber E (1980) Phenotypic diversity as an early property of putative preneoplastic hepatocyte populations in liver carcinogenesis. Cancer Res 40:725–733
4. Enomoto K, Ying TS, Griffin M, Farber E (1981) Immunohistochemical study of epoxide hydrolase during experimental liver carcinogenesis. Cancer Res 41:3281–3287
5. Rous P, Kidd JG (1941) Conditional neoplasms and subthreshold neoplastic states: A study of the tar tumors of rabbits. J Exp Med 73:369–390
6. Unger H, Adler JH (1978) The histogenesis of hepatoma occurring spontaneously in a strain of sand rats (Psammoncys obesus) Am J Pathol 90:399–410

7. Goodman DG, Ward JM, Squire RA, Chu KC, Linhart MS (1979) Neoplastic and nonneoplastic lesions in aging F344 rats. Toxicol Appl Pharmacol 48:237–248

8. Ward JM (1981) Morphology of foci of altered hepatocytes and naturally occurring hepatocellular tumors in F344 rats. Virchows Arch [A] 390:339–345

9. Harada T, Maronpot RR, Morris RW, Stitzel KA, Boorman GA (1989) Morphological and stereological characterization of hepatic foci of cellular alteration in control Fischer 344 rats. Toxicol Pathol 17:579–593

10. Oyamada M, Dempo K, Fujimoto Y, Takahashi H, Satoh MI, Mori M, Masuda R, Yoshida MC, Satoh K, Sato K (1988) Spontaneous occurrence of placental glutathione S-transferase-positive foci in the livers of LEC rats. Jpn J Cancer Res (Gann) 79:5–8

11. Takahashi H, Enomoto K, Nakajima Y, Mori M (1990) High sensitivity of the LEC rat liver to the carcinogenic effect of diethylnitrosamine. Cancer Lett 51:247–250

12. Schulte-Herman R, Timmerman-Trosiener I, Scuppler J (1983) Promotion of spontaneous preneoplastic cells in rat liver as a possible explanation of tumor production by nonmutagenic compounds. Cancer Res 43:830–844

33 — High Sensitivity of LEC Rats to Carcinogens Based Upon a Short-Term Carcinogenicity Assay

Yasuo Nakajima, Katsuhiko Enomoto, Hidetoshi Takahashi, Mutsomi I. Satoh, Masahito Oyamada, and Michio Mori[1]

Introduction

A high incidence of spontaneous liver tumors has been reported in the LEC rat, a new mutant strain, which has been recently established at the Center for Experimental Plants and Animals of Hokkaido University.

Our previous studies on the process of spontaneous liver cancer development in LEC rats have revealed that the concept of multistep carcinogenesis is also applicable to the spontaneous liver carcinogenesis of LEC rats [1]. The first step in chemically induced carcinogenesis, initiation, has been considered to be genetic changes in the target cells caused by DNA-carcinogen interaction. Since little is known about the initiation phase of spontaneous cancer development, in the present paper, we focused upon the initiation phase of spontaneous liver carcinogenesis in the LEC rat. We had initially examined spontaneous oncogene activation in the liver of the LEC rat, but there was no evidence of any activation of oncogenes. We now examined whether the LEC rat is sensitive to a low dose of liver carcinogen, diethylnitrosamine, using a modified Solt and Farber's selection protocol [2]. The results indicated a high sensitivity by LEC rats to the initiation effects of the chemical carcinogen. We followed this by examining whether or not the LEC rat is sensitive to the initiation effect of other chemical carcinogens. The mechanism(s) of spontaneous initiation in the LEC rat liver in relation to its high sensitivity to carcinogens and the possible application of LEC rats to the in vivo short-term assay of weak hepatocarcinogens available in the environment are discussed.

---

[1] Department of Pathology, Sapporo Medical College, Sapporo, 060 Japan

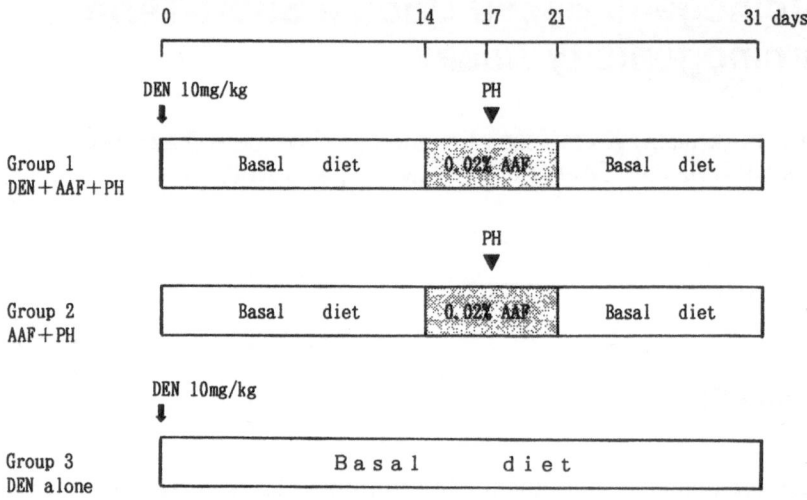

Fig. 1. Experimental protocol used in the present study are shown. Group 1 (DEN + AAF + PH), 14 days after i.p. administration of 10 mg/kg of diethylnitrosamine (DEN), rats were treated with the modified Solt-Farber protocol. After completion of the AAF diet, they were sacrificed at 31 days after initial DEN treatment. Two control groups were prepared, i.e., group 2 (AAF + PH) and group 3 (DEN alone)

Sensitivity of LEC rats to Diethylnitrosamine

Figure 1 summarizes the regimen for detecting initiated hepatocytes in the livers of LEC and LEA rats at the 8th week after birth by a modified protocol of Solt and Farber as assayed by glutathione S-transferase placental form (GST-P) positive foci. In group 1, 14 days after a single i.p. adminis-tration of 10 mg/kg diethylnitrosamine (DEN), rats were fed a diet con-taining 0.02% 2-acethylaminofluorene (AAF) for 7 days. On the 4th day of the AAF feeding, they were subjected to partial hepatectomy (PH). After completion of the AAF diet, they were placed on a basal diet for 10 days and sacrificed at 31 days after the initial DEN treatment. Initiated cells in the liver were assayed by GST-P positive foci. Two control groups were prepared, i.e., group 2 (AAF + PH) and group 3 (DEN alone) (Fig. 1).

The liver was fixed with ice-cold acetone for hematoxylin and eosin staining and immunohistochemical examination for GST-P. The GST-P-positive foci larger than 0.01 mm^2 were counted. The numbers per square centimeter of the liver specimen were measured by a Personal Image Analysis System LA-555 (PIAS, Japan).

LEC rats in group 1 showed a tenfold greater number of GST-P positive foci in the liver than LEA rats for both male and female subjects (Table 1). The average area of the focus in LEC rats was also larger than that in LEA rats. Thus, the results of the present study clearly indicated that the

Table 1. GST-P positive foci in the livers of LEC and LEA rats after selection of a modified Solt and Farber protocol.

Sex	(Group) Treatment[a]	Strain	Animals[b] (n)	Number of foci (/cm²)	Average size of foci (mm²)
Male	(1) DEN + AFF + PH	LEC	10	15.2 ± 2.2[c]	0.071 ± 0.011[c]
		LEA	11	1.4 ± 0.4	0.063 ± 0.014
	(2) AAF + PH	LEC	13	1.8 ± 0.3[c]	0.066 ± 0.017[c]
		LEA	8	0.6 ± 0.3	0.027 ± 0.001
	(3) DEN alone	LEC	14	0	0
		LEA	11	0	0
Female	(1) DEN + AFF + PH	LEC	6	19.2 ± 3.4[c]	0.047 ± 0.007[c]
		LEA	13	0.4 ± 0.1	0.036 ± 0.008
	(2) AAF + PH	LEC	11	0.7 ± 0.5[c]	0.019 ± 0.001[c]
		LEA	5	0.2 ± 0.1	0.019 ± 0.004
	(3) DEN alone	LEC	15	0	0
		LEA	15	0	0

Data are mean ± SE values
[a] Each treatment is shown in Fig. 1
[b] All of the rats were sacrificed at 12 weeks
[c] Significantly different from LEA rats at $P < 0.01$

hepatocytes of LEC rats are highly susceptible to the initiation effects of DEN, when compared with those of LEA rats.

Then, we examined whether or not such a high sensitivity of LEC rats to DEN is an age-associated phenomenon. Four- and eight-week-old LEC rats were subjected to the experimental protocol shown in Fig. 1. Age-matched Fischer 344 rats were used as control. The results clearly show that both LEC and Fischer rats at 4 weeks of age have a rather high sensitivity to DEN, and that there was no significant difference in the number of GST-P positive foci between the two strains (Table 2). However, 8-week-old Fischer rats showed a greater decrease in the number of GST-P positive foci compared with 4-week-old Fischer rats. On the other hand, 8-week-old LEC rats showed almost the same number of GST-P positive foci and thus exhibited a sixfold greater number of GST-P positive foci than those seen in Fischer rats of the same age. These results suggested that the LEC rat retains a high sensitivity to the initiation effect of DEN at least until 8 weeks after birth, whereas the control Fischer rat rapidly loses sensitivity to DEN by 8 weeks after birth, probably in accordance with the decrease in the growth activity of hepatocytes.

Although the mechanism(s) involved in such a high sensitivity to the initiation effect of DEN is not yet understood, the following possibilities should be considered. First, an altered metabolism of DEN due to alterations of the drug-metabolizing enzymes in the liver of LEC rats [3] is conceivable. Second, a reduced ability of hepatocytes to repair the DNA damages induced by DEN can also be postulated, since we recently found a reduced ability of LEC rat hepatocytes to repair the damage of DNA induced with ultraviolet light exposure. Further studies on the relation between the DNA-repairing ability and high sensitivity of the LEC rat to the initiation effects of DEN are necessary.

Sensitivity of LEC Rats to Other Carcinogens

As mentioned above, it becomes clear that 8-week-old LEC rats are highly susceptible to the initiation effects of a small dose of DEN compared with Fischer and LEC rats.

In order to explore the possibilities of application of this rat to an in vivo short-term carcinogenicity assay, we investigated the sensitivity of LEC rats to other known liver carcinogens using the modified protocol of Solt and Farber.

The carcinogens used in this study were benz(a)pyrene (BP), N-methyl-N-nitrosourea (MNU), and 2-acetylaminofluorene (AAF), which were chosen from the polycyclic aromatic hydrocarbons, N-nitroso compounds and aromatic amines, respectively. In an attempt to determine the applicability of the LEC rat for the detection of weak carcinogens, the doses used in this study were one-tenth of those reported by Tsuda et al. [4].

Table 2. Number of the GPT-P-positive foci in the livers of 4- and 8-week-old LEC and Fischer rats.

Sex	Strain	4-Week-old rats		8-Week-old rats	
		Animals (n)	Number of foci (/cm^2)	Animals (n)	Number of foci (/cm^2)
Male	LEC	11	12.6 ± 1.3	6	10.8 ± 1.4[a]
	Fischer	8	10.5 ± 2.4	12	2.7 ± 0.5[b]
Female	LEC	ND	ND	4	6.5 ± 0.5[c]
	Fischer	ND	ND	12	1.8 ± 0.5

Each value represents the mean ± SE. *ND*, not done
[a] Significantly different from male Fischer rats at $P < 0.001$
[b] Significantly different from 4-week-old Fischer rats at $P < 0.01$
[c] Significantly different from female Fischer rats at $P < 0.05$

Table 3. Number of GST-P-positive foci in the livers of 8-week-old LEC and Fischer rats treated with 3 carcinogens.

Carcinogens	Dose (mg/kg)	Route	Strain	Animals (n)	Number of foci (/cm^2)
BP[a]	20	i.p.[d]	LEC	10	2.6 ± 0.8[f]
			Fischer	12	0.3 ± 0.1
MNU[b]	10	i.p.	LEC	11	2.2 ± 0.4[f]
			Fischer	10	0.3 ± 0.1
2-AAF[c]	10	i.g.[e]	LEC	10	2.4 ± 0.5[f]
			Fischer	10	0.6 ± 0.1

Each value represents the mean ± SE
[a] *BP*, benzo (a) pyrene
[b] *MNU*, N-methyl-N-nitrosourea
[c] *2-AAF*, 2-acetylaminofluorene
[d] *i.p.*, intraperitoneally
[e] *i.g.*, intragastrically
[f] Significantly different from Fischer rats at $P < 0.01$

The results indicated that significantly higher numbers of GST-P positive foci were induced in the liver of the LEC rat than those found in control Fischer rats, indicating a high sensitivity of the LEC rat to these carcinogens (Table 3). However, the number of foci induced by these carcinogens was relatively low compared with that induced by DEN treatment. This may be because of the rather low doses of carcinogens which were administrated. The original doses employed by Tsuda et al. were at the minimal levels effective for inducing sizable numbers of enzyme-altered foci after partial hepatectomy. Kitagawa et al. [5] also showed that this low dose of BP induces enzyme-altered foci only when administered after partial hepatectomy. Thus, further experiments using different doses are necessary in order to determine the optimal doses of each carcinogen in the LEC rat.

However, the results of the present study clearly suggested the usefulness of LEC rats for in vivo short-term tests of liver carcinogens. There are several assay systems which have been developed for the detection of environmental carcinogens [6]. The long-term in vivo carcinogenicity test using rodents has been shown to be the most reliable among these systems for the prediction of carcinogenic potentials in our environment.

Recently, short-term and medium-term in vivo assay systems for liver carcinogens have been developed utilizing the modified method of Solt and Farber with Fischer rats [7]. The results of the present study suggested that the application of LEC rats in these systems might provide a more sensitive short-term in vivo assay system for the detection of environmental carcinogens.

The mechanism(s) responsible for the spontaneous development of hepatocellular carcinomas in LEC rats has not yet been fully understood. However, with respect to initiation of spontaneous liver tumor in the LEC rat liver, the data obtained in this study may lead to the conclusion that LEC rat hepatocytes are readily initiated by the weak carcinogens available in the environment. The initiated hepatocytes proliferate selectively in the presence of spontaneous chronic hepatitis and subsequently develop into hepatocellular carcinomas. Thus, LEC rats may also be utilized as a useful model for analyzing the mechanisms of initiation of liver carcinogenesis.

Acknowledgments. The authors are grateful to Ms. K. Kagami and Ms. N. Kawano for their careful breeding of rats. This work was supported in part by a Grant-in-Aid for Cancer Research from the Ministry of Health and Welfare, Japan.

References

1. Sawaki M, Enomoto K, Takahashi H, Nakajima Y, Mori M (1990) Phenotype of preneoplastic and neoplastic liver lesions during spontaneous liver carcinogenesis of LEC rats. Carcinogenesis 11:1857–1861
2. Solt D, Farber E (1976) New principle for the analysis of chemical carcinogenesis. Nature 263:701–703
3. Sugiyama T, Takeichi N, Kobayashi H, Yoshida MC, Sasaki M, Taniguchi N (1988) Metabolic predisposition of a novel mutant (LEC rats) to hereditary hepatitis and hepatoma: Alterations of the drug metabolizing enzymes. Carcinogenesis 9:1569–1578
4. Tsuda H, Lee G, Farber E (1980) Induction of resistant hepatocytes as a new principle for a possible short-term in vivo test for carcinogenesis. Cancer Res 40:1157–1164
5. Kitagawa T, Hirakawa T, Ishikawa T, Nemoto N, Takayama S (1980) Induction of hepatocellular carcinoma in rat liver by initial treatment with benzo(a)pyrene

after partial hepatectomy and promotion by phenobarbital. Toxicol Lett 6: 167–171

6. Montesano R, Bartsch H, Vainio H, Wilbourn J, Yamasaki H (eds) (1986) Long-term and short-term assays for carcinogens: A critical appraisal. IARC Scientific Publications, Lyon

7. Ito N, Tsuda H, Tatematsu M, Inoue T, Tagawa Y, Aoki T, Uwagawa S, Kagawa M, Ogiso T, Masui T, Imaida K, Fukushima S, Asamoto M (1988) Enhancing effect of various hepatocarcinogens on induction of preneoplastic glutathione S-transferase placental form positive foci in rats — an approach for a new medium-term bioassay system. Carcinogenesis 9:387–394

34 — Replicative and Unscheduled DNA Synthesis of LEC Rat Hepatocytes: Relevance to Natural Development of Hepatocellular Carcinoma

Norimasa Sawada, Hirohumi Sakamoto, Hidetoshi Takahashi, Katsuhiko Enomoto, Yumiko Oyamada, and Michio Mori[1]

Introduction

The LEC rat is a new mutant inbred strain which suddenly displays coagulative necrosis of hepatocytes at around 4 months after birth [1], for which a single autosomal recessive gene (hts gene, [2]) is responsible. Those LEC rats surviving with chronic hepatitis eventually develop hepatocellular carcinomas as they become old [1,3–5]. Since this hepatitis-hepatocellular carcinoma sequence is quite similar to the development of human liver cancer, LEC rats are expected to serve as an excellent animal model for the study of human hepatocarcinogenesis.

A rapid increase in the number and size of preneoplastic liver lesions occurs without any carcinogen treatment in LEC rats with the passage of time after the onset of hepatitis [4]. Although the mechanisms of naturally developing hepatocellular carcinomas in LEC rats are not fully understood, extremely high sensitivity of the LEC rat to chemical carcinogens has been reported [6]. Since spontaneous preneoplastic lesions rapidly develop in the liver of LEC rats, in association with continuous liver cell necrosis, the resulting generation of growth-stimulating foctors seems to be responsible for the promotion of initiated hepatocytes. The activities of biotransformation of carcinogens are low in the LEC rat due to a decrease in phase I drug-metabolizing enzymes in the liver [7], whereas the activities of detoxication remain high. Thus, we expect that the changes in the potential for replicative and unscheduled DNA synthesis might take place in the hepatocytes of the LEC rat.

Potential for Cell Proliferation of LEC Rat Hepatocytes

Cell proliferation plays an important role in carcinogenic processes and cell transformation by chemicals [8]. Both the initiative and promotive effects of chemical carcinogens are enhanced by the proliferation of

---

[1] Department of Pathology, Sapporo Medical College, Sapporo, 060 Japan

Table 1. Recovery of liver weight of LEC rats after two-thirds partial hepatectomy.

	Days after two-thirds partial hepatectomy			
	1	2	3	7
LEC, 8-week-old	1.84 ± 0.14* (n = 6)	2.60 ± 0.25 (n = 5)	3.19 ± 0.19 (n = 3)	3.41 ± 0.18 (n = 4)
LEA, 8-week-old	1.73 ± 0.07 (n = 4)	2.45 ± 0.02 (n = 3)	3.29 ± 0.24 (n = 3)	3.37 ± 0.22 (n = 4)
LEC, 25-week-old	1.26 ± 0.12 (n = 3)	1.57 ± 0.11 (n = 4)	1.95 ± 0.15 (n = 5)	1.95 ± 0.12 (n = 3)
LEA, 25-week-old	1.26 ± 0.06 (n = 3)	1.62 ± 0.03 (n = 3)	1.90 ± 0.08 (n = 5)	2.16 ± 0.11 (n = 6)

* Means of percentage of liver weight to body weight ± S.D.

Table 2. Response of LEC rat hepatocytes to EGF in primary culture.

	Labeling indexes
LEC rat hepatocytes, 8-week-old,	55.1%**
LEA rat hepatocytes, 8-week-old	53.3%
LEC rat hepatocytes, 20-week-old,	20.1%
LEA rat hepatocytes, 20-week-old	47.6%

* Primary cultures of the rat hepatocytes were treated with 10 ng EGF/ml and then incubated in BrdU-supplemented medium from the 36th h to the 72nd h after plating. After fixation and immunohistochemical staining, the labeling index was determined
** Means of triplicate

hepatocytes [9,10] experimentally induced by partial hepatectomy. In particular, hepatocytes at the S phase of the cell cycle are shown to be sensitive to carcinogens [11], and the regeneration of hepatocytes is also known to be necessary to convert reversible DNA damage to inheritable genetic alterations [12]. Thus, the continuous regeneration of hepatocytes observed in the LEC rat liver with chronic hepatitis not only exhibits promotive effects on the initiated hepatocytes, but also causes greater efficiency in the initiation of hepatocytes by chemicals.

Table 1 shows the recovery rate of liver weight in 16-week-old LEC rats after two-thirds partial hepatectomy. There was no difference in the restoration of liver weight between control (LEA) rats and LEC rats before the onset of hepatitis. On the other hand, in 25-week-old LEC rats, oval cells mainly responded to partial hepatectomy and turned into hepatocytes during the 2 weeks following partial hepatectomy, suggesting that mature hepatocytes lose their responsiveness to growth stimuli. In order to further investigate the potential of LEC rat hepatocytes for proliferation, LEC rat hepatocytes in primary culture were treated with 10 ng epidermal growth factor (EGF)/ml to induce replicative DNA synthesis. The results are summarized in Table 2. Before the onset of hepatitis, the responsiveness of LEC rat hepatocytes to EGF was almost comparable to that of the control.

On the other hand, a remarkable decrease in the responsiveness of hepatocytes isolated from 25-week-old LEC rats is demonstrated. These results revealed that, in the LEC rat liver, proliferation of hepatocytes after suffering from hepatitis was impaired, and the replacement of hepatocytes occured through oval cell proliferation and/or frequent cell division of a limited population of hepatocytes maintaining growth activity.

Potential for DNA Repair of LEC Rat Hepatocytes

Since DNA damage may result in neoplastic transformation, the potential for repairing DNA damage is an important parameter in the initiation stage of carcinogenesis [13]. Thus, in order to elucidate the potential for DNA repair of LEC rat hepatocytes, UV(254 nm)-irradiation, which induces DNA damage independently of drug-metabolizing enzymes, was carried out on primary cultured LEC rat and Fischer 344 rat hapatocytes. The results obtained from our experiments are summarized in Table 3. It shows that the level of DNA repair of hepatocytes isolated from 32-week-old LEC rats was significantly low compared with that of control rat hepatocytes, although there was no difference in the level of unscheduled DNA synthesis between 8-week-old LEC and age-matched control rat hepatocytes. These results clearly indicate that the hepatocytes of LEC rats with chronic hepatitis were more sensitive to carcinogens than the hepatocytes of LEC rat before suffering from hepatitis.

LEC rat hepatocytes were already shown to be highly sensitive to the initiative effect of diethylnitrosamine before the onset of hepatitis [6]. However, hepatocytes isolated from 8-week-old LEC rats showed a comparable level of DNA repair to that observed in the hepatocytes isolated from age-matched Fischer 344 rats. With respect to the high sensitivity of LEC rats before the onset of hepatitis, the possibility of an altered metabolism of the carcinogen might remain as an explanation.

Table 3. Measurement of potential for DNA repair of 2-h-cultured LEC rat hepatocytes by uptake of ^{3}H-thymidine into DNA after UV (254 nm)-irradiation.

	Doses of UV-irradiation (J/m^2)			
	0	0.32	1.92	9.6
LEC rats, 8-week-old, (n = 5)[a]	0	2.0 ± 0.4[b]	3.1 ± 0.5	3.5 ± 0.7
F 344 rats, 8-week-old, (n = 5)	0	1.9 ± 0.3	2.9 ± 1.0	3.0 ± 0.4
LEC rats, 32-week-old, (n = 3)	0	0.7 ± 0.1	1.3 ± 0.3	1.4 ± 0.1
F 344 rats, 32-week-old, (n = 3)	0	2.7 ± 0.5	3.9 ± 0.3	4.4 ± 0.3

[a] One experiment consists of triplicate determination
[b] CPM/mg protein $\times 10^{-3} \pm$ S.D.

Mechanisms of Natural Development of Hepatocellular Carcinomas in LEC Rats

From these findings, the following putative mechanisms in the development of spontaneous hepatocellular carcinomas in LEC rats should be considered.

Initiation Stage

During the natural course of the development of hepatocellular carcinomas in LEC rats, the number and size of preneoplastic lesions, such as enzyme-altered foci and hyperplastic nodules, increases with time after the onset of hepatitis, although the enzyme levels of LEC rats for activating carcinogens are low, even in the neonatel period, while the levels of detoxifying enzymes are relatively high. Additionally, as described above, the potentials for both replicative and unscheduled DNA synthesis of hepatocytes are significantly low in the LEC rat with chronic hepatitis. Taken together, it seems to be reasonable to consider that the process of initiation takes place after the onset of hepatitis. Furthermore, since a great majority of hepatocytes in LEC rat wich chronic hepatitis loses responsiveness to growth stimuli, a limited cell population in the liver can respond effectively to the growth stimulation endogenously induced by continuous loss of hepatocytes due to hepatitis, and therefore go through several cell cycles, thus becoming more susceptible to the initiation effects of environmental carcinogens. With regard to the kind of cells to be initiated, both oval cells (bipotential progenitor cells [14,15]) and hepatocytes possessing growth activity could be considered as candidates.

Promotion Stage

After the onset of hepatitis, loss of hepatoctyes persistently occurs during the life span of the LEC rats, resulting in the production of growth-stimulating factors to initated hepatocytes. Since the proliferative activity of a great majority of hepatocytes in LEC rats with chronic hepatitis is markedly reduced, such a growth-stimulating force is considered to act as a potent promoter for the initiated cells [9,16,17].

Conclusions

We outlined the mechanisms of natural occurrence of hapatocellular carcinomas in LEC rats from the aspects of the potentials for replicative and unscheduled DNA synthesis. We consider that most, if not all, of the process of initiation of hepatocytes occurs after the onset of hepatitis, and that the initiated cells selectively proliferate under the condition of chronic hepatitis, resulting in the development of hepatocellular carcinomas in LEC rats. Since the hepatitis-hepatocellular carcinomas sequence observed in the LEC rat is quite similar to that observed in human hepatocarcinogenesis, studies on the mechanisms of natural development of hepatocellular carcinomas in LEC rats are expected to provide us with new insights into the understanding of human liver cancer.

References

1. Yoshida MC, Masuda R, Sasaki M, Takechi N, Kobayashi H, Dempo K, Mori M (1987) New mutation causing hereditary hepatitis in the laboratory rat. J Hered 78:361–365
2. Masuda R, Yoshida MC, Sasaki M, Dempo K, Mori M (1988) Hereditary hepatitis of LEC rats is controlled by a single autosomal recessive gene. Lab Anim 22:166–169
3. Masuda R, Yoshida MC, Dempo K, Mori M (1988) High susceptibility to hepatocallular carcinoma development in LEC rats with hereditary hepatitis. Jpn J Cancer Res 79:825–835
4. Oyamada M, Dempo K, Fujimoto Y, Takahashi H, Satoh MI, Mori M, Masuda R, Yoshida MC, Satoh K, Sato K (1988) Spontaneous occurrence of placental glutathion S-transferese-positive foci in the livers of LEC rats. Jpn J Cancer Res 79:5–8
5. Sawaki M, Enomoto K, Takahashi H, Nakajima Y, Mori M (1990) Phenotype of preneoplastic and neoplastic liver lesions during spontaneous liver carcinogenesis of LEC rats. Carcinogenesis 11:1875–1861
6. Takahashi H, Enomoto K, Nakajima Y, Mori M (1990) High sensitivity of the LEC rat liver to the carcinogenic effect of diethylnitrosamine. Cancer Lett 51:247–250
7. Sugiyama T, Takeichi N, Kobayashi H, Yoshida MC, Sasaki M, Taniguchi N (1988) Metabolic predisposition of a novel mutant (LEC rats) to hereditary hepatitis and hepatomas; Alterations of the drug metabolizing enzymes. Carcinogenesis 9:1569–1572
8. Grisham JW, Kaufmann, WK, Kaufman DG (1983) The cell cycle and chemical carcinogenesis. Surv Synth Pathol Res 1:49–66
9. Farber E (1980) The sequential analysis of liver cancer induction. Biochim Biophys Acta 605:149–166
10. Pitot HC Sirica AE (1980) The stages of initiation and promotion in hepatocarcinogenesis. Biochim Biophys Acta 605:191–215
11. Craddock VM Frei JV (1974) Induction of liver cell adenomata in the rat by single treatment with N-methyl-N-nitresourea given at various times after partial hepatectomy. Br J Cancer 30:503–511
12. Ishikawa T, Takayama S, Kitagawa T (1980) Correlation between time of partial hepatectomy after a single treatment with diethylnitrosamine and induction of adenosinetriphosphatase-deficient islands in rat liver. Cancer Res 40:4261–4264
13. Setlow RB (1978) Repair deficient disorders and cancer. Nature 271:713–717
14. Grisham JW (1980) Cell types in long-term propagable cultures of rat liver. Ann NY Acad Sci 394:128–137

15. Marceau, N. (1990) Cell lineages and differentiation programs in epidermal, urothelial and hepatic tissues and their neoplasmas. Lab Invest 63:4–20
16. Ogawa K, Mukai H, Mori M (1985) Effect of aging on proliferative activity of normal and carcinogen-altered hepatocytes in rat liver after a two-thirds partial hepatectomy. Jpn J Cancer Res 76:779–784
17. Sawada N, Ishikawa T (1988) Reduction of potential for replicative but not unscheduled DNA synthesis in hepatoytes isolated from aged as compared to aging rats. Cancer Res 48:1617–1622

... o Hashimoto L, Berlin, and M. Machihara, ...

... Abrams IM, ... 19... Ion-exchange ... allied uses; ... processes K 10 and ... media ... M, ... reprint, ... K M Co., Inc., ... Lab. processes ... 3 ... and ...

Oren R, Wood, Reiner M... (1989) ... of ... on ... ... Chem. ... ... per Water, J. ...

Int. Soc. ... for [Water Sci., ... 250.

Houweling K, ... (1988) Evaluation of processes for ... ... rinsing ... in ... Water, ... for ... water ... from ... 13 ... in ... 1-... ... ... water, ... Res., 19(3) ... 257-...

3. Biochemistry

35 — Hepatoma-Associated Alterations of Serum α_1-Antitrypsin in LEC Rats

RYUICHI MASUDA[1], TOSHIHIRO SUGIYAMA[2], NAOYUKI TANIGUCHI[2], MICHIHIRO C. YOSHIDA[1], and MOTOMICHI SASAKI[3]

Introduction

LEC rats have been established as a new mutant strain which develops hereditary hepatitis [1–3] and spontaneous hepatocellular carcinomas (hepatomas) [4]. However, the mechanisms of the development of the sequential diseases in LEC rats are not yet known precisely. Hepatic cirrhosis in human infancy or early childhood is known to be associated with alpha$_1$-antitrypsin (α_1AT) deficiency [5]. In adults, α_1 AT deficiency was described in association with cirrhosis and portal fibrosis of the liver [6–8]. Furthermore, α_1AT deficiency showed a high risk for cirrhosis and primary liver cancer [9]. This deficiency indicates an autosomal recessive mode of inheritance [5,9]. Experimental rat α_1AT deficiency produced by galactosamine-treatment was characterized previously [10,11]. However, the relation between rat α_1AT and liver disease has not been reported, although rat α_1AT is known to be a glycoprotein which acts as a liver protease inhibitor in plasma and to have several forms produced by sialylation in parental molecules [12–14]. Therefore, our interest was focused on the α_1AT of LEC rats which develop hereditary hapatitis and liver cancer. In this study, characteristics of serum α_1AT in LEC rats are described.

Quantitation of Serum α_1 AT in LEC Rats

For the immunological quantitation of serum α_1AT, anti-rat α_1AT serum was obtained from a rabbit immunized with α_1AT purified from the plasma of Wistar strain rat [15]. Using this anti-rat α_1AT serum, the serum α_1AT concentration in LEC rats at different stages of hepatic lesions was measured by the method of Mancini et al. [16]. The results were compared

[1] Chromosome Research Unit, Faculty of Science, Hokkaido University, Sapporo, 060 Japan
[2] Department of Biochemistry, Osaka University Medical School, Suita, Osaka, 530 Japan
[3] Sasaki Cancer Institute, Chiyoda-ku, Tokyo, 101 Japan

Table 1. Serum α_1AT level in LEC and LEA rats by immunodiffusion method. (Modified from [15] with permission).

Age of LEC rats (hepatic condition)	α_1AT Level (mg/100 ml) Mean ± SE		Age of LEA rats (hepatic condition)
	LEC	LEA	
2 Months (Normal)	288 ± 18 (95%)[a] (n = 4)	304 ± 17 (n = 4)	2 Months (Normal)
4 Months (Hepatitis)	320 ± 11[b] (86%) (n = 7)	370 ± 18 (n = 6)	4 Months (Normal)
Over 12 months (Hepatoma)	391 ± 33 (123%) (n = 6)	318 ± 11 (n = 6)	12 Months (Normal)

n, tested number
[a] Percentage to the value of age-matched LEA rats
[b] Statistically significant compared with age-matched LEA rats ($P < 0.05$, t-test)

with age-matched LEA rats which did not show any hepatic lesion [15] (Table 1). The level of α_1AT in LEC rats at 4 months of age (hepatitis) was significantly reduced to a level 86% of that in LEA rats ($P < 0.05$). Although quantitative analysis of rat serum α_1AT has not been reported, the values of serum α_1AT in normal human are reported between 160 and 350 mg/100 ml of serum and differ in various laboratories because of variations in available standards [17]. No significant difference was observed between LEC and LEA rats at 2 months of age and between hepatoma-bearing LEC rats and 12-month-old LEA rats.

Trypsin Inhibitory Capacity of Serum in LEC Rats

Trypsin inhibitory capacities of serum from LEC rats at different stages of hepatic lesions were assayed compared with those of age-matched LEA rats [15] (Table 2). No significant difference was observed between the levels of LEC and LEA rats at 2 months of age. The level of hepatitis rats at 4 months of age was significantly reduced to a level 83% of that of LEA rats ($P < 0.005$). Hepatoma-bearing rats showed significantly higher levels (118%) than LEA rats ($P < 0.005$). Although enzymatic analysis of rat serum α_1AT has not been reported, trypsin inhibitory capacities in normal human serum are between 2.1 and 3.8 µmol/min per ml [17]. In human α_1AT deficiency, the level is 10%–60% of the normal value. Serum α_1AT levels of LEC rats before and after the onset of hepatitis are almost within the normal range of human data. Although changes of serum α_1AT levels were observed in hepatitis and hepatoma-bearing LEC rats, they seem to be one of the biochemical reactions to hepatic disorders as reported in normal human subjects with acute or chronic liver diseases [18,19]. LEC rats did not show emphysema which tends to develop in the lung of human α_1AT deficiency. The present results indicate that no correlation was found between hepatic lesions of LEC rats and α_1AT deficiency.

Table 2. Serum trypsin inhibitory capacity in LEC and LEA rats by enzymatic method (Modified from [15] with permission).

Age of LEC rats (hepatic condition)	Trypsin inhibitory capacity (μmol/min/ml) Mean ± SE		Age of LEA rats (hepatic condition)
	LEC	LEA	
2 Months (Normal)	3.7 ± 0.1 (97%)[a] ($n = 4$)	3.8 ± 0.1 ($n = 4$)	2 Months (Normal)
4 Months (Hepatitis)	3.0 ± 0.1[b] (83%) ($n = 7$)	3.6 ± 0.1 ($n = 6$)	4 Months (Normal)
Over 12 months (Hepatoma)	3.9 ± 0.1[c] (118%) ($n = 6$)	3.3 ± 0.1 ($n = 6$)	12 Months (Normal)

n, tested number
[a] Percentage to the value of age-matched LEA rats
[b,c] Statistically significant as compared with age-matched LEA rats ($P < 0.005$, t-test)

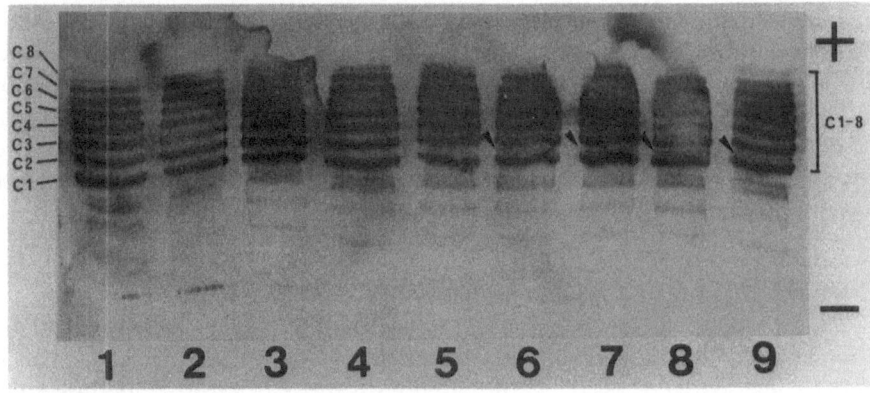

Fig. 1. Separation of hepatitis rat serum α_1AT by isoelectric focusing with ampholyte of pH 4–5, followed by immunoblotting. *Bands C_{1-8}* are separated bands of α_1AT. Each sample was 10 μl of serum. *Lane 1*, 2-month-old LEA rat; *2*, 2-month-old LEC rat; *3–9*, fulminant hepatitis LEC rats with severe jaundice at the age of 4 months. In each of lanes *6–9*, a very faint band is seen between C_1 and C_2 (*arrows*). (From [15] with permission)

Heterogeneity of Serum α_1AT in Hepatoma-Bearing LEC Rats

Serum α_1AT was clearly separated on a gel after isoelectric focusing with ampholyte [15] (Fig. 1). The α_1AT of 2-month-old LEC rats, which had not yet developed hepatitis consisted of eight common bands (C_{1-8}, in the order from basic to acidic band) (Fig. 1, *lane 2*). The α_1AT of age-matched LEA also had bands C_{1-8}, of which C_8 was very weak (Fig. 1, *lane 1*). In LEC rats with fulminant hepatitis (Fig. 1, *lanes 3–9*), the α_1AT types

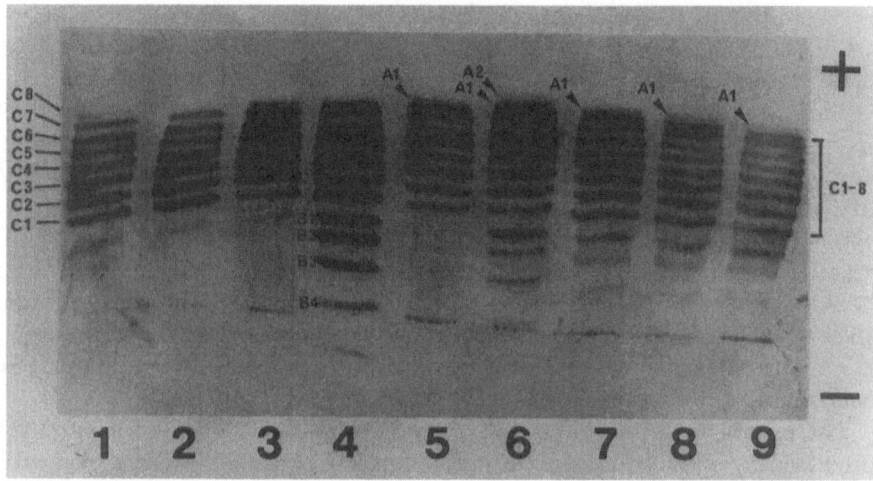

Fig. 2. Separation of hepatoma-bearing rat serum α₁AT by isoelectric focusing with ampholyte of pH 4–5, followed by immunoblotting. *Bands C₁₋₈* correspond to those of Fig. 1. *A₁* and *A₂* are more acidic forms and *B₁₋₄* are more basic forms of α₁AT. Each sample was 10 μl of serum. *Lane 1*, 2-month-old LEA rat; *2*, 12-month-old LEA rat; *3*, 2-month-old LEC rat; *4–9*, hepatoma-bearing LEC rats at the age of over 12 months. (From [15] with permission)

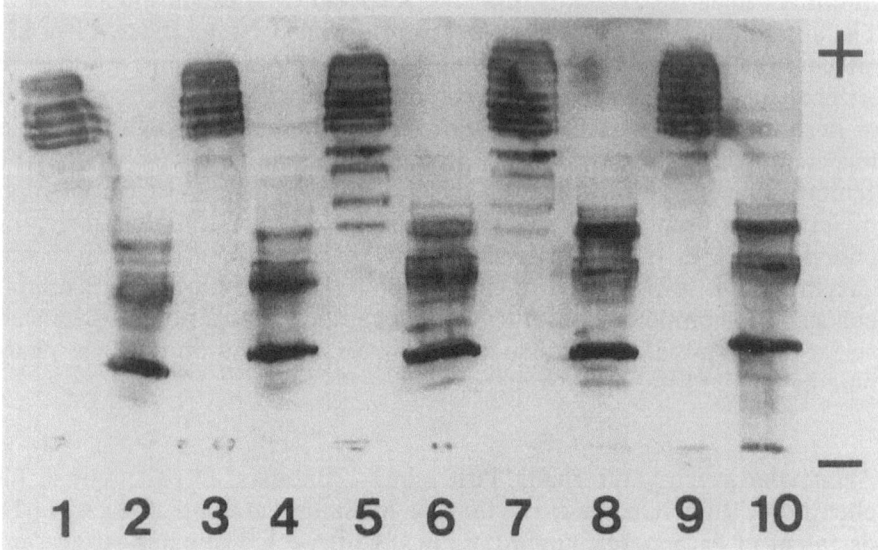

Fig. 3. Separation of rat serum α₁AT by isoelectric focusing with ampholyte of pH 4–6.5, followed by immunoblotting. Each sample of *lanes 1, 3, 5, 7*, and *9* was 10 μl of serum. Each sample of *lanes 2, 4, 6, 8*, and *10* was 5 μl neuraminidase-treated serum. *Lanes 1 and 2*, 2-month-old LEA rats; *3 and 4*, 2-month-old LEC rats, *5–10* hepatoma-bearing LEC rats at the age of over 12 months. (From [15] with permission)

were similar to that of 2-month-old LEC rats, except for the appearance of a very faint band between C_1 and C_2 (Fig. 1, *lanes 6–9*). By contrast, the α_1AT of hepatoma-bearing LEC rats was composed of more acidic bands (A_1 and A_2) and from one to four more basic bands (B_{1-4}) in addition to C_{1-8} (Fig. 2, *lanes 4–9*). A_1 was detected in five out of six animals, and faint A_2 was detected only in one of them. There were variations of A_1 intensity and B_{1-4} patterns among hepatoma-bearing rats. Very faint B_{1-4} bands were also seen in sera of 2-month-old hepatitis LEC rats and in LEA rats. Thus, A_1, A_2, and strong B_{1-4} bands were characteristics of α_1AT in hepatoma-bearing LEC rats. The α_1AT of sera treated with neuraminidase showed one main band and several minor bands in isoelectric focusing (Fig. 3). A similar pattern was observed among 2-month-old and hepatoma-bearing LEC rats and in control LEA rats.

The present results indicate that the heterogeneity of α_1AT seems to be produced by sialylation in α_1AT molecules. At least five forms of purified rat plasma α_1AT were reported by several investigators [12–14]. Among them, Ikehara et al. [13] proposed that native α_1AT forms are produced by sialylation in three parental forms. According to the degree of sialylation of the three parental forms, main five and minor two forms are arranged in order from the basic to the acidic ones. In the present study, the main eight bands (C_{1-8}) were detected as common forms of α_1AT in LEC rats, and two more acidic (A_1 and A_2) and four more basic (B_{1-4}) forms as strong bands in hepatoma-bearing LEC rats. These additional forms were not observed in fulminant hepatitis LEC rats. LEA rats also had C_{1-7} bands and a weak C_8. The difference in the number of detectable forms between the α_1AT of LEC rats and the purified α_1AT reported by Ikehara et al. [13] may be due to the different degree of sialylation of parental forms. The α_1AT heterogeneity of hepatoma-bearing LEC rats seems to be produced by high sialylation in parental forms during hepatocarcinogenesis, showing unchanged antigenicity of α_1AT molecules. Cancer-associated changes in carbohydrate moieties of glycoprotein have been extensively studied. Sialylation, phosphorylation, and other post-translational modifications occur in several enzymes [20]. Among them, sialylation is one of the most common changes. As commonly observed in glycoproteins, variations in the sialic acid content provide an adequate explanation for the presence of charge heterogeneity of the α_1AT molecule.

Acknowledgments. We thank Professor H. Sinohara, Department of Biochemistry, Kinki University School of Medicine, and Dr. K. Dempo, Department of Pathology, Sapporo Medical College, for valuable suggestions. R.M. was a recipient of a Fellowship for Japanese Junior Scientists from the Japan Society for the Promotion of Science. This work was supported in part by Grants-in-Aid for Cancer Research from the Ministry of Education, Science and Culture of Japan.

References

1. Sasaki M, Yoshida MC, Kagami K, Takeichi N, Kobayashi H, Dempo K, Mori M (1985) Spontaneous hepatitis in an inbred strain of Long-Evans rats. Rat News Lett 14:4–6
2. Yoshida MC, Masuda R, Sasaki M, Takeichi N, Kobayashi H, Dempo K, Mori M (1987) New mutation causing hereditary hepatitis in the laboratory rat. J Hered 78:361–365
3. Masuda R, Yoshida MC, Sasaki M, Dempo K, Mori M (1988) Hereditary hepatitis of LEC rats is controlled by a single autosomal recessive gene. Lab Anim 22:166–169
4. Masuda R, Yoshida MC, Sasaki M, Dempo K, Mori M (1988) High susceptibility to hepatocellular carcinoma development in LEC rats with hereditary hepatitis. Jpn J Cancer Res 79:828–835
5. Sharp HL, Bridges RA, Krivit W, Freier EF (1969) Cirrhosis associated with alpha-1-antitrypsin deficiency: A previously unrecognized inherited disorder. J Lab Clin Med 73:934–939
6. Berg NO, Eriksson S (1972) Liver disease in adults with alpha$_1$-antitrypsin deficiency. New Engl J Med 287:1264–1267
7. Cohen KL, Rubin PE, Echevarria RA, Sharp HL, Teague PO (1973) Alpha-1 antitrypsin deficiency, emphysema, and cirrhosis in an adult. Ann Intern Med 78:227–232
8. Palmer PE, Wolfe HJ, Gherardi GJ (1973) Hepatic changes in adult α_1-antitrypsin deficiency. Gastroenterology 65:284–293
9. Eriksson S, Carlson J, Velez R (1986) Risk of cirrhosis and primary liver cancer in alpha$_1$-antitrypsin deficiency. New Engl J Med 314:736–739
10. Bolmer S, Kleinerman J (1984) Serum glycoproteins in galactosamine-induced alpha$_1$-antiprotease deficiency. Am Rev Respir Dis 129:A307
11. Bolmer S, Kleinerman J (1986) Isolation and characterization of α_1-antitrypsin in PAS-positive hepatic granules from rats with experimental α_1-antitrypsin deficiency. Am J Pathol 123:377–389
12. Takahara H, Nakayama H, Sinohara H (1980) Purification and characterization of rat plasma α-1-antitrypsin. J Biochem 88:417–424
13. Ikehara Y, Miyasato M, Ogata S, Oda K (1981) Multiple forms of rat-serum α_1-protease inhibitor: Involvement of sialic acid in the multiplicity of three original forms. Eur J Biochem 115:253–260
14. Roll DE, Glew RH (1981) Isolation and characterization of rat α-1-antitrypsin. J Biol Chem 256:8190–8196
15. Masuda R, Sugiyama T, Taniguchi N, Yoshida MC, Sasaki M (1988) Hepatoma-associated alterations of serum α_1-antitrypsin in hereditary hepatitis LEC rats as a new animal model of liver disease. Int J Biochem 20:1171–1176
16. Mancini G, Carbonara AO, Heremans JF (1965) Immunochemical quantitation of antigens by single radical immunodifusion. Immunochemistry 2:235–254
17. Dietz AA, Rubinstein HM, Hodges L (1974) Measurement of alpha$_1$-antitrypsin in serum, by immunodiffusion and by enzymatic assay. Clin Chem 20:396–399
18. Fagerhol MK, Laurell CB (1970) The Pi system — inherited variants of serum α_1-antitrypsin. Prog Med Genet 7:96–111

19. Meliconi R, Parracino O, Facchini A, Morselli-Labate AM, Bortolotti F, Tremolada F, Martuzzi M, Miglio F, Gasbarrini G (1988) Acute phase proteins in chronic and malignant liver diseases. Liver 8:65–74
20. Makita A, Gasa S, Narita M, Fujita M, Taniguchi N (1983) Alterations of lysosomal hydrolases in human lung cancer. Jpn J Cancer Res 29 (monogram):231–240

36 — High Expression of Hexokinase Isozyme B During Hepatocarcinogenesis in LEC Rats

SADHANA JAIN, SURESH K. JAIN[2], TOSHIHIRO SUGIYAMA, and NAOYUKI TANIGUCHI[1]

Introduction

In rat liver, the phosphorylation of glucose by ATP is catalyzed by two distinct enzymes, glucokinase (GK) and hexokinase (HK). HK has high affinity for glucose (the K_m value is below 0.5 mM) and GK has low affinity for glucose (an apparent K_m value of 100 mM). The enzyme HK is known to consist of three isozymes (A, B, and C) separable from each other and from GK by starch gel electrophoresis [1–3] and by chromatography on DEAE-cellulose [2,4,5]. In normal tissues, the distribution of isozymes of HK is variable and depends upon glucose utilization [5,6].

Physiologically, the activity of liver GK is influenced by fasting and diabetic conditions and also by insulin, while HK remains unaltered [7,8]. However, the activity of HK is markedly enhanced in livers bearing tumors with a simultaneous decrease in GK [9–11]. Recent studies on pre-neoplastic lesions of rat liver indicate that most of the activity of the glucose phosphorylation enzyme is contributed by the B isozyme of HK [12]. Parry and Pedersen [13] have similarly shown high activity of HK and absence of GK in Novikoff ascites cells. Increased levels of B isozymes of HK are also observed in fetal liver [14]. It is postulated that HK may be used as an indicator of the early stages of liver carcinogenesis [12]. However, no data is available regarding the age-related distribution of different isozymes of HK and their expression during the various stages of hepatocarcinogenesis. The aim of this study was to provide information on the potential role of HK B in liver carcinogenesis. We have analyzed different pathological stages during the progression of hepatocarcinogenesis in LEC rats representing important steps in liver cell transformation [15–17].

[1] Department of Biochemistry, Osaka University Medical School, Suita, Osaka, 565 Japan,
[2] Department of Molecular Pharmacology, Albert Einstein College of Medicine, Bronx, NY 10461, USA

In the present study we report the age-related isozymic pattern of HK and the expression of mRNAs for GK and HK during the progression of hepatitis and hepatoma in LEC rats.

Activity of Glucose-ATP Phosphorylating Enzyme in LEC Rats

Table 1 shows mean activity of HK, GK, and glucose-ATP phosphorylating enzymes during the different stages of hepatocarcinogenesis including hepatitis in LEC rats. The activity of total glucose-ATP phosphorylating enzymes increased from three- to sevenfold at the time of hepatoma and during the benign stages of liver pathogenesis in LEC rats. The LEC rats are known to develop spontaneous hepatitis at around 16 weeks of age and advance chronic hepatitis at around 20 weeks of age which is followed by hepatoma in survivors. The highest activity of HK is seen during chronic hepatitis (20 weeks), when compared to the other stages during the progression of hepatocarcinogenesis.

The activities of GK and HK are maintained almost at a constant level up to 52 weeks of age in normal LEA rats. However, in the case of 10-week-old LEC rats, the HK activity is less than that in corresponding LEA rats and this is associated with a simultaneous increase in the activity of GK. Apparently, at 10 weeks of age, HK activity in LEC rats is similar to that of LEA rats. This is also true with several other biochemical markers such as Mn-superoxide dismutase, γ-glutamyl transpeptidase and P-450 in LEC rats [17]. Enzyme profiles in hepatocarcinoma showed a general tendency toward approaching the undifferentiated patterns in LEC rats.

Distribution of HK Isozymes in LEC Rats

The isozymes of HK were separated by high-pressure liquid chromatography (HPLC) using a DEAE-cellulose (diethylaminoethyl-cellulose) column from the livers of LEA and LEC rats at different time intervals and identified as A, B, and C by their differential velocities at low (0.5 mM) or a high (100 mM) glucose concentrations in parallel assays. High glucose/low glucose activity ratios are typically 1.0, 1.3, and 0.5 for HK A, B, and C, respectively. In purified fractions, we observed that the total HK activity is contributed by isozyme A in LEA rats (Table 2) and the presence of isozymes B and C at different stages during the progression of hepatocarcinogenesis in LEC rats. The appearance of HK B is a characteristic of hepatocarcinoma, however, HK B is detectable in LEC rats as early as 4 weeks of age. Activities of HK A and C could not be detected during the advanced chronic hepatitis (20 weeks) and hepatocarcinoma (52 weeks) in LEC rats. The levels of HK B activity during chronic hepatitis and

Table 1. Age-dependent GK and HK activities (units/gm protein) in livers of LEA and LEC rats

Age (Weeks)	Total glucose-ATP phosphotransferase		HK		GK	
	LEA	LEC	LEA	LEC	LEA	LEC
4	5.1	16.8	5.1	16.8	ND	ND
10	7.3	8.8	7.0	5.6	0.27	3.2
16	4.8	20.7	3.9	17.7	0.93	3.0
20	5.6	33.0	4.2	31.0	1.4	2.0
52	8.0	14.6	7.3	12.9	0.67	1.7

Each value is the mean of three experiments. *ND*, not detectable

Table 2. Enzyme activities (units/gm protein) of major HK isozymes recovered after HPLC fractionation in livers of LEA and LEC rats

Age (Weeks)	LEA HK Isozymes			LEC HK Isozymes		
	A	B	C	A	B	C
	(Units/g protein)			(Units/g protein)		
4	17.9	ND	ND	27.7	13.5	5.1
10	16.0	ND	ND	14.2	5.7	Trace
16	5.7	ND	ND	31.4	12.6	5.9
20	11.2	ND	ND	ND	49.2	Trace
52	10.7	ND	ND	ND	38.9	ND

Each value is the mean of three experiments. *ND*, not detectable

hepatoma increased from three- to ninefold compared to asymptomatic livers in LEC rats (Table 2).

Expression of GK and HK Messenger RNAs During Spontaneous Hepatocarcinogenesis in LEC Rats

We have analyzed the GK and HK mRNA levels in liver samples from different age groups of LEA and LEC rats. Typical mRNA levels after Northern blotting are shown in Fig. 1. Prominent components of 2.5 and 2.4 kb for HK and GK, respectively, are present in all age groups of LEA and LEC rats. Hybridization with HK cDNA showed a progressive increase of mRNA at the onset of hepatitis and during chronic hepatitis and hepatoma, with a concomitant decrease in the levels of GK message in LEC rats (Fig. 1, *lanes 1–8*). In normal rats, the major activity of liver glucose-ATP phosphorylating enzyme is contributed through GK. Our results (Fig. 1, *lanes 9–14*) from normal LEA rats indicated constant levels

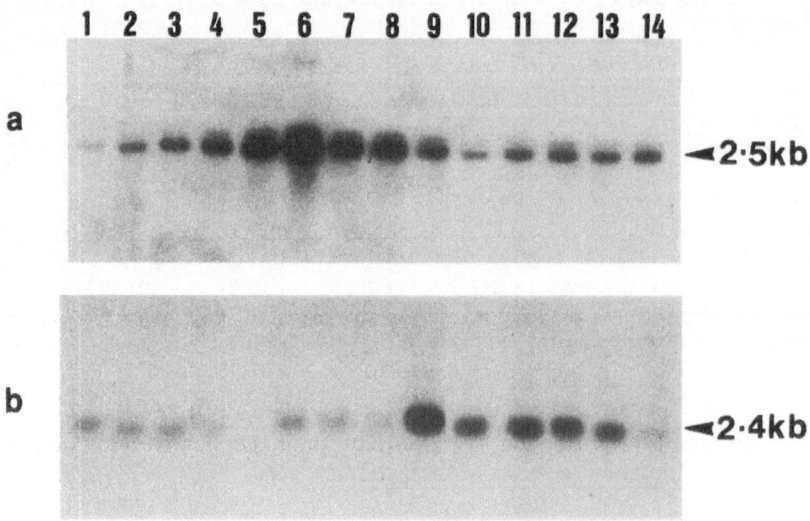

Fig. 1. a Alterations in the expression of mRNAs of HK and **b** GK during the progression of hepatocarcinogenesis in the livers of LEC and LEA rats. *Lanes 1–8* contain poly (A$^+$) RNA from livers of LEC rats at 1, 4, 8, 12, 16, 20, 32, and 52 weeks of age, respectively and *lanes 9–14* contain poly (A$^+$) RNA from livers of LEA rats at 4, 8, 16, 20, 32, and 52 weeks of age, respectively

of GK and HK mRNAs through 1–52 weeks of age. However, on densitometeric quantitation of autoradiograms after normalization with β actin message, the mRNA levels for GK were found to be from eight- to tenfold higher than HK. The expression patterns of HK and GK mRNA, in fact, represent a mirror image of each other in LEA and LEC rats.

Conclusions and Perspectives

It is well known that liver specific isozymes, e.g., GK and pyruvate kinase (PK), are decreased during the later stages of hepatocarcinoma [18,19]. The present study, however, demonstrated that the decrease in the liver-specific enzyme GK was initiated even at the early stages and continued throughout the further steps of carcinogenesis.

The distribution and expression of HK isozymes during hepatocarcinogenesis were examined in the genetically predisposed LEC rats. We found increased activity of low K_m hexokinase in the livers of LEC rats at the onset of hepatitis and during advanced chronic hepatitis and hepatoma, with a concomitant decrease in the activity of high K_m GK. We have also purified the different isozymes of HK at different stages during the progression of hepatocarcinogenesis using reverse phase HPLC, and noted the appearance of B isozyme in LEC rats at 4 weeks of age. Our HPLC data indicate that 90% of the activity of glucose-ATP phosphorylating enzyme is contributed through HK B during advanced chronic hepatitis and hepatoma in LEC rats. We demonstrated a parallel increase in the levels of HK mRNA during hepatocarcinogenesis with a simultaneous decrease in the level of GK mRNA on Northern blotting analysis. From the present data, however, it appears that the increased enzyme activity is a result of increased transcription of the HK gene. In recent studies [5,10] it was suggested that all hexokinases, including glucokinase, may be products of a single gene. It would, therefore, be interesting to explore the possible mechanism of the turning on or off of the products of hexokinase gene during the progression of carcinogenesis. Regardless of the still unknown mecnanism for the activation of HK gene, our results confirm a shift in the carbohydrate metabolism from gluconeogenesis to glucose utilization and a pentose-phosphate pathway for the biosynthesis of nucleic acids. Our data suggest that HK may be used along with other oncofetal markers as an indicator of the early stages of liver carcinogenesis.

Acknowledgments. This work was supported by Grants-in-Aid for Cancer Research from the Ministries of Education, Science and Culture, and of Health and Welfare, Japan. We thank Dr. Tamio Noguchi Osaka University Medical School for providing us plasmids containing cDNA probes for GK, HK, and β-actin.

S.K.J. thankfully acknowledges the Ministry of Education, Science and Culture, Japan for providing a Monbusho Scholarship during the tenure of this work.

References

1. Shatton JB, Morris HP, Weinhouse S (1969) Kinetic, electrophoretic and chromatographic studies on glucose-ATP phosphotransferase in rat hepatoma. Cancer Res 29:1161–1171
2. McLean P, Brown J (1966) Some properties of rat liver glucose-adenosine triphosphate phosphotransferase. Biochem J 100:793–800
3. Katzen HM, Schimke RT (1965) Multiple forms of hexokinase in rat: Tissue distribution, age dependency and properties. Proc Natl Acad Sci USA 54: 1218–1225
4. Stocchi B, Magnani M, Novelli G, Dacha M, Fornaini G (1983) Pig red blood cell hexokinase: Evidence for the presence of hexokinase types I and II and their purification and characterization. Arch Biochem Biophys 226:365–376
5. Radojkovic J, Reta T (1987) Hexokinase isozymes from Novikoff hepatoma. Biochem J 242:895–903
6. Ballard FJ, Oliver IT (1964) The effect of concentration on glucose phosphorylation and incorporation into glycogen in the livers of rats and sheep. Biochem J 92:131–136

7. Iynedjian PB, Pilot PR, Nouspikel T, Milburn JL, Quade C, Hughes S, Ucla C, Newgard CB (1989) Differential expression and regulation of the glucokinase gene in liver and islets of Langerhans. Proc Natl Acad Sci USA 86:7837–7842

8. Matschinsky FM (1990) Glucokinase on glucose sensor and metabolic signal generator in pancreatic beta-cells and hepatocytes. Diabetes 39:647–652

9. Taketa K, Shimamura J, Ueda M, Shimada Y, Kosada K (1988) Profiles of carbohydrate-metabolizing enzymes in human hepatocellular carcinomas and preneoplastic liver. Cancer Res 48:467–474

10. Arora KK, Fanciulli M, Pedersen PL (1990) Glucose phosphorylation in tumor cells: Cloning, sequencing and overexpression in active from of a full-length cDNA encoding a mitochondrial bindable form of hexokinase. J Biol Chem 265:6481–6488

11. Kabir F, Nelson BD (1989) Synthesis and targeting of hexokinase to mitochondria in hepatoma cells. Arch Biochem Biophys 274:94–99

12. Fischer G, Ruschenburg I, Eigenbrodt E, Katz N (1987) Decrease in glucokinase and glucose-6-phosphatase and increase in hexokinase in putative preneoplastic lesions of rat liver. J Cancer Res Clin Oncol 113:430–436

13. Parry DM, Pedersen PL (1983) Intracellular localization and properties of particulate hexokinase in the Novikoff ascites tumor. J Biol Chem 258:10904–10912

14. Wako Y, Suzuki K, Isobe A, Kimura S (1989) Increased hexokinase activity in fetuses of rats developed under maternal hyperglycemia. Tohoku J Exp Med 159:139–145

15. Yoshida MC, Masuda R, Sasaki M, Takeichi N, Kobayashi H, Dempo K, Mori M (1987) new mutation causing hereditary hepatitis in laboratory rat. J Hered 78:361–365

16. Masuda R, Sugiyama T, Taniguchi N, Yoshida MC, Sasaki M (1988) Hepatoma-associated alterations of serum α_1-antitrypsin in hereditary hepatitis LEC rats as a new animal model of liver disease. Int J Biochem 20:1171–1176

17. Sugiyama T, Takeichi N, Kobayashi H, Yoshida MC, Sasaki N, Taniguchi N (1988) Metabolic predisposition of a novel mutant (LEC rats) to hereditary hepatitis and hepatoma: Alterations of the drug metabolizing enzymes. Carcinogenesis 9:1569–1572

18. Lawrence GM, Beesley AC, Jepson MA, Waleker DG (1989) Thioacetamide-induced changes in hepatic hexokinase isozymes. Toxicology 58:21–31

19. Chien CT, Tauler A, Lange AJ, Chan K, Printz RL, el-Maghrabi MR, Granner DK, Pilkis SJ (1988) Expression of rat hepatic glucokinase in Escherichia coli. Biochem Biophys Res Commun 165:817–825

37 — Chromosomal Mapping of the Placental Glutathione S-Transferase Gene and Its Expression in Livers of LEC Rats

Ryuichi Masuda[1], Michihiro C. Yoshida[1], and Motomichi Sasaki[2]

Introduction

The LEC strain rat is a new mutant which suddenly suffers from fulminant hepatitis at about 4 months of age [1,2]. A crossing test of LEC rats showed that the hepatitis has an autosomal recessive mode of inheritance ruled by a single gene designated *hts* [3]. About 30% of the animals died of the disease within 1 week after onset. The remaining 70% survived with chronic hepatitis for more than 1 year and developed well-differentiated hepatocellular carcinomas (hepatomas) together with cholangiofibrosis at a remarkably high incidence [4]. Therefore, it is important to clarify what are the characteristics of hepatic lesions in LEC rats.

Recently, placental glutathione S-transferase (GST-P) became well-known as a new marker enzyme of preneoplastic lesions of rat chemical hepatocarcinogenesis [5–8]. Sugioka et al. [9] cloned a cDNA (pGP5) of rat GST-P from a cDNA library prepared from poly(A)$^+$ RNA of 2-acetylaminofluorene-induced rat hepatoma by screening with synthetic DNA probes designed on the basis of a partial amino acid sequence of a GST-P subunit. The rat GST-P gene was found to be about three kilobase (kb) pairs long and contained seven exons and six introns [10]. Previous reports indicated that GST-P was induced at a very high frequency (almost 100%) and was constitutively expressed in hyperplastic nodules and hepatoma caused by carcinogenic treatment, although this enzyme was rarely detected in normal hepatocytes. The mechanism of activation of the GST-P gene during rat chemical hepatocarcinogenesis is not known, but Northern blotting analysis suggested that GST-P gene expression is regulated for the most part at the transcriptional level [9]. A previous immunohistochemical analysis showed that GST-P-positive foci appeared in livers of LEC rats at the age of 5 months, that is, after the onset of

[1] Chromosome Research Unit, Faculty of Science, Hokkaido University, Sapporo, 060 Japan
[2] Sasaki Cancer Institute, Chiyoda-ku, Tokyo, 101 Japan

341

age, suggesting that the occurrence of foci may be related to spontaneous development of hepatoma [11]. Therefore, it is worthwhile to further investigate the GST-P expression at the molecular level in serial stages of hepatic lesions of LEC rats.

In this study, in order to better understand genomic organization of the rat GST-P gene, we first assigned its gene locus using the chromosomal *in situ* hybridization method. Next, the GST-P gene expression through normal hepatocytes to hepatitis and subsequent lesions in LEC rats was examined with Northern blotting analysis.

Chromosomal Assignment of RAT GST-P Gene by *In Situ* Hybridization

One of the unique intron fragments, the 0.6 kb *SmaI-SmaI* fragment in the fifth intron of a rat GST-P genomic clone [10], was used as a probe of chromosomal *in situ* hybridization [12], because some processed-type pseudogenes of GST-P were known in the rat genome [10]. Chromosomal *in situ* hybridization with the ^{3}H-labeled probe resulted in specific labeling of rat chromosome 1 [12] (Fig. 1). Of the 58 metaphases examined, 24 metaphases (41%) had silver grains on the long arm of chromosome 1. An example of grain localization is shown in Fig. 2. Of a total of 94 grains, 14 (15%) were clustered on the portion 1q43-q51 with most grains at 1q43 (Fig. 3). This result indicates that the GST-P gene is located on the band q43 of rat chromosome 1.

Expression of GST-P Gene in Hepatic Lesions of LEC Rats

Liver tissues were obtained from LEC rats with various hepatic lesions and from LEA rats as controls (Table 1). These two inbred strains, LEC and LEA, are maintained at the Center for Experimental Plants and Animals of Hokkaido University [1,2]. A histopathological description of these hepatic lesions in LEC rats was given in our previous reports [2,4]. A transplantable LSH206G cell line derived from spontaneous hepatoma of an LEC rat [13] was also examined. Total RNAs purified from the above tissues were examined by Northern blotting using a ^{32}P-labeled cDNA pGP5 probe of rat GST-P. The results showed a single signal of GST-P of about 0.8 kb with different expression levels among hepatic lesions [14] (Fig. 4). The signals were densitometrically scanned to quantify the relative levels of GST-P expression in different hepatic lesions (Fig. 5). Expression levels of 4- and 12-month-old LEA rats (cases 18 and 19, respectively) were similar to or less than that of 2-month-old (young) LEC rats (cases 1 and 2). The comparison of the average level of each hepatic lesion with that of the young LEC rats indicated that the GST-P expression in fulminant hepatitis

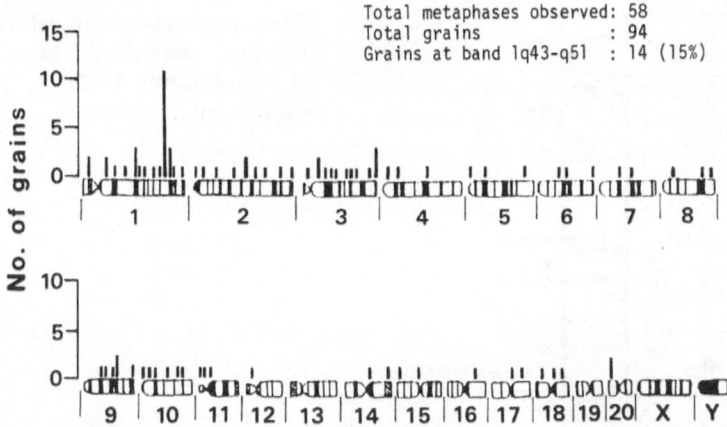

Fig. 1. Diagram showing the distribution of labeled sites with a GST-P probe in 58 rat metaphases. A high concentration of grains is seen in the long arm of chromosome 1. (From [12] with permission)

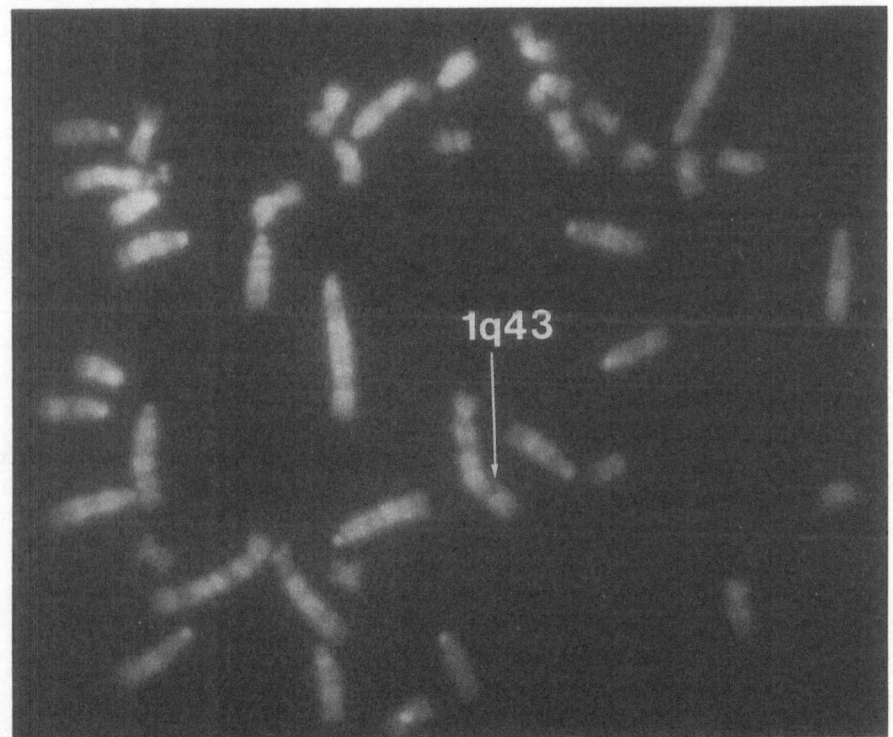

Fig. 2. Hybridization of ^{3}H-labeled GST-P probe to chromosomes of a rat metaphase, followed by Q-band staining. A silver grain is seen on 1q43 (*arrow*). (From [12] with permission)

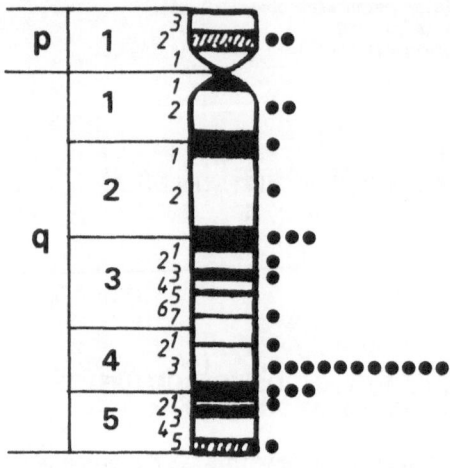

Fig. 3. Distribution of silver grains showing a peak on the band *1q43* of rat chromosome 1. (From [12] with permission)

Table 1. Profile of LEC rats with various hepatic lesions. (From [14] with permission).

Case	Sex	Age (months)	Hepatic lesions[a]
1	F	2	Normal liver
2	F	2	Normal liver
3	M	4	Fulminant hepatitis
4	M	4	Fulminant hepatitis
5	F	4	Fulminant hepatitis
6	M	4	Fulminant hepatitis
7	M	5	Chronic hepatitis
8	F	7	Chronic hepatitis
9	M	8	Chronic hepatitis
10	M	15	T: Hepatoma
11	M	15	T: Hepatoma, N: Nontumorous tissue
12	M	17	T: Hepatoma, N: Nontumorous tissue
13	F	17	T: Hepatoma, N: Nontumorous tissue
14	M	17	Transplantable LSH206G cell line
15	F	17	Cholangiofibrosis
16	M	17	Cholangiofibrosis
17	F	15	Cholangiofibrosis
18	F	4	Normal liver from control LEA rat
19	M	12	Normal liver from control LEA rat

[a] Hepatomas in cases 10-13 showed a well-differentiated type without metastasis

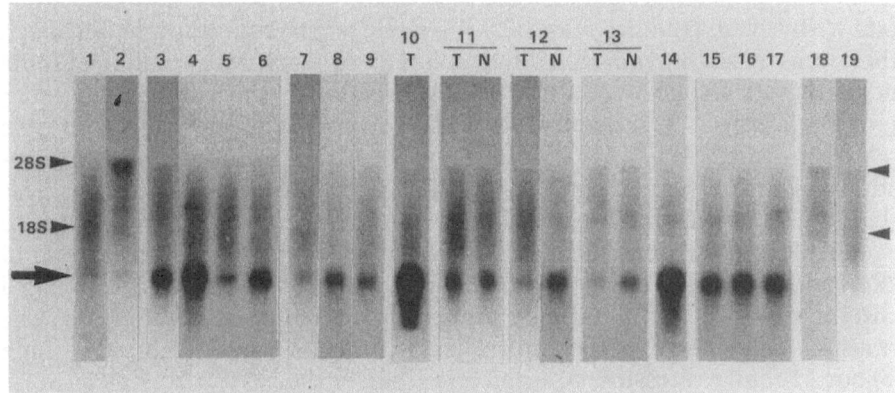

Fig. 4. Northern blot analysis of total RNAs from liver tissues of LEC rats with various hepatic lesions. GST-P bands were present at about 0.8 kb (*large arrow*), calculated from the positions of 18S (2.0 kb) and 28S (5.1 kb) rRNAs. Each *lane number* corresponds to the case number of Table 1. (From [14] with permission)

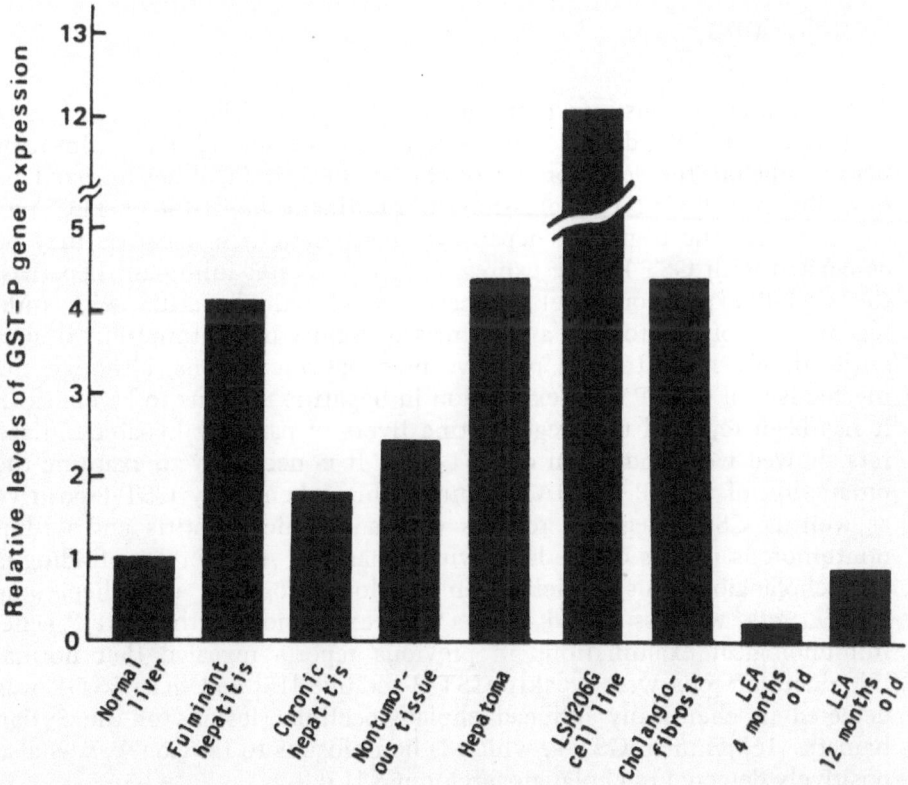

Fig. 5. Relative levels of GST-P gene expression. A histogram indicates an average level of each hepatic lesion relative to that of normal LEC rats at 2 months of age. (From [14] with permission)

rats with severe jaundice (cases 3–6) was elevated about fourfold, although there was a slight variation of expression levels among them. Chronic hepatitis rats also showed the GST-P expression at the ages of 5, 7, and 8 months (cases 7–9, respectively). However, the average level in chronic hepatitis decreased to 44% of fulminant hepatitis. Hepatomas in four long-surviving LEC rats (cases 10T–13T) showed various expression levels (less than equal in case 13T to about 13-fold greater in case 10T), with an average level of about fourfold greater, while relatively constant levels of expression were observed in nontumorous liver tissues which included chronic hepatitis and putatively preneoplastic foci (cases 11N–13N). The transplantable LSH206G cell line (case 14) showed a remarkably high (about 12-fold) expression. Similar variations in the GST-P expression were also reported in chemically induced primary hepatomas and in the transplantable hepatoma cell line [7]. The average expression level in cholangiofibrosis (cases 15–17) was more than fourfold higher than that in the young LEC rats.

Conclusions

These results demonstrate that the GST-P gene in LEC rats was highly expressed not only during hepatocarcinogenesis but also in fulminant hepatitis before the development of chronic hepatitis and hepatoma. This new finding of GST-P expression in fulminant hepatitis of LEC rats suggests that the degree of hepatocyte regeneration in hepatitis may be associated with GST-P gene expression. In fact, after fulminant hepatitis, the GST-P expression level decreased in chronic hepatitis with mild regeneration of hepatocytes and increased slightly in nontumorous tissues with chronic hepatitis and putative preneoplastic lesions, although the mechanism of GST-P gene expression in hepatitis remains to be clarified. It has been reported that regenerating livers of partially hepatectomized rats showed weak induction of GST-P [7]. It is necessary to examine the production of GST-P mRNA in immunohistochemically GST-P-positive as well as GST-P-negative regions within chronic hepatitis and within nontumorous tissues of the liver with hepatoma. Another new finding is that cholangiofibrosis, which often developed together with hepatoma in LEC rats, was associated with a high expression of the GST-P gene. Immunological examinations in previous reports revealed that normal bile ductular cells were weakly GST-P-positive [15] and that GST-P was detected in chemically induced cholangiocellular lesions of the Syrian hamster [16]. Human GST-π, which is homologous to rat GST-P, was also positively detected in cholangiocarcinomas [15].

Thus, LEC rats associated with spontaneous development of serial hepatic diseases are a promising model for elucidating the mechanism of GST-P gene expression.

Acknowledgments. The authors are grateful to Professor Masami Muramatsu, Department of Biochemistry, Faculty of Medicine, University of Tokyo, for providing GST-P probes, pGP5, and the *Sma*I-*Sma*I fragment. R.M. was a recipient of a Fellowship for Japanese Junior Scientists from the Japan Society for the Promotion of Science. This work was supported in part by Grants-in-Aid for Scientific Research and Cancer Research from the Ministry of Education, Science and Culture of Japan.

References

1. Sasaki M, Yoshida MC, Kagami K, Takeichi N, Kobayashi H, Dempo K, Mori M (1985) Spontaneous hepatitis in an inbred strain of Long-Evans rats. Rat News Lett 14:4–6
2. Yoshida MC, Masuda R, Sasaki M, Takeichi N, Kobayashi H, Dempo K, Mori M (1987) New mutation causing hereditary hepatitis in the laboratory rat. J Hered 78:361–365
3. Masuda R, Yoshida MC, Sasaki M, Dempo K, Mori M (1988) Hereditary hepatitis of LEC rats is controlled by a single autosomal recessive gene. Lab Anim 22:166–169
4. Masuda R, Yoshida MC, Sasaki M, Dempo K, Mori M (1988) High susceptibility to hepatocellular carcinoma development in LEC rats with hereditary hepatitis. Jpn J Cancer Res 79:828–835
5. Kitahara A, Satoh K, Nishimura K, Ishikawa T, Ruike K, Sato K, Tsuda H, Ito N (1984) Changes in molecular forms of rat hepatic glutathione *S*-transferase during chemical hepatocarcinogenesis. Cancer Res 44:2698–2703
6. Sato K, Kitahara A, Satoh K, Ishikawa T, Tatematsu M, Ito N (1984) The placental form of glutathione *S*-transferase as a new marker protein for preneoplasia in rat chemical hepatocarcinogenesis. Jpn J Cancer Res 75:199–202
7. Satoh K, Kitahara A, Soma Y, Inaba Y, Hatayama I, Sato K (1985) Purification, induction, and distribution of placental glutathione transferase: A new marker enzyme for preneoplastic cells in the rat chemical hepatocarcinogenesis. Proc Natl Acad Sci USA 82:3964–3968
8. Sugioka Y, Fujii-Kuriyama Y, Kitagawa T, Muramatsu M (1985) Changes in polypeptide pattern of rat liver cells during chemical hepatocarcinogenesis. Cancer Res 45:365–378
9. Sugioka Y, Kano T, Okuda A, Sakai M, Kitagawa T, Muramatsu M (1985) Cloning and the nucleotide sequence of rat glutathione *S*-transferase P cDNA. Nucleic Acids Res 13:6049–6057
10. Okuda A, Sakai M, Muramatsu M (1987) The structure of the rat glutathione *S*-transferase P gene and related pseudogenes. J Biol Chem 262:3858–3863
11. Oyamada M, Dempo K, Fujimoto Y, Takahashi H, Satoh MI, Mori M, Masuda R, Yoshida MC, Satoh K, Sato K (1988) Spontaneous occurrence of placental glutathine *S*-transferase-positive foci in the livers of LEC rats. Jpn J Cancer Res 79:5–8
12. Masuda R, Yoshida MC, Sasaki M, Okuda A, Sakai M, Muramatsu M (1986) Localization of the gene for glutathione *S*-transferase P on rat chromosome 1 at band q43. Jpn J Cancer Res 77:1055–1058

13. Masuda R, Yoshida MC, Sasaki M, Dempo K, Mori M (1988) A transplantable cell line derived from spontaneous hepatocellular carcinoma of the hereditary hepatitis LEC rat. Jpn J Cancer Res 79:250–254
14. Masuda R, Yoshida MC, Sasaki M (1989) Gene expression of placental glutathione S-transferase in hereditary hepatitis and spontaneous hepatocarcinogenesis of LEC strain rats. Jpn J Cancer Res 80:1024–1027
15. Sato K (1988) Glutathione S-transferases and hepatocarcinogenesis. Jpn J Cancer Res 79:556–572
16. More MA, Fukushima S, Ichihara A, Sato K, Ito N (1986) Intestinal metaplasia and altered enzyme expression in propylnitrosamine-induced Syrian hamster cholangiocellular and gallbladder lesions. Virchows Arch [B] 51:29–38

Subject Index